FDA警告信
回顾与案例解读

2023版

主　　编　　李香玉　张金巍　王　冰　许华平

执行主编　　朱子丰　何　辉　吴文惠　杨　清

副 主 编　　黄　哲　吴耀卫　刘　颖　陈　超　李　峰

中国健康传媒集团

中国医药科技出版社

图书在版编目（CIP）数据

FDA 警告信回顾与案例解读：2023 版 / 李香玉等主编 . -- 北京：中国医药科技出版社，2024. 9. -- ISBN 978-7-5214-4717-0

Ⅰ .R954

中国国家版本馆 CIP 数据核字第 20248PL464 号

策划编辑 于海平	**责任编辑** 高雨濛　王　梓
美术编辑 陈君杞	**版式设计** 也　在

出版　**中国健康传媒集团** ｜ 中国医药科技出版社

地址　北京市海淀区文慧园北路甲 22 号

邮编　100082

电话　发行：010-62227427　邮购：010-62236938

网址　www.cmstp.com

规格　710 × 1000 mm $\frac{1}{16}$

印张　26 $\frac{3}{4}$

字数　617 千字

版次　2024 年 9 月第 1 版

印次　2024 年 9 月第 1 次印刷

印刷　河北环京美印刷有限公司

经销　全国各地新华书店

书号　ISBN 978-7-5214-4717-0

定价　**120.00 元**

获取新书信息、投稿、为图书纠错，请扫码联系我们。

本书编委会

顾　　问　陈　敦　　刘厚佳　　韩国华　　王春华
　　　　　　邹林昆　　顾　凯

主　　编　李香玉　　张金巍　　王　冰　　许华平

执行主编　朱子丰　　何　辉　　吴文惠　　杨　清

副 主 编　黄　哲　　吴耀卫　　刘　颖　　陈　超
　　　　　　李　峰

编　　委（以姓氏拼音为序）

　　　　　　陈建新　　韩　进　　焦红江　　李雪峰
　　　　　　潘一峰　　盛建新　　史瑞文　　孙　朗
　　　　　　谭培龙　　唐传勇　　万龙岩　　王欣明
　　　　　　吴　桐　　谢海燕　　徐　铁　　叶　非
　　　　　　由庆睿　　张松梅　　赵勇杰　　朱自红

指导单位　上海药品审评核查中心

　　　　　　上海市生物医药产业促进中心

出　　品　蒲公英

　　　　　　上海临港产业大学生物医药产业学院

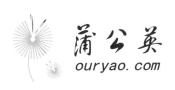

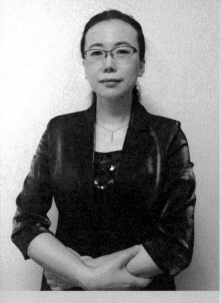

李香玉

—

上海药品审评核查中心副主任高级工程师，国家药品监督管理局药品 GMP 境外检查员，上海市专家级药品检查员，沈阳药科大学兼职副教授，美国 Georgetown University 访问学者。长期从事药品检查、审评和执法工作。著有《人用重组单克隆抗体制品的检查与实践》等，主持并参与了多项药品监管科学研究课题，主要起草《免疫细胞治疗产品生产用质粒生产质量管理指南》《除菌级过滤器生产质量管理指南》《生物制品连续制造指南》等标准。

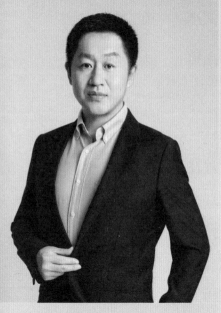

张金巍

—

博士（在读），蒲公英创始人，国际制药项目管理协会（IPPM）中国区首席代表，生物制药国产化推进联合会（BLA）发起人，PPMP（制药项目管理专家）国际 C 级认证课程开发人。深耕制药行业 20 余年，曾任职知名上市药企高管，现任多家企业高级战略顾问及生物药园区产业顾问，曾作为主编出版小说《制药人那点儿事》。

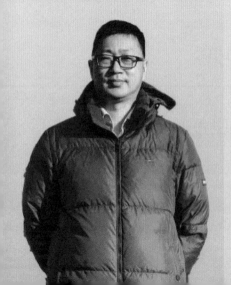

王冰

—

副主任药师，留学英国，重点实验室主任，在中国中药协会、深圳市药学会等多个学术团体任职，被多个高校聘为药学客座教授、硕士生导师，在药品质量管理和检验领域具有 20 年工作经历，主编或参编著作 4 部，发表论文 20 余篇。

许华平

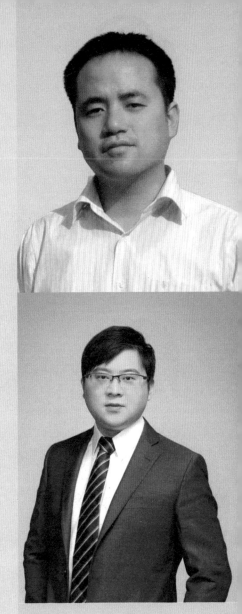

美国质量协会认证六西格玛黑带，美国项目管理学会项目管理专家，生物化学硕士，MBA（在读）。曾任职于西安杨森、中美史克和北美知名药企，在药品生产管理和质量技术方面具有 17 年的工作经验，多次参与迎接美国 FDA和加拿大卫生部的检查工作。曾作为编委会成员之一，出版《世界最新英汉双解生物学词典》。

朱子丰

明捷医药副总经理，《FDA 警告信回顾与案例解读（2022版）》执行主编。长期从事药品质量研究技术平台建设和运营工作，拥有超过 15 年药物质量研究及 CRO 运营管理经验，带领团队多次通过 FDA 现场审计，熟悉国内外药品质量标准相关法规和技术标准。擅于使用多种分析技术手段，解决药物质量研究中的复杂问题，对多种色谱分离原理及实践有丰富的经验，已发表多篇分析化学类论文和发明专利。

吴文惠

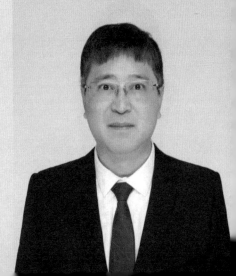

浦江学者，上海海洋大学教授，博士生导师，兼任上海市药学会海洋药物专业委员会主任委员、中国生物化学与分子生物学学会海洋分会副主任委员、中国海洋学会海洋中药专业委员会副主任委员、中华医学会航海医学分会海洋生物工程专业委员会副主任委员。从事海洋药物化学和心脑血管药理学的教育教学和科学研究，在溶栓候选药物的理论观点和实践技术方面进行了创新，先后获得上海药学科技奖和国家海洋科学技术奖。

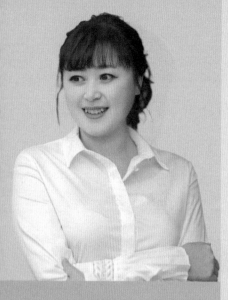

黄哲

—

管理学博士后，教授，博士研究生导师，沈阳药科大学工商管理学院副院长，沈阳药科大学药品监管科学研究院副院长。辽宁省优秀教师，辽宁省"百千万人才工程"人选百人层次，沈阳市高层次人才领军人才，沈阳市优秀研究生导师。长期从事药品监管科学、药物政策与法规、医药企业管理等教学和科研工作。主持 50 余项国家级、省部级、医药企业委托等科研项目。作为主编或副主编参编10 本教材著作，其中主编普通高等教育"十一五"国家级规划教材 1 部。

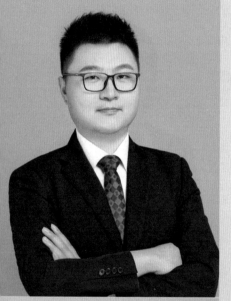

陈超

—

微生物控制及检测领域专家，上海临港产业大学生物医药学院客座专家，十三五国家重点研发计划课题《应急食品微生物检测》项目负责人。参与《中国药典》通则部分内容修订，参与多项制药领域无菌、微生物等行业标准的制定。拥有发明专利 3 项，实用新型专利 43 项，软件著作权 6 项。

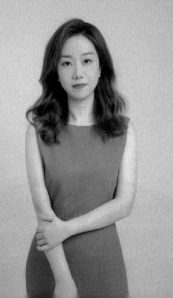

杨清

—

蒲公英合伙人，蒲公英生物制药板块负责人，蒲公英上海医药服务共创平台主理人。国际制药项目管理协会（IPPM）中国区首席运营官，生物制药国产化推进联合会（BLA）发起人，国内无菌保证体系推进者。曾任职知名上市制药集团生物制药商业化公司，超过 10 年生物制药产业化管理经历，在无菌保证、质量及生产技术型管理方面具有丰富的实战经验。

尊敬的读者：

系列丛书《FDA警告信回顾与案例解读》意在为制药行业从业者提供一个详尽的资源，帮助我们深入了解美国食品药品管理局（FDA）的监管要求，特别是关于现行药品生产质量管理规范（cGMP）的各个方面。2022版出版以来，得到了制药行业同仁的大力支持和积极反馈，这激励我们继续编纂2023版。本版汇编了2023年FDA发出的44封与cGMP相关的警告信，结合实例对这些警告信进行了解读和探讨。

《FDA警告信回顾与案例解读》（2023版）的编撰，是在中国医药产业蓬勃发展的大背景下的一次尝试。作为全球最权威的药品监管机构之一，FDA肩负着确保药品、医疗器械、兽药、化妆品、食品等产品的安全性和有效性的重任。为了实现这一目标，FDA对在美国市场销售的产品实施了严格的监管，以确保它们遵守相关法规和标准。通过批准前检查、cGMP例行检查、批准后合规性跟进检查和有因检查等多种方式，FDA评估并保障了产品的质量和安全性。检查后其发出的警告信，不仅代表了对药品品质和安全的严格要求，也是对整个行业的质量水平和合规性的集中体现。

在过去的半个世纪，特别是21世纪以来，生命科学领域实现了一系列重大技术突破。生物技术产品和服务以更亲民的价格、更接地气的形态走进了普通家庭，与此同时，生物资源保护、生物技术创新及应用的制度体系也日趋完善。在这样的大背景下，《"十四五"生物经济发展规划》的发布，为我国在生物经济时代的发展带来了新的机遇和挑战。中国医药产业正站在这个生物经济时代的风口浪尖。我们希望，通过这本书向中国医药企业提供关于FDA警告信的详尽信息，助力行业深入理解FDA的规定，从而更好地适应国际市场。

当FDA在检查过程中发现不符合规定的行为时，会向相关生产商发出警告信。这些警告信不仅是对违规行为的指正，更是对整个行业的提醒，引导其他企业规避相似的风险。警告信中详细列出了违规事项，并提供了整改建议和措施。这些信件揭示了药品生产中的常见问题，对于提升企业质量管理水平具有不可或缺的参考价值。警告信体现了 FDA 对产品质量和安全的严格标准，为制药企业提供了宝贵的学习机会。通过对这些案例的学习，我们能够更深入地理解国际医药行业所面临的挑战和问题，致力于提升药品品质，确保全球患者的用药安全。本书的编撰，旨在为制药企业开启一扇窗口，提供一个参考，帮助行业更好地理解和遵循 GMP 规定。通过对实际案例的分析，企业可以洞察到常见的质量管理和合规性问题及其解决方案，从而提升自身的质量管理能力，确保产品的安全性和有效性。

本书共分为七部分，涉及 FDA 警告信的各个主题，每一封警告信都经过了仔细的翻译和编排，内容包括原料药、外包活动、生物制品、无菌制剂、其他成品制剂以及特殊类型的警告信等。我们相信，对 FDA 警告信的深入了解，对于中国医药产业的科研机构和生产企业来说，都将是一笔宝贵的财富。

在本书的编纂过程中，我们得到了许多业内专家的支持与帮助。他们的专业意见和实际经验为本书的内容提供了重要的参考和借鉴。在此，向所有参与本书编写和审阅工作的专家和同仁表示衷心的感谢。特别感谢明捷医药和维科生物在本书撰写过程中提供的支持和帮助。明捷医药，持续致力于建立和完善符合全球医药健康产品政策法规的质量研究技术平台，2023 年顺利完成美国 FDA 的检查，展示了其在药物质量研究领域的领先地位。明捷医药的成功经历为中国医药产业树立了良好的典范，也为本书提供了有力的背景性支持。维科生物，是一家专业提供环境微生物控制整体解决方案的国家高新技术企业，在空间消杀、消杀剂、隔离器生产 / 检验、微生物检测方面都有极其丰富的经验。感谢以上两家公司在推动医药品质提升和国际化进程中的积极贡献。

在全球药品监管环境日益变化的今天，制药企业面临的挑战也日渐增多。我们希望本书能成为制药行业的得力助手，协助企业在复杂的监管环境中保持合规，不断提升药品质量，守护公众健康。药品质量事关亿万人的生命安全，作为制药行业的一分子，我们肩负着崇高的责任和使命。秉承"制药技术的传播者，GMP 理论的践行者"的蒲公英理念，我们期待本版继续能为广大制药企业提供实用的指导，助力行业的健康发展，共同守护每一个人的健康与安全。

本书经再三斟酌，不足之处，切望指正，衷心感谢！

蒲公英创始人　　张金巍

2024 年 2 月

美国食品药品管理局（FDA）是一个联邦政府机构，其职责是确保药品、医疗器械、动物药品、化妆品、食品添加剂等产品的安全。为了保证在美国市场推出的产品的安全性和质量，FDA 会调查这些公司是否遵守法规。为此，FDA 开展四种不同类型的检查，包括批准前检查、现行药品生产质量管理规范（cGMP）例行检查、批准后合规性跟进检查和有因检查。

FDA 在检查期间观察到违规情况时，会向生产商发出警告信。警告信被定义为"就 FDA 在其检查或调查期间记录的违规情况，通知受监管行业的信函"。在发出警告信之前，FDA 要求生产商对 483 表格中通常列出的缺陷做出回应。如果发现这些回应不令人满意，并且违规情况具有重要的监管意义并可能影响产品的安全和质量，FDA 会以警告信的形式向生产商发出正式的缺陷通知。收到警告信后，公司应采取适当措施整改警告信中列出的问题，以获得 FDA 办公室的关闭信。在警告信中，针对观察到的违规情况所需采取的纠正措施，FDA 还会向生产商提供建议和指导。

可以说，其中 FDA 所指出的缺陷项很大程度上代表了制药公司在 cGMP 方面的重大问题。为此，本书对其进行了翻译汇编，供业内参考。在本汇编的第一部分中，就 FDA 对 cGMP 的解释进行了回顾总结；在第二到第七部分中收录了 2023 年 FDA 发出的 44 封 cGMP 相关的警告信。对于每封警告信，编写时提炼每封警告信的特别之处作为标题，但需要注意的是，由于各企业面临的问题很多且企业之间可能有很多相似之处，标题的概括难以做到全面，仅供读者参考。

第一部分：从 FDA 视角看 cGMP

FDA 始终致力于通过对药品质量的严格监管，确保消费者的用药安全。cGMP 法规是保证药品质量的主要监管标准。消费者期望每批药品都符合质量标准，以确保安全和有效性。然而，大多数普通消费者对 cGMP 并不了解，也不清楚 FDA 如何确保药品生产过程符合基本要求。为此，FDA 对 cGMP 的概念进行了解释，涉及的问题有：cGMP 是什么？为什么 cGMP 如此重要？FDA 如何确定公司是否遵守 cGMP 法规？当出现 cGMP 违规情况时，FDA 如何保护公众？从这些问题中可以一窥 FDA 监管的目的和初衷。

第二部分：原料药

中国目前已经成为仅次于印度的美国第二大原料药进口国，有越来越多的中国药企在美国申报原料药。本部分收录了 2023 年有关原料药的两封 FDA 警告信，分别针对美国和中国原料药公司。

#	标题	签发日期	公司名称	签发机构	公司所在国家／地区
1	窄治疗窗药物的工艺验证问题	2023-03-30	ALI Pharmaceutical Manufacturing，LLC-645781-03/30/2023	FDA	药品质量业务三处	美国
2	原料药厂家拒绝向 FDA 提供记录和资料	2023-06-20	Chengdu KeCheng Fine Chemicals Co.，Ltd.	药物审评与研究中心	CDER	中国

第三部分：外包活动

本部分共收录了 14 家企业，涉及不同类型的外包活动。对于外包活动，FDA 表示许多药品生产商使用独立合同商，例如生产设施、检验实验室、包装商和贴标商。FDA 将合同商视为生产商的延伸。无论产品所有者与其外包设施签订了何种协议，产品所有者都要对药品质量负责。

#	标题	签发日期	公司名称	签发机构	外包活动
1	质量部门未能履责	2023-01-20	Atlantic Management Resources LTD dba. Claire Ellen Products	药品质量业务一处	合同生产商
2	未能提供生产工艺的验证数据	2023-02-01	Profounda，Inc.	药品质量业务二处	合同生产商
3	与非药用产品的共线生产问题	2023-02-22	Dunagin Pharmaceuticals Inc. dba Massco Dental	药品质量业务二处	使用 CMO 生产产品
4	原辅料鉴别方面存在疏漏	2023-03-01	Formology Lab Inc.	药品质量业务四处	合同生产商
5	水系统未经充分设计与监控	2023-03-10	Cosmetic Science Laboratories LLC	药品质量业务四处	使用 CMO 生产产品
6	未能进行充分的放行检验	2023-03-13	NuGeneration Technologies LLC	药品质量业务四处	使用 CMO 生产产品
7	建议聘请顾问，对公司进行全面审计	2023-03-20	Omega Packaging Corp	药品质量业务一处	合同生产商

#	标题	签发日期	公司名称	签发机构	外包活动
8	未验证药品微生物检验方法	2023-03-24	Sure-Biochem Laboratories, LLC	药品质量业务一处	委托检验实验室
9	产品苯污染，未能充分调查	2023-04-20	Accra-Pac, Inc. dba Voyant Beauty	药品质量业务二处	合同生产商
10	未能建立有胜任力的质量部门	2023-07-17	LXR Biotech, LLC	药品质量业务三处	合同生产商
11	机械润滑剂的污染风险	2023-07-26	Denison Pharmaceuticals, LLC	药品质量业务一处	合同生产商
12	批生产记录存在倒记问题	2023-08-11	Cosmobeauti Laboratories & Manufacturing Inc.	药物审评与研究中心 | CDER	合同生产商
13	实验室设备缺乏权限控制	2023-08-17	Lex Inc.	药品质量业务二处	合同生产商
14	MAH 未能对委托生产进行充分监督	2023-10-20	Elemental Herbs Inc. dba ALL good	药品质量业务四处	使用 CMO 生产产品

第四部分：生物制品

　　FDA 将人用药品大致分为了 4 大类，分别为处方药、非处方药、植物药以及生物制品。生物制品作为特殊的药品，其获得 FDA 许可（license）需满足《公共卫生服务法案》（PHS 法案）第 351 部分的相关要求。其中，美国将细胞治疗归为生物制品范畴，由 FDA 的生物制品审评与研究中心（CBER）统一负责审批监管。本部分收录了四封针对细胞治疗产品和一封血液相关产品生产企业的警告信。

#	标题	签发日期	公司名称	签发机构	公司所在国家/地区
1	生物制品上市前未进行审批	2023-06-05	Stratus Biosystems, LLC dba CellGenuity Regenerative Science	药品质量业务二处	美国
2	细胞产品的无菌保证问题	2023-06-21	Row1 Inc. dba Regenative Labs	生物制品业务一处	美国
3	未通过无菌检验，产品依然放行	2023-06-01	RenatiLabs Inc.	生物制品业务一处	美国
4	偏差调查不完善	2023-09-14	Fresenius Kabi AG	生物制品业务一处	德国
5	培养基模拟灌装的灌装数量不足	2023-09-18	Signature Biologics, LLC	药品质量业务二处	美国

缺陷即意味着存在对患者的风险。而从患者的角度看，无菌制剂无疑是风险较高的一种产品类型，因此对于无菌制剂的检查自然成为 FDA 工作的重点之一。那么，对于常见的缺陷项，无菌制剂企业通常遇到了什么问题？企业的实践和 FDA 的视角有哪些差距？FDA 提出了什么样的期望？从以下的警告信中或许可以得到答案。

#	标题	签发日期	公司名称	签发机构	公司所在国家 / 地区
1	眼科药品未满足无菌要求	2023-04-28	Pharmedica USA, LLC	药品质量业务四处	美国
2	无菌洁净室的压差问题	2023-07-20	Iso-Tex Diagnostics, Inc.	药品质量业务二处	美国
3	注射剂药品的颗粒物检查存在缺陷	2023-07-25	Baxter Healthcare Corporation	药物审评与研究中心 | CDER	美国
4	烟雾研究未充分模拟实际生产条件	2023-08-03	K.C. Pharmaceuticals Inc.	药品质量业务四处	美国
5	培养基灌装中模拟的干预次数不足	2023-09-11	Similasan AG	药物审评与研究中心 | CDER	瑞士
6	无菌操作技术存在问题	2023-10-16	Sun Pharmaceutical Industries Ltd.	药物审评与研究中心 | CDER	印度
7	美国多州暴发细菌感染，触发 FDA 检查	2023-10-20	Global Pharma Healthcare Private Limited	药物审评与研究中心 | CDER	印度
8	投诉比例，不是产品质量指标	2023-11-17	Cipla Limited	药物审评与研究中心 | CDER	印度

针对其他成品制剂，本部分收录了 9 封 2023 年的 FDA 警告信。

#	标题	签发日期	公司名称	签发机构	公司所在国家 / 地区
1	质量部门未能履行职责	2023-01-23	Skyless, LLC	药品质量业务二处	波多黎各
2	OOS 调查不充分	2023-04-06	Zermat International S.A. de C.V.	药物审评与研究中心 | CDER	美国
3	清洁验证未考虑转运容器	2023-04-13	Pharmaplast S.A.E.	药物审评与研究中心 | CDER	埃及

#	标题	签发日期	公司名称	签发机构	公司所在国家/地区
4	标识为"已清洁"的设备不洁净	2023-05-26	NeilMed Pharmaceuticals Inc.	药品质量业务四处	美国
5	不良卫生条件下生产	2023-07-13	Jamol Laboratories, Inc.	药品质量业务一处	美国
6	判定OOS结果无效，依据不充分	2023-07-20	Medgel Private Limited	药物审评与研究中心 | CDER	印度
7	药品存在交叉污染风险	2023-07-25	Centaur Pharmaceuticals Private Ltd.	药物审评与研究中心 | CDER	印度
8	对于脆弱患者存在重大安全风险	2023-08-15	Gadal Laboratories Inc.	药品质量业务二处	美国
9	生产线清场不充分，有导致药品混淆的风险	2023-09-05	Safecor Health, LLC	药品质量业务一处	美国

第七部分：特殊类型的警告信

在新冠病毒流行期间，当现场检查不可行时，FDA 依赖于记录要求，以此评估药品生产商对 cGMP 的持续遵守情况。根据《联邦食品、药品和化妆品法案》（FD&C 法案）第 704（a）（4）条，FDA 可以要求企业提供记录，这一要求可以在检查之前提出，也可以代替检查。拒绝访问或复制 704（a）（4）要求的任何记录，将构成 FDCA 规定的禁止行为。此外，设施未能及时提供所要求的记录或拒绝提供未经允许的不合理编辑记录，将被视为检查的"延迟"或"限制"。对于任何在延迟、拒绝、限制或拒绝检查的设施中生产、加工、包装或储存的药品，均被视为掺假。除了记录要求外，FDA 越来越依赖产品样品的分析检验，以此评估产品质量。在后新冠时代，FDA 还在继续使用这些现场检查的替代工具。本部分收录了 6 封这些特殊类型的警告信。

#	标题	签发日期	公司名称	签发机构	公司所在国家/地区
1	FDA 检验发现婴幼儿产品存在微生物污染	2023-01-18	Buzzagogo, LLC	药物审评与研究中心 | CDER	美国
2	记录审查：显示放行前未对成品进行检验	2023-01-19	B & J Group	药品质量业务一处	美国
3	记录审查：显示稳定性数据不充分	2023-01-30	Fei Fah Medical Manufacturing Pte. Ltd.	药物审评与研究中心 | CDER	新加坡

#	标题	签发日期	公司名称	签发机构	公司所在国家/地区
4	记录审查：显示未进行原料鉴别检验	2023-11-15	Xiamen Wally Bath Manufacture Co., Ltd.	药物审评与研究中心 | CDER	中国
5	未能提供信息	2023-08-03	Sangleaf Pharm., Co. Ltd.	药物审评与研究中心 | CDER	韩国
6	拒绝提供对记录的访问和复制	2023-09-18	Zhao Qing Longda Biotechnology Co. Ltd.	药物审评与研究中心 | CDER	中国

本书编委会

2024 年 2 月

目　录

1 **第一部分**

从 FDA 视角看 cGMP

9 **第二部分**

原料药

1　窄治疗窗药物的工艺验证问题 ················· 10

2　原料药厂家拒绝向 FDA 提供记录和资料 ············· 25

28 **第三部分**

外包活动

1　质量部门未能履责 ····················· 29

2　未能提供生产工艺的验证数据 ················ 36

3　与非药用产品的共线生产问题 ················ 52

4　原辅料鉴别方面存在疏漏 ·················· 71

5　水系统未经充分设计与监控 ················· 79

6　未能进行充分的放行检验 ·················· 87

7　建议聘请顾问，对公司进行全面审计 ············· 94

8　未验证药品微生物检验方法 ················ 100

9　产品苯污染，未能充分调查 ················ 108

10　未能建立有胜任力的质量部门 ··············· 117

11　机械润滑剂的污染问题 ·················· 122

12　批生产记录存在倒记问题 ················· 134

13　实验室设备缺乏权限控制 ················· 142

14　MAH 未能对委托生产进行充分监督 ············ 157

162 第四部分
生物制品

1 生物制品上市前未进行审批 ················· 163
2 细胞产品的无菌保证问题 ················· 173
3 未通过无菌检验，产品依然放行 ················· 178
4 偏差调查不完善 ················· 185
5 培养基模拟灌装的灌装数量不足 ················· 192

197 第五部分
无菌制剂

1 眼科药品未满足无菌要求 ················· 198
2 无菌洁净室的压差问题 ················· 205
3 注射剂药品的颗粒物检查存在缺陷 ················· 215
4 烟雾研究未充分模拟实际生产条件 ················· 225
5 培养基灌装中模拟的干预次数不足 ················· 234
6 无菌操作技术存在问题 ················· 243
7 美国多州暴发细菌感染，触发 FDA 检查 ················· 258
8 投诉比例，不是产品质量指标 ················· 285

303 第六部分
其他成品制剂

1 质量部门未能履行职责 ················· 304
2 OOS 调查不充分 ················· 312
3 清洁验证未考虑转运容器 ················· 321
4 标识为"已清洁"的设备不洁净 ················· 326
5 不良卫生条件下生产 ················· 332
6 判定 OOS 结果无效，依据不充分 ················· 339
7 药品存在交叉污染风险 ················· 348
8 对于脆弱患者存在重大安全风险 ················· 357
9 生产线清场不充分，有导致药品混淆的风险 ················· 373

特殊类型的警告信

1 FDA 检验发现婴幼儿产品存在微生物污染 ················ 382

2 记录审查：显示放行前未对成品进行检验 ··············· 386

3 记录审查：显示稳定性数据不充分 ·················· 392

4 记录审查：显示未进行原料鉴别检验 ················· 398

5 未能提供信息 ························· 404

6 拒绝提供对记录的访问和复制 ··············· 407

第一部分

从 FDA 视角看 cGMP

Pharmaceutical Quality affects every American. The Food and Drug Administration (FDA) regulates the quality of pharmaceuticals very carefully. The main regulatory standard for ensuring pharmaceutical quality is the Current Good Manufacturing Practice (cGMP) regulations for human pharmaceuticals. Consumers expect that each batch of medicines they take will meet quality standards so that they will be safe and effective. Most people, however, are not aware of cGMP, or how FDA assures that drug manufacturing processes meet these basic objectives. Recently, FDA has announced a number of regulatory actions taken against drug manufacturers based on the lack of cGMP. This paper discusses some facts that may be helpful in understanding how cGMP establishes the foundation for drug product quality.

药品质量关乎每个人的健康与安全。美国食品药品管理局（FDA）严格监管着药品的生产质量，其中主要的监管标准是现行药品生产质量管理规范（cGMP）。消费者期望每一批药品都符合质量标准，以确保其安全性和有效性。然而，对于大多数人来说，他们并不了解 cGMP，也不清楚 FDA 如何确保药品生产过程满足这些基本要求。最近，FDA 针对药品生产商采取了多项监管行动，这些行动基于对 cGMP 的缺失进行了审查。本文旨在讨论一些关键事实，帮助理解 cGMP 如何建立药品质量的基础。

What is cGMP? | 什么是 cGMP？

cGMP refers to the Current Good Manufacturing Practice regulations enforced by the FDA. cGMP provides for systems that assure proper design, monitoring, and control of manufacturing processes and facilities. Adherence to the cGMP regulations assures the identity, strength, quality, and purity of drug products by requiring that manufacturers of medications adequately control manufacturing operations. This includes establishing strong quality management systems, obtaining appropriate quality raw materials, establishing robust operating procedures, detecting and investigating product quality deviations, and maintaining reliable testing laboratories. This formal system of controls at a pharmaceutical company, if adequately put into practice, helps to prevent instances of contamination, mix-ups, deviations, failures, and errors. This assures that drug products meet their quality standards.

cGMP 是指 FDA 执行的现行药品生产质量管理规范。cGMP 系统确保了生产工艺和设施的正确设计、监控和控制。cGMP 要求制药公司充分控制生产操作，以确保药品的鉴别、规格、质量和纯度。这涵盖了多方面的要求，包括建立稳健的质量管理体系、获取适当的优质原料、建立健全操作程序、检测和调查产品质量偏差，以及维护可靠的检验实验室。制药公司的这种正式控制系统，如果得到充分实施，有助于预防污染、混淆、偏差、不合格和错误的发生。这一过程确保了药品符合其质量标准。

The cGMP requirements were established to be flexible in order to allow each manufacturer to decide individually how to best implement the necessary controls by using scientifically sound design, processing methods, and testing procedures. The flexibility in these regulations allows companies to use modern technologies and innovative approaches to achieve higher quality through continual improvement. Accordingly, the "C" in cGMP stands for "current," requiring companies to use technologies and systems that are up-to-date in order to comply with the regulations. Systems and equipment that may have been "top-of-the-line" to prevent contamination, mix-ups, and errors 10 or 20 years ago may be less than adequate by today's standards.

cGMP 要求的制定具有灵活性，这样每个制药公司都能够独立决定如何通过科学合理的设计、加工方法和检验程序来最好地实施必要的控制。这种灵活性使得制药公司能够充分利用现代技术和创新方法，通过持续改进来实现更高的质量水平。因此，cGMP 中的"c"代表着"现行"，要求制药公司采用最新的技术和系统以符合法规。10 或 20 年前被视为防止污染、混淆和错误的"顶级"系统和设备，按照今天的标准可能已经不够了。

It is important to note that cGMP regulations for drugs contain the minimum requirements. Many pharmaceutical manufacturers are already implementing comprehensive, modern quality systems and risk management approaches that exceed these minimum standards.

值得注意的是，药品 cGMP 包含最低要求。很多制药公司已经在实施超出这些最低标准的全面、现代化的质量体系和风险管理方法。

Why is cGMP so important? | 为什么 cGMP 如此重要？

A consumer usually cannot detect (through smell, touch, or sight) that a drug product is safe or if it will work. While cGMP requires testing, testing alone is not adequate to ensure quality. In most instances testing is done on a small sample of a batch (for example, a drug manufacturer may test 100 tablets from a batch that contains 2 million tablets), so that most of the batch can be used for patients rather than destroyed by testing. Therefore, it is important that drugs are manufactured under conditions and practices required by the cGMP regulations to assure that quality is built into the design and manufacturing process at every step. Facilities that are in good condition, equipment that is properly maintained and calibrated, employees who are qualified and fully trained, and processes that are reliable and reproducible, are a few examples of how cGMP requirements help to assure the safety and efficacy of drug products.

消费者通常无法（通过嗅觉、触觉或视觉）识别药品是否安全或有效。虽然 cGMP 要求进行检验，但仅靠检验是不足以确保质量的。在大多数情况下，检验是针对批次中的少量样品进行的（例如，药品生产商可能会对包含 200 万片的批次中的 100 片进行检验），以保证该批次中的大部分药品可供患者使用，而不是被检验消耗掉。因此，药品在 cGMP 要求的条件和实践下生产非常重要，以确保设计和生产工艺的每一步都能保证质量。拥有状态良好的设施、正确维护和校准的设备、有资质且经过充分培训的员工，以及可靠且可重现的工艺，都是 cGMP 要求中确保药品安全性和有效性的关键点。

How does FDA determine if a company is complying with cGMP regulations?
FDA 如何确定制药公司是否遵守 cGMP 法规？

FDA inspects pharmaceutical manufacturing facilities worldwide, including facilities that manufacture active ingredients and the finished product. Inspections follow a standard approach and are conducted by highly trained FDA staff. FDA also relies upon reports of potentially defective drug products from the public and the industry. FDA will often use these reports to identify sites for which an inspection or investigation is needed. Most companies that are inspected are found to be fully compliant with the cGMP regulations.

FDA 检查世界各地的药品生产设施，包括生产原料药和成品的设施。检查遵循标准方法，并由训练有素的 FDA 工作人员进行。FDA 还依赖公众和行业对潜在缺陷药品的报告。FDA 经常基于这些报告来确定需要检查或调查的场所。大多数接受检查的制药公司都完全符合 cGMP 法规。

If a manufacturer is not following cGMP, are drug products safe for use
如果制药公司不遵守 cGMP，药品可以安全使用吗

If a company is not complying with cGMP regulations, any drug it makes is considered "adulterated" under the law. This kind of adulteration means that the drug was not manufactured under conditions that comply with cGMP. It does not mean that there is necessarily something wrong with the drug.

如果一家制药公司不遵守 cGMP 法规，根据法律规定，其生产的药品都将被视为"掺假"产品。这种掺假意味着该药品不是在符合 cGMP 要求的条件下生产的。这并不意味着药品一定有问题。

For consumers currently taking medicines from a company that was not following cGMP, FDA usually advises these consumers not to interrupt their drug therapy, which could have serious implications for their health. Consumers should seek advice from their health care professionals before stopping or changing medications. Regulatory actions against companies with poor cGMP are often intended to prevent the possibility of unsafe and/or ineffective drugs. In rare cases, FDA regulatory action is intended to stop the distribution or manufacturing of violative product. The impact of cGMP violations depends on the nature of those violations and on the specific drugs involved. A drug manufactured in violation of cGMP may still meet its labeled specifications, and the risk that the drug is unsafe or ineffective could be minimal. Thus, FDA's advice will be specific to the circumstances, and health care professionals are best able to balance risks and benefits and make the right decision for their patients.

对于目前从不遵守 cGMP 的制药公司购买药品的消费者，FDA 通常建议这些消费者不要中断药品治疗，这可能对其健康产生严重影响。消费者在停止或更换药品之前应寻求医疗健康专业人员的建议。针对 cGMP 执行较差的公司的监管行动通常是为了防止出现不安全和（或）无效药品的可能性。在极少数情况下，FDA 的监管行动旨在阻止违规产品的流通或生产。cGMP 违规情况的影响取决于这些违规情况的性质以及所涉及的具体药品。违反 cGMP 生产的药品仍可能符合其标识的质量标准，并且该药品不安全或无效的风险可能很小。因此，FDA 的建议将根据具体情况而定，医疗健康专业人员最有能力平衡风险和收益，并为患者做出正确的决定。

What can FDA do to protect the public when there are cGMP violations?
当出现 cGMP 违规行为时，FDA 可以采取哪些措施来保护公众？

If the failure to meet cGMP results in the distribution of a drug that does not offer the benefit as labeled because, for example, it has too little active ingredient, the company may subsequently recall that product. This protects the public from further harm by removing these drugs from the market. While FDA cannot force a company to recall a drug, companies usually will recall voluntarily or at FDA's request. If a company refuses to recall a drug, FDA can warn the public and can seize the drug.

如果公司因不符合 cGMP 要求，导致上市销售的药品达不到标示的疗效（如药品含量低于标准），则公司随后会启动召回。通过将这些药品从市场上撤下，可以保护公众免受进一步的伤害。虽然 FDA 不能强迫公司召回药品，但公司通常会主动召回或应 FDA 要求启动召回。如果一家公司拒绝召回某种药品，FDA 可以警告公众并扣押该药品。

FDA can also bring a seizure or injunction case in court to address cGMP violations even where there is no direct evidence of a defect affecting the drug's performance. When FDA brings a seizure case, the agency asks the court for an order that allows federal officials to take possession of "adulterated" drugs. When FDA brings an injunction case, FDA asks the court to order a company to stop violating cGMP. Both seizure and injunction cases often lead to court orders that require companies to take many steps to correct cGMP violations, which may include repairing facilities and equipment, improving sanitation and cleanliness, performing additional testing to verify quality, and improving employee training. FDA can also bring criminal cases because of cGMP violations, seeking fines and jail time.

即使没有直接证据表明存在影响药品性能的缺陷，FDA 也可以向法庭提起扣押或禁令案件，以解决 cGMP 违规问题。当 FDA 提起扣押案件时，FDA 会要求法院发布命令，允许联邦官员扣押"掺假"药品。当 FDA 提起禁令案件时，FDA 要求法院命令一家公司停止违反 cGMP 的行为。扣押和禁令案件通常都会导致法院下令，要求公司采取很多措施整改 cGMP 违规情况，其中可能包括修复设施和设备、改善卫生和清洁、进行额外检验以确认质量，以及加强员工培训。FDA 还可以因违反 cGMP 行为对公司提起刑事诉讼，进行罚款和监禁。

How would a new drug company learn about cGMP and about FDA's expectations on complying with them?
新制药公司如何了解 cGMP 以及 FDA 对遵守这些法规的期望？

FDA publishes regulations and guidance documents for industry in the Federal Register. This is how the federal government notifies the public of what we are doing and why. FDA's website, www.fda.gov also contains links to the cGMP regulations, guidance documents, and various resources to help drug companies comply with the law. FDA also conducts extensive public outreach through presentations at national and international meetings and conferences, to discuss and explain the cGMP requirements and the latest policy documents.

FDA 在《联邦公报》上发布行业法规和指南。这就是联邦政府向公众通报我们正在做什么及其原因的方式。FDA 的网站 www.fda.gov 还包含 cGMP 法规、指南和各种资源的链接，以帮助制药公司遵守法律。FDA 还通过在国内和国际会议上的演讲进行广泛的公众宣传，讨论和解释 cGMP 要求和最新政策文件。

Current Good Manufacturing Practice（cGMP）Regulations
现行药品生产质量管理规范（cGMP）要求

FDA ensures the quality of drug products by carefully monitoring drug manufacturers' compliance with its Current Good Manufacturing Practice（cGMP）regulations. The cGMP regulations for drugs contain minimum requirements for the methods, facilities, and controls used in manufacturing, processing, and packing of a drug product. The regulations make sure that a product is safe for use, and that it has the ingredients and strength it claims to have.

FDA 通过仔细监控药品生产商是否遵守现行药品生产质量管理规范（cGMP）要求，来确保药品质量。药品 cGMP 要求包含药品生产、加工和包装中使用的方法、设施和控制的最低要求。这些法规确保产品使用安全，并且具有其声称的原辅料和规格。

The approval process for new and generic drug marketing applications includes a review of the manufacturer's compliance with the cGMP. FDA assessors and investigators determine whether the firm has the necessary facilities, equipment, and ability to manufacture the drug it intends to market.

新药和仿制药上市申请的审批流程包括审查生产商是否遵守 cGMP。FDA 评估人员和调查员确定该公司是否拥有必要的设施、设备和能力来生产其打算上市的药品。

Code of Federal Regulations（CFR）| 联邦法规（CFR）

FDA's portion of the CFR is in Title 21, which interprets the Federal Food, Drug and Cosmetic Act and related statutes, including the Public Health Service Act. The pharmaceutical or drug quality-related regulations appear in several parts of Title 21, including sections in parts 1–99, 200–299, 300–499, 600–799, and 800–1299.

FDA 的 CFR 部分位于第 21 篇，该章解释了《联邦食品、药品和化妆品法案》及相关法规，包括《公共卫生服务法案》。与药品或药品质量相关的法规出现在第 21 篇的多个部分中，包括第 1–99、200–299、300–499、600–799 和 800–1299 部分中的章节。

The regulations enable a common understanding of the regulatory process by describing the requirements to be followed by drug manufacturers, applicants, and FDA.

这些法规通过描述药品生产商、申请人和 FDA 需要遵循的要求，使人们能够对监管流程达成共识。

- *21 CFR Part 314 For FDA approval to market a new drug.*
- 21 CFR Part 314 FDA 批准新药上市。
- *21 CFR Part 210. Current Good Manufacturing Practice in Manufacturing Processing, packing, or Holding of Drugs.*
- 21 CFR 第 210 部分。现行药品生产加工、包装或储存的药品生产质量管理规范。
- *21 CFR Part 211. Current Good Manufacturing Practice for Finished Pharmaceuticals.*
- 21 CFR 第 211 部分。现行成品制剂的药品生产质量管理规范。

● *21 CFR Part 212. Current Good Manufacturing Practice for Positron Emission Tomography Drugs.*

● 21 CFR 第 212 部分。正电子发射断层扫描药品的现行药品生产质量管理规范。

● *21 CFR Part 600. Biological Products：General.*

● 21 CFR 第 600 部分。生物制品：一般通则。

第二部分

原料药

1 窄治疗窗药物的工艺验证问题

警告信编号: MARCS-CMS 645781

签发时间: 2023-3-30; 公示时间: 2023-10-31

签发机构: 药品质量业务三处 (Division of Pharmaceutical Quality Operations III)

公　　司: ALI Pharmaceutical Manufacturing, LLC

所在国家/地区: 美国

主　　题: cGMP/原料药 (API)/掺假 [cGMP/Active Pharmaceutical Ingredient (API)/Adulterated]

简　　介: FDA 在 2022 年 9 月到 10 月对该公司进行了检查,发现了多项违反原料药 cGMP 的重大缺陷。其中第一条强调未能验证猪甲状腺的生产工艺。猪甲状腺用于治疗甲状腺功能减退症,产品治疗窗窄,需要通过工艺验证评估中间体混合和生产正确性,以避免患者剂量接受不足或过量的风险。公司回复称猪甲状腺是其唯一原料药,已实施最差情况取样程序,因此可以规避工艺验证的风险。然而,FDA 认为该公司的回应不充分,其指出公司未解决已流通批次的微生物风险,并未提供充分证明这些批次提供了代表性样本量,以进行工艺评估。此外,公司也未提供详细的计划细节来整改其工艺验证计划。

The U.S. Food and Drug Administration (FDA) inspected your drug manufacturing facility, ALI Pharmaceutical Manufacturing, LLC, FEI 1920841, at 4410 S. 102nd Street, Omaha, from September 26 to October 3, 2022.

2022 年 9 月 26 日至 10 月 3 日,美国食品药品管理局(FDA)检查了你公司的药品生产设施 ALI Pharmaceutical Manufacturing, LLC (FEI 1920841),其地址为美国(略,见上)。

This warning letter summarizes significant deviations from current good manufacturing practice (cGMP) for active pharmaceutical ingredients (API).

本警告信总结了与原料药（API）现行药品生产质量管理规范（cGMP）相关的重大偏差。

Because your methods, facilities, or controls for manufacturing, processing, packing, or holding do not conform to cGMP, your API are adulterated within the meaning of section 501（a）（2）（B）of the Federal Food, Drug, and Cosmetic Act（FD&C Act）, 21 U.S.C. 351（a）（2）（B）.

由于你公司用于生产、加工、包装或储存的方法、设施或控制措施不符合 cGMP，因此根据 FD&C 法案第 501（a）（2）（B）条、21 U.S.C. 351（a）（2）（B）的规定，你公司的原料药被认为是掺假。

We reviewed your October 21, 2022, response to our Form FDA 483 in detail and acknowledge receipt of your subsequent correspondence.

我们详细审查了你公司于 2022 年 10 月 21 日对 FDA 483 表格的回复，并确认收到你们随后的来函。

During our inspection, our investigators observed specific deviations including, but not limited to, the following.

在检查过程中，我们的调查员发现了具体偏差，包括但不限于以下内容。

未能验证生产工艺

1. Failure to demonstrate that your manufacturing process can reproducibly manufacture an intermediate and API meeting its predetermined quality attributes.

1. 未能证明你们的生产工艺可以重现地生产满足其预定质量属性的中间体和原料药。

You failed to adequately validate your porcine thyroid API manufacturing processes, including the（b）（4）of（b）（4）intermediates. Additionally, the（b）（4）process validation was not representative of your current manufacturing process. For example：

你公司未能充分验证猪甲状腺 API 生产工艺，包括（b）（4）工艺中的（b）（4）中间体。此外，（b）（4）工艺验证并不代表你公司当前的生产工艺。例如：

● You based your（b）（4）process for（b）（4）intermediates on your（b）（4）room temperature mapping report. However, you performed the study with（b）（4）porcine thyroid which lacked evidence to address possible variation when（b）（4）intermediates are（b）（4）. Further, this report indicated that your target material temperature was only reached after（b）

（4）of（b）（4）. Your report also lacked information about the material of construction（e.g., thickness and composition）of the drums, whether liner bags were used in the drums, and the quantity of intermediate in each drum.

● 你公司的（b）（4）中间体的（b）（4）工艺是基于（b）（4）室温绘图报告。然而，你们使用（b）（4）猪甲状腺进行了研究，但缺乏证据来解决（b）（4）中间体为（b）（4）时可能出现的变异。此外，该报告表明，你公司的目标物料温度仅在（b）（4）的（b）（4）之后达到。报告还缺乏有关桶的结构物料（如厚度和成分）、桶中是否使用内衬袋，以及每个桶中中间体数量的信息。

● You determined the（b）（4）room processing time for（b）（4）porcine thyroid intermediate based on a retrospective evaluation of data obtained from previously（b）（4）lots. You concluded that a single log reduction of microbes takes（b）（4）in the（b）（4）room. However, your raw data show multiple instances of less than one log reduction in more than（b）（4）.

● 对于（b）（4）猪甲状腺中间体，你公司确定了（b）（4）房间处理时间，这是基于对之前（b）（4）批次获得数据的回顾性评估。你们得出的结论是，微生物的一个对数减少在（b）（4）房间中需要花费（b）（4）时间。但是，原始数据显示多个实例下，在超过（b）（4）的情况下，对数减少量少于一个。

● Your（b）（4）process performance qualification（PPQ）report failed to sufficiently correlate test data for the initial microbial load with the total time each lot was in the（b）（4）room. Further, you lacked justification for only sampling（b）（4）of each PPQ lot. You did not demonstrate material uniformity, including chemical and microbiological attributes.

● 你公司的（b）（4）工艺性能确认（PPQ）报告未能将初始微生物负荷的检验数据与每批在（b）（4）房间中的总时间充分关联起来。此外，你们仅对每个 PPQ 批次进行（b）（4）取样，对此缺乏论证。你公司没有证明物料的均匀性，包括化学和微生物属性。

● You lacked justification for holding times between stages of（b）（4）, and final blend of porcine thyroid API. You stored（b）（4）intermediate in the（b）（4）room for up to（b）（4）.

● 你公司对（b）（4）各阶段之间的存放时间以及猪甲状腺 API 的最终混合缺乏论证。你们将（b）（4）中间体存储在（b）（4）房间，最长放置了（b）（4）时间。

The porcine thyroid, USP API you manufactured is used to produce drug products to treat hypothyroidism. Because of the narrow therapeutic range of these products, proper blending and manufacture of your intermediate that is appropriately evaluated through process validation is essential to prevent patients from receiving insufficient or excessive doses.

你公司的猪甲状腺（USP API）用于生产治疗甲状腺功能减退症的药品。由于这些药品的治疗范围较窄，因此需要通过工艺验证适当评估中间体的正确混合和生产，对于防止患者剂量接受不足或过量，这至关重要。

In your response, you provide a retrospective evaluation of your microbiological results for the full-strength porcine thyroid API that you state is the only API you currently manufacture. You state that you implemented a worst-case interim sampling procedure to obtain samples from the top, middle and bottom of each container. You also commit to implement a fixed length of time of the (b)(4) by applying a worst-case analysis from the results of the (b)(4) intermediate.

在回复中，你公司对全规格猪甲状腺 API 的微生物学结果进行了回顾性评估，你们声称这是目前生产的唯一原料药。你公司声称实施了最差情况的临时取样程序，从每个容器的顶部、中部和底部获取样品。你公司还承诺，通过应用（b）（4）中间结果的最差情况分析来实现（b）（4）的固定时间长度。

Your response is inadequate. You do not address the impact of microbial results on your other distributed porcine thyroid API ((b)(4)) that may still be within their reevaluation date. Although you commit to evaluate intra-batch variability for (b)(4) intermediates, you do not provide sufficient rationale to demonstrate that (b)(4) lots provides a representative sample size to evaluate your process. These studies will be conducted for in-process (b)(4) and in-process (b)(4) samples and do not include final blended API. You do not provide sufficient details of your plans to assess and remediate your validation program.

你公司的回应不够充分。针对其他已流通的猪甲状腺 API [（b）（4）]，你公司没有解决微生物结果的影响，这些 API 可能仍在再验期内。尽管承诺评估（b）（4）中间体的批次内变异性，但你公司没有提供充分的论证，来证明（b）（4）批次提供了具有代表性的样本量，以评估工艺。这些研究将针对过程（b）（4）和过程（b）（4）样品进行，而不包括最终混合 API。你公司没有提供充分的计划细节，来评估和整改验证计划。

In response to this letter, provide：

在回复本函时，请提供：

● A comprehensive, independent assessment of the design and control of your firm's manufacturing operations, with a detailed and thorough review of all hazards that may impact chemical and microbiological attributes of your API. Regarding microbiological attributes, the assessment should include, but not be limited to, total counts and objectionable microorganisms such as *Bacillus cereus*.

● 对你公司生产操作的设计和控制进行全面、独立的评估，并对可能影响 API 化学和微生物属性的所有危害进行详细、彻底的审查。关于微生物属性，评估应包括但不限于总计数和有害微生物，例如蜡样芽孢杆菌。

● A detailed risk assessment addressing the hazards posed by distributing API with potentially objectionable contamination. Specify actions you will take in response to the risk assessment, such as customer notifications and product recalls.

● 详细的风险评估，以解决流通具有潜在有害污染的 API 所带来的危害。指定你公司将针对风险评估采取的行动，例如客户通知和产品召回。

● Complete investigations into all lots with potential objectionable microbial contamination or an out-of-specification（OOS）microbiological result whether or not later invalidated. The investigations should detail your findings regarding the root causes of the contamination.

● 对所有可能存在有害微生物污染或超标（OOS）微生物结果（无论之后是否无效）的批次进行全面调查。调查应详细说明你公司对污染根本原因的调查结果。

● Appropriate microbiological lot release specifications（i.e., total counts, identification of bioburden to detect objectionable microbes）for each of your API.

● 为你公司的每种 API，制定适当的微生物批放行质量标准（即总计数、微生物鉴别，以检测有害微生物）。

● A list of chemical and microbial specifications, including test methods, used to analyze each lot of your intermediate and API before lot disposition decision.

● 化学和微生物质量标准清单，包括检验方法，用于在批次处置决定之前分析每批中间体和原料药。

● A summary of results from testing retain samples of all API lots within expiry. You should test all appropriate quality attributes including, but not limited to, identity and strength of active ingredients and microbiological quality（total counts and identification of bioburden to detect any objectionable microbes）of each lot. If testing yields an OOS result, indicate the corrective actions you will take, including notifying customers and initiating recalls.

● 就所有仍效期内所有 API 批次的留样，提供检验结果汇总。你公司应检验所有适当的质量属性，包括但不限于每批次的原料药的鉴别和规格以及微生物质量（总计数和微生物鉴别，以检测有害微生物）。如果检验产生 OOS 结果，请说明你公司将采取的纠正措施，包括通知客户和发起召回。

● A detailed summary of your validation program for ensuring a state of control throughout the product lifecycle, along with associated procedures. Describe your program for process performance qualification, and ongoing monitoring of both intra-lot and inter-lot variation to ensure a continuing state of control. This should include the process for selecting API lots to achieve the final API blend.

● 用于确保整个产品生命周期控制状态的验证计划的详细总结以及相关程序。描述你公司的工艺性能确认计划，以及对批次内和批次间变化的持续监控，以确保持续的控制状态。这应包括选择 API 批次的流程，以实现最终 API 混合。

● A timeline for performing appropriate（PPQ）for each of your marketed API.

● 对每种上市 API 执行工艺性能确认（PPQ）的时间表。

● Include your process performance protocol（s）, and written procedures for qualification of equipment and facilities.

● 包括你公司的工艺性能方案，以及设备和设施确认的书面程序。

● An assessment of each API process to ensure that there is a data-driven and scientifically sound program that identifies and controls all sources of variability, such that your production processes, and will consistently meet appropriate specifications and manufacturing standards. This includes, but is not limited to, evaluating suitability of equipment for its intended use, sufficiency of detectability in your monitoring and testing systems, quality of input materials, and reliability of each manufacturing process step and control.

● 对每种原料药生产工艺的评估，以确保有一个数据驱动和科学合理的程序，来识别和控制所有可变性来源，以便使你公司的生产工艺始终如一满足相应的质量标准和生产标准。这包括但不限于评估设备对其预期用途的适用性、监测和检验系统中可检验性的充分性、输入物料的质量、每个生产工艺步骤和控制的可靠性。

● Timelines for completed process performance qualification for marketed porcine thyroid API（b）（4）and（b）（4）processed.

● 针对已上市并进行（b）（4）和（b）（4）处理的猪甲状腺 API，提供完成工艺性能确认的时间表。

偏差调查不力

2. Failure to establish and follow written procedures for investigating critical deviations or the failure of intermediates and API lots to meet specifications.

2. 未能建立并遵循书面程序，来调查关键偏差或中间体和原料药批次不符合质量标准的情况。

You failed to adequately investigate OOS results. For example：

你公司未能充分调查 OOS 结果。例如：

● You received a customer complaint for an OOS microbial result for full-strength porcine thyroid API. The complaint lot was composed of（b）（4）sublots of（b）（4）intermediate，two of which were reprocessed due to potential *Escherichia coli*（*E. coli*）contamination. Your investigation consisted mainly of a retrospective evaluation of similar complaints received at your firm. You did not sufficiently extend your investigation to the manufacturing process and there is no evidence that you evaluated retain samples.

● 你公司收到了关于全规格猪甲状腺 API 微生物结果 OOS 的客户投诉。投诉批次由（b）（4）中间体的（b）（4）个亚批组成，其中两个亚批由于潜在的大肠埃希菌（*E. coli*）污染而被返工。你公司的调查主要包括对收到的类似投诉进行回顾性评估，而没有充分地将调查扩展到生产工艺，也没有证据表明你们评估了留样。

● You reported an OOS microbiological result，of six times the allowable limit，for a porcine thyroid API lot manufactured for stability studies. Your limited phase 2 investigation concluded the OOS result was most probably due to a contamination during sampling. The manufacturing process of the lot was not sufficiently evaluated as part of the investigation and no additional actions were taken.

● 对于为稳定性研究而生产的一批猪甲状腺 API，你公司报告的微生物 OOS 结果是允许限度的六倍。你们有限的第 2 阶段调查得出的结论是，OOS 结果很可能是由于取样过程中的污染造成的。该批次的生产工艺没有作为调查的一部分得到充分评估，也没有采取其他措施。

● You initiated two OOS investigations into high（b）（4）results for porcine thyroid API. You did not identify a root cause for each investigation. Your investigations did not sufficiently extend to manufacturing operations that could affect the OOS lots as well as other lots of porcine thyroid API. Although the investigations were both associated with similarly high OOS（b）（4）results，the conclusions of each investigation were different. In the May 2021 investigation，you stated that the lot could not be further processed and should be rejected. However，the August 2021 investigation concluded that the lot could be reworked. No corrective action and preventive action（CAPA）was opened for either investigation. In addition，the lot associated with the August 2021 investigation was rejected during our inspection，one year after the investigation was closed and without establishing a documented reason for its rejection.

● 针对猪甲状腺 API 的（b）（4）过高结果，你公司启动了两项 OOS 调查。你们没有确定每项调查的根本原因。调查没有充分扩展到可能影响 OOS 批次，以及其他猪甲状腺 API 批次的生产操作。尽管两项调查都与相似的（b）（4）过高 OOS 结果相关，但每项调查的结论都不同。在 2021 年 5 月的调查中，你公司表示该批次无法进一步处理，应被拒放。然而，2021 年 8 月的调查得出的结论是，该批次可以进行返工。两项调查均未采取纠正和预防措施（CAPA）。此外，与 2021 年 8 月调查相关的批次是在调查结束一年后，在我们的检查期间被拒放的，并且没有建立拒放原因的记录。

In your response, you state that you revised your investigation procedures to include trend analysis, bracketing, and a more robust root cause determination, including operator interviews. You initiated multiple CAPAs to further investigate the root cause of the（b）（4）failures and to provide additional information for microbial OOS results.

在回复中，你公司表示你们修订了调查程序，以包括趋势分析、分组和更可靠的根本原因确定（包括操作员访谈）。你公司启动了多项 CAPA，以进一步调查（b）（4）不合格的根本原因，并为微生物 OOS 结果提供更多信息。

Your response is inadequate. Your response to the complaint investigation does not address your failure to adequately evaluate your manufacturing process. It also does not include any commitment to evaluate retain samples. Although you commit to further investigate the root cause for your microbial and（b）（4）OOS results you fail to provide the evidence. It is not clear if you evaluated the manufacturing process and extended the investigations to other lots that may have been potentially impacted.

你公司的回应不充分。你公司对投诉调查的回复并未阐明你们未能充分评估生产工艺的问题。就评估留样，也未能包括任何承诺。尽管承诺进一步调查微生物和（b）（4）OOS 结果的根本原因，但你们未能提供证据。目前尚不清楚你公司是否评估了生产工艺，并将调查范围扩大到可能受到潜在影响的其他批次。

In response to this letter, provide：

在回复本函时，请提供：

● A comprehensive, independent assessment of your overall system for investigating deviations, discrepancies, complaints, OOS results, and failures. Provide a detailed action plan to remediate this system. Your action plan should include, but not be limited to, significant improvements in investigation competencies, scope determination, root cause evaluation, CAPA effectiveness, quality unit oversight, and written procedures. Address how your firm will ensure all phases of investigations are appropriately conducted.

● 对调查偏差、差异、投诉、OOS 结果和不合格的整个系统进行全面、独立的评估。提供一个详细的行动计划来整改该系统。你公司的行动计划应包括但不限于在调查能力、范围确定、根本原因评估、CAPA 有效性、质量部门监督和书面程序方面的显著提高。说明你公司将如何确保适当地进行所有阶段的调查。

● A retrospective, independent review of all invalidated OOS（including in-process and release/stability testing）results for porcine thyroid API lots manufactured and release in the last three years and a report summarizing the findings of the analysis, including the following for each OOS：

● 就过去三年中生产和放行的猪甲状腺 API 批次，针对所有无效 OOS 结果（包括中控和放行 / 稳定性检验），提供回顾性的独立审查报告，以及一份总结分析结果的报告，就每个 OOS 包括以下内容：

○ Determine whether the scientific justification and evidence relating to the invalidated OOS result conclusively or inconclusively demonstrates causative laboratory error.

○ 对于与无效 OOS 结果相关的科学论证和证据，确定其是否确凿或不确凿地证明了实验室相关的错误。

○ For investigations that conclusively establish laboratory root cause, provide rationale, and ensure that all other laboratory methods vulnerable to the same or similar root cause are identified for remediation.

○ 对于最终确定实验室为根本原因的调查，提供论证，并确定所有其他易受相同或类似根本原因影响的实验室方法，以进行整改。

○ For all OOS results found by the retrospective review to have an inconclusive or no root cause identified in the laboratory, include a thorough review of production（e.g., lot manufacturing records, adequacy of the manufacturing steps, suitability of equipment/ facilities, variability of raw materials, process capability, deviation history, complaint history, lot failure history）. Provide a summary of potential manufacturing root causes for each investigation, and any manufacturing operation improvements.

○ 在回顾性审查中，对于发现 OOS 结果在实验室中没有确定的根本原因，或没有根本原因的情况，应包括对生产的全面检查（例如，批生产记录、生产步骤是否适当、设备 / 设施的适用性，原料的可变性、工艺能力、偏差历史、投诉历史和批次不合格历史）。就每次调查的潜在生产根本原因，以及任何生产操作改进，提供总结。

混批质量控制

3. Failure to ensure that API lots meet specifications prior to blending with other lots.

3. 在与其他批次混合之前，未能确保 API 批次符合质量标准。

You failed to perform analytical testing prior to the final blend of (b)(4) intermediate lots. Your final blend consisted of up to (b)(4) intermediate lots. This practice may result in the blending of lots not meeting specifications and unreliable results reported for your finished API.

在最终混合（b）（4）个中间批次之前，你公司未能执行分析检验。最终混合由多达（b）（4）个中间批次组成。这种实践可能会导致混合批次不符合质量标准，且使得成品 API 报告的结果不可靠。

In your response, you commit to implement top, middle, and bottom sampling of each container for in-process (b)(4) intermediates of your finished full strength porcine thyroid API.

在回复中，针对全规格猪甲状腺 API 成品的（b）（4）中间体，你公司承诺进行容器的顶部、中部和底部取样。

Your response is inadequate because you do not sufficiently explain why you will only test (b)(4) intermediates for microbial load and (b)(4). You did not commit to perform full testing of (b)(4) intermediate lots prior to blending. In addition, your response lacks a commitment to evaluate lot uniformity of other strengths of distributed porcine thyroid API previously manufactured at your firm that may still be on the market.

你公司的回应不充分，因为没有充分解释为何仅将对（b）（4）中间体进行微生物负荷和（b）（4）检验。你公司也没有承诺在混合之前对（b）（4）中间批次进行全面检验。此外，针对之前生产的、已流通并可能仍在市场上的其他规格的猪甲状腺 API，你公司的回复缺乏对其批次一致性评估的承诺。

In response to this letter, provide:

在回复本函时，请提供：

● A comprehensive, independent assessment of your in-process monitoring and sampling operations, focusing on each upstream process step that can introduce variability. Provide your remediation plan to improve: (1) in-process detection of variation; (2) upstream controls; and (3) sampling plans.

● 对过程中监控和取样操作进行全面、独立的评估，重点关注可能引入变异性的每个上游工艺步骤。提供你公司的整改计划以改进：①过程中变异检测；②上游控制；③取样计划。

● An action plan and timelines for conducting full chemical and microbiological testing of retain samples to determine the quality of all lots of API distributed to the United States that are within expiry as of the date of this letter.

● 行动计划和时间表：对留样进行全面的化学和微生物检验，对于流通给美国的所有效期内（本函发出之日计）API 批次，确定其质量。

● A summary of all results obtained from testing retain samples from each lot. If such testing reveals substandard quality API, take rapid corrective actions, such as notifying customers and product recalls.

● 所有批次的留样检验总结。如果此类检验表明 API 质量不合格，请迅速采取整改措施，例如通知客户和产品召回。

Process Validation | 工艺验证

Process validation evaluates the soundness of design and state of control of a process throughout its lifecycle. Each significant stage of a manufacturing process must be designed appropriately and assure the quality of raw material inputs, in-process materials, and finished drugs. Process qualification studies determine whether an initial state of control has been established.

工艺验证评估工艺在其整个生命周期内的设计合理性和控制状态。生产工艺中的每个重要阶段都必须进行适当的设计，并确保原料输入、中间体和成品制剂的质量。工艺确认研究确定是否已建立初始控制状态。

Successful process qualification studies are necessary before commercial distribution. Thereafter, ongoing vigilant oversight of process performance and product quality is necessary to ensure you maintain a stable manufacturing operation throughout the product lifecycle.

在商业流通之前，必须进行成功的工艺确认研究。此后，有必要对工艺性能和产品质量进行持续的警戒性监控，以确保你们在整个产品生命周期内保持稳定的生产操作。

Process Controls | 过程控制

Your firm lacks an ongoing program for monitoring process control to ensure stable manufacturing operations and consistent drug quality. See FDA's guidance document *Process Validation：General Principles and Practices* for general principles and approaches that FDA considers appropriate elements of process validation at https://www.fda.gov/regulatory-information/search-fda-guidance-documents/process-validation-general-principles-and-practices.

你公司缺乏用于监控过程控制的持续计划，以确保稳定的生产操作和一致的药品质量。有关 FDA 认为适当的工艺验证要素的一般原则和方法，请参阅 FDA 的指南，工艺验证：一般原则和实践，网址（略，见上）。

Quality Systems | 质量体系

Your firm's quality systems are inadequate. For guidance on establishing and maintaining cGMP-compliant quality systems, see FDA's guidances: *Q8（R2）Pharmaceutical Development* at https://www.fda.gov/regulatory-information/search-fda-guidance-documents/q8r2-pharmaceutical-development, *Q9 Quality Risk Management* at https://www.fda.gov/regulatory-information/search-fda-guidance-documents/q9-quality-risk-management and *Q10 Pharmaceutical Quality System* at https://www.fda.gov/regulatory-information/search-fda-guidance-documents/q10-pharmaceutical-quality-system.

你公司的质量体系不完善。有关建立和维护符合 cGMP 的质量体系的指南，请参阅 FDA 的指南：Q8（R2）药物开发，网址（略，见上），Q9 质量风险管理，网址为（略，见上）和 Q10 药品质量体系，网址（略，见上）。

Test Results Out-of-Specification | 检验结果不符合质量标准

For more information about handling failing, out-of-specification, out-of-trend, or other unexpected results and documentation of your investigations, see FDA's guidance document *Investigating Out-of-Specification（OOS）Test Results for Pharmaceutical Production* at https://www.fda.gov/regulatory-information/search-fda-guidance-documents/investigating-out-specification-oos-test-results-pharmaceutical-production-level-2-revision.

有关处理不合格、OOS、超常或其他非预期结果以及你公司的调查记录的更多信息，请参阅 FDA 的指南，调查药品生产的不合格（OOS）检验结果，网址（略，见上）。

A possible laboratory error is insufficient to close an investigation at Phase 1. Whenever an investigation lacks conclusive evidence of laboratory error, a thorough investigation of potential manufacturing causes must be performed.

实验室错误的可能性不足以结束第一阶段的调查。当调查缺乏实验室错误的确凿证据时，就必须对潜在的生产原因进行彻底调查。

Contractor's Responsibilities | 合同商的责任

During the inspection, a review of microbiological results for five porcine thyroid API lots showed identical results, which is not typical for microbial testing. Your firm did not perform an evaluation of the validity of these atypical results. It is your responsibility to use a qualified contract testing laboratory that produces accurate and reliable results.

在检查过程中，对五个猪甲状腺原料药批次的微生物学结果进行审查显示出相同的结果，这对于微生物检验来说并不常见。对于这些非典型结果的有效性，你公司没有进行评估。你们有责任使用有资质的委托检验实验室来产生准确可靠的结果。

We also noted that your contract laboratory provided you with certificates of analysis （COA）that you used to release your lots, even though the COA stated, "results are not suitable for GMP release for clinical or commercial use." This testing does not support the release of your API for human use.

我们还注意到，你公司的委托实验室向你们提供了用于放行批次的分析证书（COA），尽管 COA 声明"结果不适合用于临床或商业用途的 GMP 放行"。此检验不支持放行你公司的 API 供人用。

FDA considers contractors, such as contracted laboratories, as extensions of the manufacturer's own facility. Your failure to comply with cGMP may affect the quality, safety, and efficacy of the drugs you test for your clients. It is essential that you understand your responsibility to operate in full compliance with cGMP, and that you inform all your customers of any out-of-specification results or significant problems encountered during the testing of these drugs.

FDA 将合同方（例如委托实验室）视为生产商自己设施的延伸。你公司未能遵守 cGMP 可能会影响你们为客户检验的药物的质量、安全性和有效性。你公司必须了解自己的责任，即完全按照 cGMP 进行操作，并就在检验这些药物期间遇到的任何不符合质量标准的结果或重大问题，告知所有客户。

Additional API cGMP Guidance | 其他原料药 cGMP 指南

FDA considers the expectations outlined in ICH Q7 when determining whether API are manufactured in conformance with cGMP. See FDA's guidance document *Q7 Good Manufacturing Practice Guidance for Active Pharmaceutical Ingredients* for guidance regarding cGMP for the manufacture of API at https://www.fda.gov/regulatory-information/search-fda-guidance-documents/guidance-industry-q7a-good-manufacturing-practice-guidance–active–pharmaceutical–ingredients.

在确定原料药的生产是否符合 cGMP 时，FDA 会考虑 ICH Q7 中概述的期望。有关原料药生产的 cGMP 指南，请参阅 FDA 的指南 Q7 原料药药品生产质量管理规范指南，网址（见上，略）。

cGMP Consultant Recommended | cGMP 顾问推荐

Based upon the nature of the deviations we identified at your firm, we strongly recommend engaging a consultant qualified to evaluate your operations to assist your firm in meeting cGMP requirements. Your use of a consultant does not relieve your firm's obligation to comply with cGMP. Your firm's executive management remains responsible for resolving all deficiencies and systemic flaws to ensure ongoing cGMP compliance

根据我们在你公司发现的偏差性质，我们强烈建议聘请有资质评估你公司运营的顾问，以协助你公司满足 cGMP 要求。聘用顾问并不能免除你公司遵守 cGMP 的义务。你公司的高级管理层仍负责解决所有缺陷和系统性问题，以确保持续遵守 cGMP。

Conclusion | 结论

The deviations cited in this letter are not intended to be an all–inclusive list of deviations that exist at your facility. You are responsible for investigating and determining the causes of any deviations and for preventing their recurrence or the occurrence of other deviations.

本信函中引用的偏差行为并非旨在列出与你公司设施相关的所有偏差行为。你公司有责任调查和确定这些偏差的原因，并防止其再次发生或发生其他偏差情况。

If you are considering an action that is likely to lead to a disruption in the supply of drugs produced at your facility, FDA requests that you contact CDER's Drug Shortages Staff immediately, at drugshortages@fda.hhs.gov, so that FDA can work with you on the most effective way to bring your operations into compliance with the law. Contacting the Drug Shortages Staff also allows you to meet any obligations you may have to report discontinuances or interruptions in your drug manufacture under 21 U.S.C. 356C(b). This also allows FDA to consider, as soon as possible, what actions, if any, may be needed to avoid shortages and protect the health of patients who depend on your products.

如果你公司考虑采取的行动会导致所生产药品的供应中断，FDA 要求你们立即联系 CDER 的药品短缺工作人员（drugshortages@fda.hhs.gov），以便 FDA 可以与你们以最有效的方式沟通，使你公司的运营符合法律规定。根据 21 U.S.C. 356C(b) 规定，与

23

药品短缺工作人员联系，还可以使你公司履行报告药品供应中断的义务。这也使 FDA 可以尽快考虑可能需要采取什么措施，以避免短缺，并保护依赖你们产品的患者的健康（如有）。

Correct any deviations promptly. Failure to promptly and adequately address this matter may result in regulatory or legal action without further notice including, without limitation, seizure, and injunction. Unresolved deviations may also prevent other Federal agencies from awarding contracts.

及时纠正任何偏差。未能及时和充分解决此问题可能会导致监管或法律行动，恕不另行通知，包括但不限于扣押和禁令。未解决的偏差也可能阻止其他联邦机构授予合同。

Failure to address deviations may also cause FDA to withhold issuance of Export Certificates. FDA may withhold approval of new applications or supplements listing your firm as a drug manufacturer until any deviations are completely addressed and we confirm your compliance with cGMP. We may re-inspect to verify that you have completed corrective actions to address any deviations.

未能解决偏差也可能导致 FDA 拒绝颁发出口证书。FDA 可能会拒绝批准将你们公司列为新药申请或补充申请的药品生产商，直到完全解决所有偏差并且我们确认你公司符合 cGMP。我们可能会再次检查，以确认你公司已完成对任何偏差的纠正措施。

This letter notifies you of our findings and provides you an opportunity to address the above deficiencies. After you receive this letter, respond to this office in writing within 15 working days. Specify what you have done to address any deviations and to prevent their recurrence. In response to this letter, you may provide additional information for our consideration as we continue to assess your activities and practices. If you cannot complete corrective actions within 15 working days, state your reasons for delay and your schedule for completion.

本信函通知你公司我们的发现，并为你公司提供解决上述缺陷的机会。收到本信函后，请在 15 个工作日内以书面形式回复本办公室。说明你公司为解决任何偏差并防止其再次发生所做的工作。在回复本信函时，你公司可以提供更多信息供我们考虑，因为我们将继续评估你们的活动和实践。如果你公司无法在 15 个工作日内完成纠正措施，请说明延误原因和完成时间表。

2 原料药厂家拒绝向 FDA 提供记录和资料

警告信编号： MARCS-CMS 659389

签发时间： 2023-6-20；**公示时间：** 2023-6-27

签发机构： 药物审评与研究中心 | CDER（Center for Drug Evaluation and Research | CDER）

公　　司： Chengdu KeCheng Fine Chemicals Co., Ltd.

所在国家 / 地区： 中国

主　　题： cGMP/ 原料药（API）/ 掺假 [cGMP/Active Pharmaceutical Ingredient（API）/Adulterated]

简　　介： FDA 表示，该公司作为 API 生产商，多次向美国出口原料药。FDA 在 2022 年 7 月和 8 月分别发出了两次记录要求，但未得到回复。尽管该公司声称不再向美国出口产品，但直到 2023 年 1 月仍在继续向美国出口 API。该公司未提供 FDA 要求的记录，导致没有迹象表明该公司生产的药品质量保证水平是可靠的。FDA 于 2023 年 6 月将该公司生产的所有药品列入进口警报，可能拒绝批准其相关的新申请或补充申请。该公司被要求在 15 个工作日内书面回复，提供信息供 FDA 考虑，并继续接受 FDA 的评估或检查。

Your firm was registered with the United States Food and Drug Administration（FDA or Agency）as a manufacturer of several active pharmaceutical ingredients（APIs）. A review of import records showed multiple shipments of API into the U.S. which declared Chengdu KeCheng Fine Chemicals Co., Ltd. as the drug manufacturer. On July 18, 2022, the FDA sent an electronic request for records and other information pursuant to section 704（a）（4）of the Federal Food, Drug, and Cosmetic Act（FD&C Act）, 21 U.S.C. 374（a）（4）, to the contact e-mail address provided in your registration file. This request went unanswered. A second request was sent via email on August 8, 2022, followed by a telephone call from the FDA to you on October 24, 2022, regarding this matter. During the telephone call, you refused to provide your full name or an alternate email address for further communication. You stated that your firm was not shipping products to the U.S. and that you would deregister your firm as a drug establishment. However, your firm has continued to ship API to the U.S. as recently as January 2023. The Agency sent a follow-up electronic request for such records and other information on March 9, 2023. You failed to respond to these attempted communications or otherwise provide the requested records or other information. Pursuant to section 704（a）（4）, FDA's request and follow-up communications included a sufficient and clear description of the records sought.

你公司已在美国食品药品管理局（FDA）注册为多种原料药（API）的生产商。进口记录审查显示，多批原料药运往美国，药品生产商为（略，见上）。2022 年 7 月 18 日，根据《联邦食品、药品和化妆品法案》（FD&C 法案）第 704（a）（4）条［21 U.S.C. 374（a）（4）］，FDA 根据你公司在注册文件中提供的电子邮件地址，以电子邮件的形式提出"提供记录和其他信息"的要求。这一要求没有得到回复。2022 年 8 月 8 日，第二次要求通过电子邮件发出；随后 FDA 于 2022 年 10 月 24 日就此事致电你公司。在电话通话期间，你公司拒绝提供你们的全名或备用电子邮件地址以进行进一步沟通。你公司表示不会将产品出口到美国，并且将注销公司作为药品企业的注册。然而，直到 2023 年 1 月，你公司还继续向美国运送原料药。2023 年 3 月 9 日，FDA 发出了后续电子要求，要求提供记录和其他信息。你公司未能回应这些沟通尝试，或以其他方式提供所要求的记录或其他信息。根据 FD&C 法案第 704（a）（4）条，FDA 的要求和后续沟通包括了对所要求记录的充分且清晰的描述。

It is a prohibited act under section 301（e）of the FD&C Act（21 U.S.C. 331（e））to refuse to permit access to or copying of any record as required by section 704（a）. Because your API firm failed to respond to the section 704（a）（4）records requests and associated communication attempts, we have no indication of the level of quality assurance for drugs listed as manufactured at your facility.

根据 FD&C 法案第 301（e）条［21 U.S.C. 331（e）］，拒绝允许访问或复制 FD&C 法案第 704（a）条要求的任何记录属于禁止行为。由于你公司未能回应 FD&C 法案第 704（a）（4）条记录要求和相关的沟通尝试，因此没有证据证明你公司设施生产的药品质量保证水平。

FDA placed all drugs and drug products manufactured by your firm on Import Alert 66-79 on June 8, 2023.

2023 年 6 月 8 日，FDA 将你公司生产的所有药品列入进口警报 66-79。

Until FDA is able to confirm compliance with cGMP and other applicable requirements, we may withhold approval of any new applications or supplements listing your firm as a drug manufacturer. In addition, shipments of articles manufactured at Chengdu KeCheng Fine Chemicals Co., Ltd., Floor 9, No. 18 Chuangye Road, Chengdu High-Tech District,

Chengdu, Sichuan into the U.S. that appear to be adulterated or misbranded are subject to being detained or refused admission pursuant to section 801（a）（3）of the FD&C Act, 21 U.S.C. 381（a）（3）.

在 FDA 能够确认符合 cGMP 和其他适用要求之前，我们可能会拒绝批准将你公司列为药品生产商的新申请或补充申请。此外，根据 FD&C 法案第 801（a）（3）条、21 U.S.C. 381（a）（3），在地址（略，见上）生产的物品运往美国时，视为掺假或标识错误的产品将会被扣留或拒绝入境。

After you receive this letter, respond to this office in writing within 15 working days. In response to this letter, you may provide information for our consideration as we continue to assess your activities and practices, and/or submit a request to schedule an FDA inspection.

你公司收到此函后，请在 15 个工作日内以书面形式回复本办公室。在回复本函时，你公司可以提供信息供我们考虑，因为我们将继续评估你公司的活动和实践、和（或）提交安排 FDA 检查的要求。

第三部分

外包活动

1 质量部门未能履责

警告信编号： MARCS-CMS 642082

签发时间： 2023-1-20；**公示时间：** 2023-3-14

签发机构： 药品质量业务一处（Division of Pharmaceutical Quality Operations I）

公　　司： Atlantic Management Resources LTD dba. Claire Ellen Products

所在国家/地区： 美国

主　　题： cGMP/成品制剂/掺假（cGMP/Finished Pharmaceuticals/ Adulterated）

简　　介： 2022 年 7 月至 8 月，FDA 对位于美国马萨诸塞州的药品生产设施进行了检查，并发现了严重的 cGMP 违规情况。警告信详细指出了质量部门建立不完善的问题，其中包括质量部门缺乏书面责任和程序，未制定物料取样、检查和检验的记录程序，以及没有供应商确认计划和顺势疗法成品检验程序。FDA 强调了质量部门的关键职责，包括批准或拒绝物料、半成品和成品，确保生产过程中的控制得到适当执行，并调查任何不符合规定的差异。另外，作为合同生产商，FDA 再次强调，无论与产品所有者达成何种协议，公司都必须对生产的药品质量负责。

本警告信以下部分与本书此前其他警告信内容类似，故略去：结论（Conclusion）。

The U.S. Food and Drug Administration（FDA）inspected your drug manufacturing facility，Atlantic Management Resources Ltd. dba. Claire Ellen Products，FEI 3014117482，located at 39 Harvey Lane，Westborough，MA，from July 26，2022 to August 10，2022.

2022 年 7 月 26 日至 8 月 10 日，美国食品药品管理局（FDA）检查了你公司的药品生产设施 Atlantic Management Resources Ltd. dba. Claire Ellen Products，FEI

3014117482，位于美国马萨诸塞州（略，见上）。

This warning letter summarizes significant violations of Current Good Manufacturing Practice（cGMP）regulations for finished pharmaceuticals. See Title 21 Code of Federal Regulations（CFR）, parts 210 and 211（21 CFR parts 210 and 211）.

本警告信总结了对成品制剂现行药品生产质量管理规范（cGMP）的严重违规情况。请参阅联邦法规（CFR）第 21 篇第 210 和 211 部分（21 CFR 第 210 和 211 部分）。

Because your methods, facilities, or controls for manufacturing, processing, packing, or holding do not conform to cGMP, your drug products are adulterated within the meaning of section 501（a）（2）（B）of the Federal Food, Drug, and Cosmetic Act（FD&C Act）, 21 U.S.C. 351（a）（2）（B）.

由于你公司用于生产、加工、包装或贮存的方法、设施或控制措施不符合 cGMP，因此根据 FD&C 法案第 501（a）（2）（B）条、21 U.S.C.351（a）（2）（B）的规定，你公司药品被认为是掺假。

Atlantic Management Resources Inc., the manufacturing business entity for Atlantic Management Resources LTD, located at the same address, was duly registered with FDA at the time of manufacturing and distributing, as required by section 510 of the FD&C Act and 21 CFR Part 207. With some limited exceptions, firms that manufacture, prepare, propagate, compound, or process drugs in the United States, or that are offered for import into the United States, must be registered with the FDA. Sections 510（b）,（c）,（d）, and（i）of the FD&C Act, 21 U.S.C. 360（b）,（c）,（d）, and（i）.

Atlantic Management Resources Inc. 是 Atlantic Management Resources LTD 的生产业务实体，位于同一地址，根据 FD&C 法案第 510 条和 21 CFR 第 207 部分的要求，在生产和流通时已在 FDA 正式注册。除一些有限的例外情况外，在美国生产、准备、扩增、调配或加工药品的公司，或者进口到美国的公司，必须向 FDA 进行注册。这是基于 FD&C 法案第 510（b）（c）（d）和（i）条，即 21 U.S.C. 360（b）（c）（d）和（i）。

Atlantic Management Resources LTD distributed under its own name and label, drugs that were not duly listed with FDA. Failure to properly list a drug product is prohibited under section 301（p）of the FD&C Act, 21 U.S.C. 331（p）, and will render a drug misbranded under section 502（o）of the FD&C Act, 21 U.S.C. 352（o）. Introduction or delivery for introduction of such products into interstate commerce is prohibited under section 301（a）of the FD&C Act, 21 U.S.C. 331（a）. These violations are described in more detail below.

Atlantic Management Resources LTD 以其自己的名称和标签流通未在 FDA 正式注册的药品。FD&C 法案第 301（p）条、21 U.S.C. 331（p）禁止未能正确注册药品，并且根据 FD&C 法案第 502（o）条，即 21 U.S.C. 352（o），这将导致药品标识错误。FD&C 法案第 301（a）条、21 U.S.C. 331（a）禁止将此类产品引入或交付到州际贸易中。下面将更详细地描述这些违规情况。

As per Atlantic Management Resources LTD's response to FDA, dated November 5, 2022, the firm agreed to cease production and distribution of all drug products, however, all products previously listed with FDA remain listed, and Atlantic Management Resources Inc, the manufacturing business entity located at the same address, renewed its registration on January 9, 2023 with FDA for the 2023 calendar year.

根据 Atlantic Management Resources LTD 于 2022 年 11 月 5 日对 FDA 的回应，该公司同意停止生产和流通所有药品，但是之前在 FDA 注册的所有产品仍在初测状态，并且生产业务实体 Atlantic Management Resources Inc 位于同一地址，于 2023 年 1 月 9 日在 FDA 更新了 2023 日历年的注册情况。

We reviewed your August 17, 2022 response to our Form FDA 483 in detail and acknowledge receipt of your subsequent correspondence. Your response is inadequate because it did not provide sufficient detail or evidence of corrective actions to bring your operations into compliance with cGMP.

我们详细审查了你公司于 2022 年 8 月 17 日对 FDA 483 表格的回复，并确认收到你们随后的来函。你公司的回复不充分，因为没有提供充分的细节或纠正措施的证据，以使你们的运营符合 cGMP。

During our inspection, our investigators observed specific violations including, but not limited to, the following.

在检查过程中，我们的调查员发现了具体的违规情况，包括但不限于以下内容。

质量部门未能履责

1. Your firm failed to establish an adequate quality unit and the responsibilities and procedures applicable to the quality control unit are not in writing and fully followed（21 CFR 211.22（a）and（d）).

1. 你公司未能建立适当的质量部门，适用于质量部门的责任和程序未以书面形式呈现且未得到完全遵守［21 CFR 211.22（a）和（d）］。

Your firm failed to establish a quality unit（QU）with the responsibilities and authority to oversee the manufacture of your homeopathic drug products.

你公司未能建立一个具有监督顺势疗法药品生产的责任和权力的质量部门（QU）。

You stated that your firm does not have any written procedures, including those that govern quality operations. For example, you failed to have written procedures to ensure documented sampling, examination, and testing of components before production. In addition, you failed to establish a program for qualifying suppliers and ensuring that your homeopathic finished drug products are tested prior to release and distribution to the customer.

你公司表示没有任何书面程序，包括管理质量运营的程序。例如，没有制定书面程序，来确保生产前对物料进行取样、检查和检验的记录。此外，你公司未能制定供应商确认计划，并确保顺势疗法成品在放行和流通给客户之前经过检验。

Quality unit responsibilities include, but are not limited to, approving or rejecting incoming materials, in-process materials, and drug products; ensuring that controls are implemented and completed satisfactorily during manufacturing operations; and reviewing production records and investigating any unexplained discrepancies.

质量部门的职责包括但不限于批准或拒放进场物料、半成品和药品；确保在生产运营期间令人满意地实施和完成控制；审查生产记录并调查任何无法解释的偏差。

These, and other basic quality responsibilities, are integral to conducting effective and appropriate oversight for the manufacturing of your drugs.

这些以及其他基本质量责任是对药品生产进行有效和适当监督的组成部分。

Your firm's quality systems are inadequate. See FDA's guidance document *Quality Systems Approach to Pharmaceutical cGMP Regulations* for help implementing quality systems and risk management approaches to meet the requirements of cGMP regulations 21 CFR, parts 210 and 211 at https://www.fda.gov/media/71023/download.

你公司的质量体系不够完善。请参阅 FDA 指南，药品 cGMP 法规的质量系统方法，以帮助实施质量系统和风险管理方法，以满足 cGMP 法规 21 CFR 第 210 和 211 部分的要求，网址（略，见上）。

储存条件

2. Your firm failed to store drug products under appropriate conditions of temperature, humidity, and light so that the identity, strength, quality, and purity are not affected (21 CFR 211.142 (b)).

2. 你公司未能在适当的温度、湿度和光线条件下储存药品，以致其鉴别、规格、质量和纯度不受影响［21 CFR 211.142（b）］。

You failed to have adequate storage and warehousing of drug products. For example, although a supplier's certificate of analysis（COA）for a bulk drug stated that the drug is sensitive to heat, sunlight, and moisture, you failed to monitor storage conditions for the drug, including for temperature and humidity. You also acknowledged that there were inadequate storage conditions for drug products, and for your containers and closures. The holding of drug products must be performed under appropriate conditions so that the identity, strength, quality, and purity are not affected.

你公司没有充分的药品储存和仓储。例如，尽管供应商的原料药分析证书（COA）表明，该药品对热、光和湿气敏感，但你公司未能监控该药品的储存条件，包括温湿度。你们还承认药品、容器和密封件的储存条件不充分。药品的保存必须在适当的条件下进行，以免影响其鉴别、规格、质量和纯度。

批生产和控制记录

3. Your firm failed to prepare batch production and control records that include documentation of the accomplishment of each significant step in the manufacture, processing, packing, or holding of the batch, for each batch of drug product（21 CFR 211.188（b））.

3. 你公司未能为每批药品准备批生产和控制记录，其中包括该批次生产、加工、包装或放置中每个重要步骤的完成情况［21 CFR 211.188（b）］。

Your firm failed to have batch and control records that document your manufacturing operations. You stated that there were no batch records and no batch numbers. Batch records are required to capture significant information to assure that your drug products have been manufactured, processed, packed, or held properly.

你公司没有记录生产操作的批次和控制记录。你们表示没有批记录，也没有批次号。批记录需要捕获重要信息，以确保药品已正确生产、加工、包装或保存。

Drug Production Ceased | 药品生产停止

On November 3, 2022, FDA held a teleconference with you. We recommended you remove any batches of drug product currently in distribution from the U.S. market and also consider ceasing further distribution.

2022 年 11 月 3 日，FDA 与你公司召开了电话会议。我们建议你们从美国市场上下架目前正在流通的所有批次药品，并考虑停止进一步流通。

On November 5, 2022, you communicated your firm's commitment to cease distribution of the drug product on the website, cease production and distribution of all drug products, and consider a voluntary recall all drug products.

2022 年 11 月 5 日，你公司承诺停止在网站上流通药品，停止生产和流通所有药品，并考虑自愿召回所有药品。

On November 21, 2022, you issued a voluntary nationwide recall of all drug products.

2022 年 11 月 21 日，你公司发布了在全国范围内自愿召回所有药品的决定。

We acknowledge your commitment to cease production and distribution of all drug products.

我们知晓，你公司承诺停止生产和流通所有药品。

In response to this letter, confirm whether you intend to resume manufacture of any drugs at this facility or any other facility in the future. If you plan to resume any manufacturing regulated under the FD&C Act, notify this office prior to resuming your manufacturing operations. If you resume cGMP activities, you are responsible for resolving all deficiencies and systemic flaws to ensure your firm is capable of ongoing cGMP compliance. In addition, based upon the nature of the violations we identified at your firm, you should engage a consultant qualified as set forth in 21 CFR 211.34, to assist your firm in meeting drug cGMP requirements. The qualified consultant should also perform a comprehensive six-system audit of your entire operation for cGMP compliance and evaluate the completion and efficacy of all corrective actions and preventive actions before you pursue resolution of your firm's compliance status with FDA.

在回复本函时，请确认你公司将来是否打算在该设施或任何其他设施恢复任何药品的生产。如果计划恢复任何受 FD&C 法案监管的生产，请在恢复生产运营之前通知本办公室。如果恢复 cGMP 活动，你公司有责任解决所有缺陷和系统问题，以确保你公司能够持续遵守 cGMP。此外，根据我们发现的违规情况的性质，你公司应聘请符合 21 CFR 211.34 规定的有资质的顾问，以协助你公司满足药品 cGMP 要求。有资质的顾问还应对你们的整个运营进行全面的六大系统审核，以确保 cGMP 合规性，并在你们寻求解决公司与 FDA 的合规状态之前，评估所有纠正和预防措施的完成情况和有效性。

Owner's Responsibilities｜产品所有人的责任

Drugs must be manufactured in conformance with cGMP. FDA is aware that many drug manufacturers use independent contractors such as production facilities, testing laboratories, packagers, and labelers. FDA regards contractors as extensions of the manufacturer.

药品必须按照 cGMP 生产。FDA 意识到很多药品生产商使用独立合同商，例如生产设施、检验实验室、包装商和贴标商。FDA 将合同商视为生产商的延伸。

You are responsible for the quality of your drugs regardless of agreements in place with a contract facility. You are required to ensure that drugs are made in accordance with section 501 (a)(2)(B) of the FD&C Act to ensure safety, identity, strength, quality, and purity. See FDA's guidance document *Contract Manufacturing Arrangements for Drugs*: *Quality Agreements* at https://www.fda.gov/regulatory-information/search-fda-guidance-documents/ contract-manufacturing-arrangements-drugs-quality-agreements-guidance-industry.

无论与产品所有者达成何种协议，作为外包设施生产，你公司应对生产的药品质量负责。你们需要确保按照 FD&C 法案第 501 (a)(2)(B) 条的规定生产药品，以确保安全性、鉴别、规格、质量和纯度。请参阅 FDA 的指南文件，药品合同生产安排：质量协议，网址（略，见上）。

Establishment Registration and Drug Listing Violations 企业注册和药品清单违规

Under section 510 (j)(1) of the FD&C Act, 21 U.S.C. 360 (j)(1), 21 CFR 207.41, and 21 CFR 207.49 (a)(5), all drugs manufactured, prepared, propagated, compounded, or processed for U.S. commercial distribution must be listed with FDA. Atlantic Management Resources LTD distributed under its own name and label, Neuroquell Plus Cream, which was not listed with FDA at the time of manufacturing and distribution. Failure to properly list a drug product is prohibited under section 301 (p) of the FD&C Act, 21 U.S.C. 331 (p), and will render a drug misbranded under section 502 (o) of the FD&C Act, 21 U.S.C. 352 (o).

根据 FD&C 法案第 510 (j)(1) 条、21 U.S.C. 360 (j)(1)、21 CFR 207.41 和 21 CFR 207.49 (a)(5)，所有为美国商业流通而生产、制备、扩增、调配或加工的产品必须在 FDA 注册。Atlantic Management Resources LTD 以自己的名称和标签，对 Neuroquell Plus Cream 进行流通，该产品在生产和流通时并未在 FDA 注册。FD&C 法案第 301 (p) 条、21 U.S.C. 331 (p) 禁止未能正确注册的药品，并且根据 FD&C 法案第 502 (o) 条、21 U.S.C. 352 (o)，将导致药品标识错误。

The introduction or delivery for introduction of a misbranded drug into interstate commerce is prohibited under section 301 (a) of the FD&C Act, 21 U.S.C. 331 (a).

FD&C 法案第 301 (a) 条、21 U.S.C. 331 (a) 禁止将标识错误药品引入或交付到州际贸易中。

2 未能提供生产工艺的验证数据

警告信编号： MARCS-CMS 642595

签发时间： 2023-2-1；**公示时间：** 2023-3-14

签发机构： 药品质量业务二处（Division of Pharmaceutical Quality Operations II）

公　　司： Profounda, Inc.

所在国家/地区： 美国

主　　题： cGMP/成品制剂/掺假（cGMP/Finished Pharmaceuticals/Adulterated）

简　　介： 2022年8月3日至8月9日，FDA对位于美国奥兰多的药品生产设施进行了检查。检查中，该公司未能提供OTC药品生产工艺的验证数据，以确认工艺状态和符合标准。FDA强调在商业流通之前，必须进行成功的工艺确认研究。随后，需要对工艺性能和产品质量进行持续的警戒性监控，以确保在整个产品生命周期内维持稳定的生产操作。最后，FDA提醒作为合同商，公司的药品必须按照cGMP生产。公司可聘请有资质的顾问改善质量体系，但聘请顾问并不免除遵守cGMP的责任。高级管理层仍需解决所有缺陷，以维持符合cGMP的状态。

本警告信以下部分与本书此前其他警告信内容类似，故略去：结论（Conclusion）。

The U.S. Food and Drug Administration（FDA）inspected your drug manufacturing facility, Profounda, Inc., FEI 3011873350, at 10501 South Orange Ave., STE 124, Orlando, from August 3 to August 9, 2022.

2022年8月3日至8月9日，美国食品药品管理局（FDA）检查了你们的药品生产设施 Profounda, Inc., FEI 3011873350，其位于美国奥兰多（略，见上）。

This warning letter summarizes significant violations of Current Good Manufacturing

Practice（cGMP）regulations for finished pharmaceuticals. See Title 21 Code of Federal Regulations（CFR）, parts 210 and 211（21 CFR parts 210 and 211）.

本警告信总结了对成品制剂现行药品生产质量管理规范（cGMP）的严重违反情况。请参见美国联邦法规（CFR）第 21 篇第 210 和 211 部分（21 CFR 第 210 和 211 部分）。

Because your methods, facilities, or controls for manufacturing, processing, packing, or holding do not conform to cGMP, your drug products are adulterated within the meaning of section 501（a）（2）（B）of the Federal Food, Drug, and Cosmetic Act（FD&C Act）, 21 U.S.C. 351（a）（2）（B）.

由于你公司用于生产、加工、包装或储存的方法、设施或控制措施不符合 cGMP，因此根据 FD&C 法案 501（a）（2）（B）条、21 U.S.C.351（a）（2）（B）的规定，你公司药品被认为是掺假。

We reviewed your August 17, 2022, response to our Form FDA 483 in detail and acknowledge receipt of your subsequent correspondence.

我们详细审查了你公司于 2022 年 8 月 17 日对 FDA 483 表格的回复，并确认收到你们随后的来函。

During our inspection, our investigators observed specific violations including, but not limited to the following.

在检查过程中，我们的调查员发现了具体违规情况，包括但不限于以下内容。

工艺验证

1. Your firm failed to establish written procedures for production and process control designed to assure that the drug products you manufacture have the identity, strength, quality, and purity they purport or are represented to possess（21 CFR 211.100（a））.

1. 公司未建立用于生产和过程控制的书面程序，以确保你公司所生产的药品具有其声称或代表拥有的鉴别、规格、质量和纯度［21 CFR 211.100（a）］。

Your firm failed to provide data to demonstrate that you have validated manufacturing processes for your over-the-counter（OTC）drug products, including but not limited to "Rhinase D." Your firm lacked qualification protocols, reports, or studies to determine if manufacturing processes were in a state of control and appropriate acceptance criteria were met.

你公司未能提供数据，来证明你们已经验证了非处方（OTC）药品的生产工艺，这些药品包括但不限于"Rhinase D"。你公司缺乏确认方案、报告或研究，来确定生产工艺是否处于受控状态，以及是否满足适当的可接受标准。

In your response, you state that you will complete a validation report for "Rhinase D" that will include results for "Rhinase" drug product.

在回复中，你公司声明将完成"Rhinase D"的验证报告，其中将包括"Rhinase"药品的结果。

Your response is inadequate. You have not demonstrated that your manufacturing processes are designed, controlled, and reproducibly yield batches of uniform character and quality. Notably, "Rhinase" does not contain the same active ingredient as "Rhinase D."

你公司的回应不够充分。你们还没有证明你们的生产工艺是经过设计、可控，并且可以重现地生产具有统一特征和质量的批次。值得注意的是，"Rhinase"不含与"Rhinase D"相同的原料药。

You also fail to provide detailed process performance qualification protocols for the validation of your different OTC drug product manufacturing processes and corrective actions.

你公司也未能提供详细的工艺性能确认方案来验证不同的 OTC 药品生产工艺，且未能提供纠正措施。

Process validation evaluates the soundness of design and state of control of a process throughout its lifecycle. Each significant stage of a manufacturing process must be designed appropriately and assure the quality of raw material inputs, in-process materials, and finished drugs. Process qualification studies determine whether an initial state of control has been established.

工艺验证评估工艺在其整个生命周期内的设计合理性和控制状态。生产工艺中的每个重要阶段都必须进行适当的设计，并确保原料输入、中间体和成品制剂的质量。工艺确认研究确定是否已建立初始控制状态。

Successful process qualification studies are necessary before commercial distribution. Thereafter, ongoing vigilant oversight of process performance and product quality is necessary to ensure you maintain a stable manufacturing operation throughout the product lifecycle.

在商业流通之前，必须进行成功的工艺确认研究。此后，有必要对工艺性能和产品质量进行持续的警戒性监控，以确保你公司在整个产品生命周期内保持稳定的生产操作。

See FDA's guidance document *Process Validation: General Principles and Practices* for general principles and approaches that FDA considers appropriate elements of process validation at https://www.fda.gov/files/drugs/published/Process-Validation--General-Principles-and-Practices.pdf.

有关 FDA 认为适当的工艺验证要素的一般原则和方法，请参阅 FDA 的指南，工艺验证：一般原则和实践，网址（略，见上）。

In response to this letter, provide：

在回复本函时，请提供：

● A list of all products released by your firm, including examples of labeling. Also include a thorough and independent evaluation of all products released by your firm that remain within expiry, to determine if they are drugs, as defined by the FD&C Act.

● 你公司放行的所有产品的清单，包括标签示例。还包括对你公司放行的所有在有效期内的产品进行彻底、独立的评估，以确定它们是否属于 FD&C 法案所定义的药品。

● A detailed summary of your validation program for ensuring a state of control throughout the product lifecycle, along with associated procedures. Describe your program for process performance qualification and ongoing monitoring of both intra-Page batch and inter-batch variation to ensure a continuing state of control. Also, include your program for qualification of your equipment and facility.

● 有关确保整个产品生命周期中控制状态的验证项目的详细总结，以及相关程序。描述你公司的程序，以进行工艺性能确认，并持续监控批内和批间变化，以确保持续的控制状态。此外，还需包括你们的设备和设施的确认计划。

● Include your process performance protocol（s）and written procedures for qualification of equipment and facilities.

● 包括你公司的工艺性能方案以及设备和设施确认的书面程序。

● A timeline for performing appropriate process performance qualification（PPQ）for each marketed drug product you manufacture.

● 为你公司生产的每种上市药品执行适当的工艺性能确认（PPQ）的时间表。

● An assessment of each drug product process to ensure that there is a data-driven and scientifically sound program that identifies and controls all sources of variability, such that your production processes will consistently meet appropriate specifications and manufacturing standards. This includes, but is not limited to, evaluating suitability of equipment for its intended use, sufficiency of detectability in your monitoring and testing systems, quality of input materials, and reliability of each manufacturing process step and control.

● 对每个药品工艺进行评估，以确保有一个数据驱动且科学合理的程序来识别和控制所有变异源，从而使你公司的生产工艺始终满足相应的质量标准和生产标准。这包括但不限于评估设备对其预期用途的适用性、监控和检验系统的可检测性的充分性、输入物料的质量，以及每个生产工艺步骤和控制的可靠性。

稳定性研究

2. Your firm failed to follow a written testing program designed to assess the stability characteristics of drug products and to use results of stability testing to determine appropriate storage conditions and expiration dates(21 CFR 211.166(a)).

2. 你公司未能建立并遵循适当的书面检验程序，以评估药品的稳定性特征；未能使用稳定性检验结果，来确定适当的储存条件和有效期［21 CFR 211.166（a）］。

Your firm failed to establish an adequate stability program and determine appropriate expiration dates for the OTC drug products that you manufacture. For example, you assigned a five-year expiry period to "Rhinase D" drug product batch 1J02（30g）. At the time of inspection, only（b）（4）of real-time and accelerated data were available. You lacked sufficient stability data to substantiate the "Rhinase D" five-year expiry period.

你公司未能为生产的非处方药制定适当的稳定性计划，并确定适当的有效期。例如，你公司为"Rhinase D"药品批次 1J02（30g）指定了五年有效期。在检查时，只有（b）（4）的实时和加速数据可及。你们缺乏充分的稳定性数据，来证实"Rhinase D"的五年有效期。

In your response, you explain that your five-year expiry date is based on the stability of "Rhinase," a different drug product that does not contain oxymetazoline hydrochloride, the active ingredient used in "Rhinase D." Furthermore, you indicated that it was your assumption that your product would be stable and（b）（4）. In addition, you commit to labeling "··· future batches only with（b）（4）data or longer but only if［you］have real time stability data."

在回复中，你公司解释说五年有效期是基于"Rhinase"的稳定性，"Rhinase"是一种不同的药品，不含盐酸羟甲唑啉（"Rhinase D"中使用的原料药）。此外，你公司表示你们的假设是药品会稳定并且（b）（4）。此外，你们承诺标识"……未来批次，仅使用（b）（4）数据或更长时间，但前提是［你公司］拥有实时稳定性数据。"

Your response is inadequate. You fail to provide data to demonstrate that the chemical and microbiological properties of your drug products will remain within specification throughout their labeled expiry period. You also fail to provide interim measures to address whether your drug products that remain on the market have adequate stability data. For products without appropriate stability studies, there is insufficient scientific evidence to support that drug products will meet established specifications and retain their quality attributes through their labeled expiry.

你公司的回应不够充分。你们未能提供数据，来证明药品的化学和微生物特性在其标签有效期内保持在质量标准范围内。也未能提供临时措施，来解决你公司留在市场上的药品是否有充分的稳定性数据。对于没有适当稳定性研究的药品，没有充分的科学证据，来支持在标签有效期内药品将符合既定质量标准、并保持其质量属性。

In response to this letter, provide:

在回复本函时，请提供：

● A comprehensive independent assessment and corrective action and preventive action (CAPA) plan to ensure the adequacy of your stability program. Your remediated program should include, but not be limited to:

● 全面、独立的评估和 CAPA 计划，以确保你公司的稳定性计划是充分的。整改计划应包括但不限于：

○ Stability indicating methods

○ 稳定性指示方法

○ Stability studies for each drug product in its marketed container-closure system before distribution is permitted

○ 在流通之前，对市售容器密闭系统中的每种药品进行稳定性研究

○ An ongoing program in which representative batches of each product are added each year to the program to determine if the shelf-life claim remains valid

○ 持续进行的计划，每年将每种产品的代表性批次添加到其中，以确定有效期声明是否仍然有效

○ Detailed definition of the specific attributes to be tested at each station(timepoint)

○ 每个点（时间点）要检验的特定属性的详细定义

● All procedures that describe these and other elements of your remediated stability program.

● 针对稳定性整改计划的这些以及其他元素，其所有相关的描述性程序。

● A comprehensive independent assessment of all drug products in the U.S. market to determine if you have data to support that they conform to specifications throughout their shelf–life, including evaluating storage conditions, differences in each formulation, packaging configurations, and all historical stability studies that have been performed. If there are gaps in the data needed to scientifically support that your drug products retain their quality attributes through their labeled shelf–life, provide a CAPA plan which will include an impact assessment for any batches that remain within their shelf–life in the market.

● 对美国市场上的所有药品进行全面的独立评估，以确定你公司是否有数据支持它们在整个有效期内符合质量标准，包括评估储存条件，每种处方、包装配置的差异，以及所有已执行的历史稳定性研究。如果支持你公司的药品在标签有效期内保持其质量属性所需的科学数据存在差距，请提供 CAPA 计划，其中包括对市场上有效期内所有批次的影响评估。

● A summary of results from testing retain samples within expiry for all drug product batches not currently in your existing stability program. Testing of each batch should be completed within 60 days of this letter. You should test all appropriate quality attributes including, but not limited to, identity and strength of active ingredients as well as microbiological quality（total counts; identification of bioburden to detect any objectionable microbes）of each batch. If testing yields an out–of–specification（OOS）result, indicate the corrective actions you will take, including notifying customers and initiating recalls.

● 就当前不在现有稳定性计划中的所有药品批次的有效期内留样，提供检验结果汇总。每批次的检验应在本函发出后 60 天内完成。你公司应检验每批的所有适当的质量属性，包括但不限于原料药的鉴别和规格以及微生物质量（总计数；微生物负荷的鉴别以检测任何有害微生物）。如果检验得出不合格（OOS）的结果，请指出你们将采取的纠正措施，包括通知客户和启动召回。

设备问题

3. Your firm failed to use equipment in the manufacture, processing, packing, or holding of drug products that is of appropriate design, adequate size, and suitably located to facilitate operations for its intended use and for its cleaning and maintenance（21 CFR 211.63）.

3. 在药品的生产、加工、包装或储存中，你公司未能使用设计合理、尺寸足够且位置适当的设备，以实现预期用途及清洁和维护操作（21 CFR 211.63）。

Your purified water system used to manufacture drug products was not designed and maintained appropriately for its intended use. For example, your water system included a dead leg and was not continuously circulating, which could foster the development of biofilms. When the water was not in use, it sat stagnant in the system except when the（b）（4）points–

of-use（POUs）were opened.

对于用于生产药品的纯化水系统，你公司未根据其预期用途进行适当的设计和维护。例如，水系统存在死角且不能持续循环，这可能会促进生物膜的形成。当水不使用时，除非（b）（4）使用点（POUs）打开，否则水会停滞在系统中。

In your response, you discuss the current controls in place for your water system and the use of testing data from your "validation report." In addition, you also indicate you employ the use of（b）（4）during production on a（b）（4）basis. You commit to increase the testing frequency to include each batch of water produced for OTC drug products and to（b）（4）.

在你公司的回复中，讨论了水系统的当前控制措施，以及"验证报告"中检验数据的使用。此外，你公司还表明，在生产工艺中基于（b）（4）的基础上使用了（b）（4）。你们承诺增加检验频率，以涵盖为 OTC 药品生产的每批水以及（b）（4）。

Your response is inadequate. You fail to describe how your water system maintenance, cleaning process, seasonal variations, and other actual conditions of use were considered during your "validation" efforts and to provide adequate justification for the sampling frequency. Your response also fails to address that you do not perform（b）（4）testing on the（b）（4）that you use during production.

你公司的回应不够充分。你们未能描述在"验证"工作期间如何考虑水系统维护、清洁工艺、季节变化和其他实际使用条件，也未能为取样频率提供充分的论证。就没有对生产过程中使用的（b）（4）执行（b）（4）检验，你公司的回复也未能解决这一问题。

In response to this letter, provide:

在回复本函时，请提供：

● A comprehensive assessment and remediation plan for the design, control, and maintenance of the water system.

● 针对水系统的设计、控制和维护的综合评估和整改计划。

● Validation report for the water system obtained after all identified system design issues have been fully remediated and any maintenance repairs have been completed. Include the system validation protocol, the complete test results, and the final validation report.

● 在所有已识别的系统设计问题得到完全整改，并且所有维护修理都已完成后，完成水系统的验证报告。包括系统验证方案、完整的检验结果和最终验证报告。

● Your total microbial count limits to monitor whether this system is producing water suitable for the intended use for each of your products.

● 你公司的微生物总计数限度，用于监控该系统是否生产适合你们每种产品预期用途的水。

● A detailed risk assessment addressing the potential effects of the water system on the quality of all drug product lots currently in the U.S. within expiry. Specify actions that you will take in response to the risk assessment, such as customer notifications and product recalls.

● 详细的风险评估，旨在解决水系统对美国目前到期的所有药品批次质量的潜在影响。指定你公司为回应风险评估将采取的措施，例如，通知客户和召回产品。

● A procedure for your water system monitoring that specifies routine microbial testing of water to ensure its acceptability for use in each batch of drug products produced by your firm. In addition, your response should describe how your sampling method will be improved to ensure purified water collection is performed in a manner that is representative of actual manufacturing conditions and does not compromise detection of microbes.

● 水系统监测程序，指定对水进行常规微生物检验，以确保其在你公司生产的每批药品中的使用可接受性。此外，你们的回复应描述如何改进取样方法，以确保纯化水收集方式能够代表实际生产条件且不影响微生物检验。

● The current action (and alert, if any) limits for total counts and objectionable organisms used for your purified water system. Ensure that the total count limits for your purified water are appropriately stringent in view of the intended use of each of the products produced by your firm.

● 当前的行动限（和警戒限，如有）纯化水系统中使用的总计数和有害微生物。鉴于你公司生产的每种产品的预期用途，确保纯化水的总计数限度适当严格。

实验室控制措施

4. Your firm failed to establish laboratory controls that include scientifically sound and appropriate specifications, standards, sampling plans, and test procedures designed to assure that components, drug product containers, closures, in-process materials, labeling, and drug products conform to appropriate standards of identity, strength, quality, and purity (21 CFR 211.160 (b)).

4. 你公司未能建立实验室控制措施，其中包括科学合理且相应的规范、标准、取样计划和检验程序，以确保物料、药品容器、密封件、在制品、标签和药品符合适当的相关规定，即鉴别、规格、质量和纯度的标准［21 CFR 211.160 (b)］。

Your firm had inadequate laboratory controls. For example:

你公司的实验室控制不充分。例如：

● Microbiological methods used for determining the quality of purified water and finished drug products were deficient. Specifically, you failed to perform growth promotion testing on every batch of ready-to-use media and to verify microbiological method suitability for each drug product you manufacture.

● 用于测定纯化水和成品制剂质量的微生物方法存在缺陷。具体来说，你公司未能对每批即用型培养基进行生长促进检验，也未能验证微生物方法对所生产药品的适用性。

● Your firm failed to conduct appropriate laboratory testing for each batch of drug product that is required to be free of objectionable microorganisms (21 CFR 211.165 (b)). In particular, your firm failed to conduct testing for Burkholderia cepacia complex (BCC) for numerous non-sterile aqueous-based dosage form drug products at release and on stability.

● 对于要求不含有害微生物的药品，你公司未能进行适当的实验室检验［21 CFR 211.165（b）］。特别是，对于多种非无菌水基剂型药品制剂，在放行和稳定性检验中，你公司未能进行洋葱伯克霍尔德菌复合体（BCC）。

For further information regarding the significance of BCC and other objectionable contamination of non-sterile, water-based drug products, see FDA's advisory notice posted on July 7, 2021, at https://www.fda.gov/drugs/drug-safety-and-availability/fda-advises-drug-manufacturers-burkholderia-cepacia-complex-poses-contamination-risk-non-sterile.

有关 BCC 和非无菌水基药品的其他不良污染的更多重要性信息，请参阅 FDA 于 2021 年 7 月 7 日发布的咨询通知，网址（见上，略）。

In your response, you state that quality control of media is performed by your supplier, who also performed a shipping study, and that positive and negative controls are not necessary. Additionally, you commit to initiating testing for BCC.

在回复中，你公司声明培养基的质量控制是由供应商进行的，他们还进行了运输研究，并且不需要阳性和阴性控制。此外，你公司承诺启动 BCC 检验。

Your response is inadequate. You fail to address the full scope and impact of the cGMP deficiencies as well as the associated risks to drug product quality, including batches in distribution. Without appropriate testing of media you cannot ensure your drug products meet appropriate microbial quality specifications.

你公司的回应不够充分。你们未能解决 cGMP 缺陷的全部范围和影响，以及药品质量的相关风险，包括流通批次。如果不对培养基进行适当的检验，你公司就无法确保药品符合适当的微生物质量标准。

In response to this letter, provide：

在回复本函时，请提供：

● A comprehensive, independent assessment of your laboratory practices, procedures, methods, equipment, documentation, and analyst competencies. Based on this review, provide a detailed plan to remediate and evaluate the effectiveness of your laboratory system.

● 对实验室实践、程序、方法、设备、文件和分析员能力进行完整、全面、独立的评估。在此审查的基础上，提供详细的计划来整改和评估你公司实验室系统的有效性。

● A comprehensive, independent assessment of the design and control of your firm's manufacturing operations, with a detailed and thorough review of all microbiological hazards.

● 对你公司生产业务的设计和控制进行全面、独立的评估，并对所有微生物危害进行详细彻底的审查。

● A detailed risk assessment addressing the hazards posed by distributing drug products with potentially objectionable contamination. Specify actions you will take in response to the risk assessment, such as customer notifications and product recalls.

● 详细的风险评估，以解决流通具有潜在有害污染的药品所带来的危害。指定你公司将针对风险评估采取的行动，例如，客户通知和产品召回。

● Complete investigations into all batches with potential objectionable microbial contamination. The investigations should detail your findings regarding the root causes of the contamination.

● 对所有可能存在有害微生物污染的批次进行全面调查。应详细说明有关污染根本原因的调查结果。

● Appropriate microbiological batch release specifications（i.e., total counts, identification of bioburden to detect objectionable microbes）for each of your drug products.

● 为你公司的每种药品制定适当的微生物批放行质量标准（即总计数、微生物鉴别以检测有害微生物）。

● All chemical and microbial test methods used to analyze each of your drug products.

● 用于分析你公司每种药品的所有化学和微生物检验方法。

● A gap assessment to ensure that all of your drug products referenced in the United

States Pharmacopeia meet compendial criteria.

● 差距评估，可确保参考《美国药典》的所有药品均符合药典标准。

● A list of chemical and microbial specifications, including test methods, used to analyze each batch of your drug products before a batch disposition decision.

● 在做出批处置决定之前，用于分析每批药品的化学和微生物质量标准（包括检验方法）清单。

物料检验

5. Your firm failed to withhold from use each lot of components, drug product containers, and closures until the lot had been sampled, tested, or examined, as appropriate, and released for use by the quality control unit(21 CFR 211.84(a)).

5. 在对批次进行取样、检验或检查（视情况而定）并质量放行以供使用之前，你公司未停止使用每批物料、药品容器和密封件［21 CFR 211.84(a)］。

You lacked testing for every shipment of every lot of components used in the manufacture of your drug products. Specifically, you lacked a specific identity test to detect diethylene glycol(DEG) and ethylene glycol(EG)in all shipments, containers, and lots of glycerin before use in manufacturing drug products. DEG contamination in glycerin has resulted in various lethal poisoning incidents in humans worldwide. In addition, we note that both glycerin and propylene glycol are ingredients used in your drug products. As a drug manufacturer, you are responsible for performing specific identity tests for all incoming shipments of component lots prior to release for use in manufacturing.

针对用于生产药品的每批物料的每批货物，你公司的检验不够充分。具体来说，缺乏专属鉴别检验，来检测用于生产药品的所有货物、容器和批次的甘油中的二甘醇（DEG）和乙二醇（EG）。在全球范围内，甘油中的 DEG 污染已导致多起人类致命中毒事件。此外，我们注意到甘油和丙二醇都是你们药品中使用的原辅料。作为药品生产商，你公司有责任在放行前对所有用于生产的进场物料批次进行专属鉴别检验。

In your response, you indicated that your firm reviewed the COA for DEG testing. You also committed to immediately begin testing glycerin for DEG using an independent outside laboratory and consider "appropriate action" in the event an OOS occurs.

在回复中，你公司表示你们审查了 DEG 检验的 COA。你们还承诺，立即使用独立的外部实验室开始检验甘油中的 DEG，并在发生 OOS 时考虑"采取适当措施"。

Your response is inadequate. As previously mentioned, you fail to address the full scope and impact of the cGMP deficiencies as well as the associated risks to drug product quality, including addressing batches already in distribution. With respect to your glycerin-containing products, you have not addressed if your evaluation will include all lots of glycerin for each drug product batch you manufactured and that remains within shelf-life in the U.S. market. Without appropriate testing of components and ingredients, you cannot ensure the quality and safety of your drug products.

你公司的回应不够充分。如前所述，你们未能解决 cGMP 缺陷的全部范围和影响，以及药品质量的相关风险，包括解决已流通的批次问题。就含甘油的产品而言，你公司并未明确表示评估是否会覆盖所生产的、在美国市场上仍在有效期内的每一批含有甘油的药品批次。如果不对原辅料进行适当的检验，你公司就无法确保药品的质量和安全性。

See FDA's guidance document *Testing of Glycerin for Diethylene Glycol* to help you meet the cGMP requirements when manufacturing drugs containing glycerin, or other ingredients at risk for DEG or EG contamination, at https://www.fda.gov/regulatoryinformation/search-fda-guidance-documents/testing-glycerin-diethylene-glycol.

请参阅 FDA 指南，甘油中的二甘醇检验，以帮助你公司在生产含有甘油或其他有 DEG 或 EG 污染风险原辅料的药品时满足 cGMP 要求，网址（略，见上）。

In response to this letter, provide：

在回复本函时，请提供：

● A comprehensive, independent review of your material system to determine whether all suppliers of components, containers, and closures are each qualified and the materials are assigned appropriate expiration or retest dates. The review should also determine whether incoming material controls are adequate to prevent use of unsuitable components, containers, and closures.

● 对物料系统进行全面、独立审查，以确定所有物料、容器和密封件的供应商是否均有资质，并为物料指定适当的有效期或复验期。审查还应确定进场物料控制是否足以防止使用不适当的物料、容器和密封件。

● The chemical and microbiological quality control specifications you use to test and release each incoming lot of components for use in manufacturing.

● 针对每批用于生产目的的进场物料，用于检验和放行的化学和微生物质控标准。

● A description of how you will test each component lot for conformity with all appropriate specifications for identity, strength, quality, and purity. If you intend to accept any results from your supplier's COA instead of testing each component lot for strength, quality, and purity, specify how you will robustly establish the reliability of your supplier's results through initial validation as well as periodic revalidation. In addition, include a commitment to always conduct at least one specific identity test for each incoming component batch.

● 说明如何检验每个批次，确定是否符合有关鉴别、规格、质量和纯度质量标准。如果你公司打算接受供应商 COA 的结果，而不是检验每个物料批次的规格、质量和纯度，请说明如何进行初始验证和定期再验证，从而稳健地确定供应商结果的可靠性。此外，还应承诺对于每个进场原辅料批次，至少进行一个专属鉴别检验。

● A summary of results obtained from testing all components to evaluate the reliability of the COA from each component manufacturer. Include your SOP that describes this COA validation program.

● 一份从所有物料检验获得的结果汇总，以评估每个物料生产商的 COA 可靠性。包括描述此 COA 验证计划的程序。

● A summary of your program for qualifying and overseeing contract facilities that test the drug products you manufacture.

● 对于检验你公司生产的药品的外包设施，进行资质审查和监督计划的汇总。

● Within 30 days, provide the results of tests for DEG and EG in retain samples of all glycerin lots used in production of your glycerin-containing drug products. Indicate whether DEG or EG are present in any glycerin lots used to manufacture your drug products, some of which are intended for use in pediatrics. In addition, perform testing of all lot retain samples of any other drug product ingredients used by your firm that are at risk for DEG or EG contamination.

● 在 30 天内，提供用于生产含甘油药品的所有甘油批次留样中 DEG 和 EG 的检验结果。说明用于生产药品的所有甘油批次中是否存在 DEG 或 EG，特别考虑到其中一些药品用于儿科。此外，就你公司使用的存在 DEG 或 EG 污染风险的任何其他药物原辅料，对其所有批次留样进行检验。

● Provide a full risk assessment for drug products that contain glycerin (and any other ingredient at risk for DEG or EG contamination) and are within expiry in the U.S. market. Take prompt and appropriate actions to determine the safety of all lots of the ingredient (s) and any related drug product that could contain DEG or EG, including customer notifications and product recalls for any contaminated lots. Identify additional appropriate corrective actions and preventive actions that secure supply chains in the future, including but not limited to ensuring that all incoming raw material lots are from fully qualified manufacturers and free from unsafe impurities. Detail these actions in your response to this letter.

● 为美国市场上含有甘油（以及任何其他有 DEG 或 EG 污染风险的原辅料）且在有效期内的药品提供全面的风险评估。立即采取适当的措施，确定所有批次的原辅料以及任何可能含有 DEG 或 EG 的相关药品的安全性，包括通知客户和召回任何受污染批次的产品。确定其他适当的纠正和预防措施，以确保未来的供应链安全，包括但不限于确保所有进场原料批次均来自完全确认的生产商且不含不安全的杂质。在你公司对本函的回复中详细说明这些行动。

Responsibilities as a Contractor | 作为合同商的责任

Drugs must be manufactured in conformance with cGMP. FDA is aware that many drug manufacturers use independent contractors such as production facilities, testing laboratories, packagers, and labelers. FDA regards contractors as extensions of the manufacturer.

药品必须按照 cGMP 生产。FDA 意识到很多药品生产商使用独立合同商，例如生产设施、检验实验室、包装商和贴标商。FDA 将合同商视为生产商的延伸。

You are responsible for the quality of drugs you produce as a contract facility regardless of agreements in place with product owners. You are required to ensure that drugs are made in accordance with section 501（a）（2）（B）of the FD&C Act for safety, identity, strength, quality, and purity. See FDA's guidance document *Contract Manufacturing Arrangements for Drugs: Quality Agreements* at https://www.fda.gov/regulatoryinformation/search-fda-guidance-documents/contract-manufacturing-arrangements-drugs-quality-agreements-guidance-industry.

无论与产品所有者达成何种协议，作为外包设施生产，你公司应对生产的药品质量负责，应确保按照 FD&C 法案第 501（a）（2）（B）条的规定生产药品，以确保安全性、鉴别、规格、质量和纯度。请参阅 FDA 的指南文件，药品合同生产安排：质量协议，网址（略，见上）。

cGMP Consultant Recommended | cGMP 顾问推荐

Based upon the nature of the violations if your firm intends to resume manufacturing drugs for the U.S. market, we strongly recommend engaging a consultant qualified as set forth in 21 CFR 211.34 to assist your firm in meeting drug cGMP requirements. Your use of a consultant does not relieve your firm's obligation to comply with cGMP. Your firm's executive management remains responsible for resolving all deficiencies and systemic flaws to ensure ongoing cGMP compliance.

根据违规的性质，如果你公司打算恢复为美国市场生产药品，我们强烈建议你公司聘请符合 21 CFR 211.34 规定的有资质的顾问，来协助你公司满足药品 cGMP 要求。聘用顾问并不能免除公司遵守 cGMP 的义务。你公司的高级管理层仍然负责解决所有缺陷和系统性问题，以确保持续符合 cGMP。

3 与非药用产品的共线生产问题

警告信编号： MARCS-CMS 644335

签发时间： 2023-2-22；**公示时间：** 2023-3-21

签发机构： 药品质量业务二处（Division of Pharmaceutical Quality Operations II）

公　　司： Dunagin Pharmaceuticals Inc. dba Massco Dental

所在国家 / 地区： 美国

主　　题： cGMP/ 成品制剂 / 掺假（cGMP/Finished Pharmaceuticals/ Adulterated）

简　　介： FDA 于 2022 年 8 月至 9 月对该药品生产设施进行了检查。 FDA 指出，该公司生产的药品与非药用物料的设备存在共线 生产，可能导致药品被非药用产品原辅料污染。FDA 要求该 公司停止使用共享设备生产药品。如果继续生产药品和非药用 产品，请提供分隔区域的计划以确保专用设备用于药品生产。 此外，FDA 要求该公司对之前在共享设备上生产的药品进行 风险评估，并提供针对潜在污染风险和药品质量的解决方案计 划，包括潜在的召回或市场撤回。

本警告信以下部分与本书此前其他警告信内容类似，故略去：前言、 cGMP 顾 问 推 荐（cGMP Consultant Recommended）、 结 论 （Conclusion）。

与非药用产品共享设备

1. Your firm failed to have separate or defined areas or such other control systems necessary to prevent contamination or mix-ups（21 CFR 211.42（c））.

1. 你公司未能设立单独或界定的区域，或其他必要的控制系统，来防止污染或混 淆 ［21 CFR 211.42（c）］。

You manufacture finished drug products, including toothpaste and mouth rinse products containing sodium fluoride, stannous fluoride, and potassium nitrate using the same equipment you use to manufacture numerous nonpharmaceutical materials in your facility, including (b)(4). This product is labeled as "Caution: Keep away from children, do not consume and avoid contact with eyes."

你公司生产的药品制剂包括含有氟化钠、氟化亚锡和硝酸钾的牙膏和漱口水产品，其所使用的设备同时用于生产你公司的多种非药用物料，包括（b）（4）。该产品标签为"注意：远离儿童，请勿食用并避免接触眼睛。"

The ingredients in your nonpharmaceutical products could contaminate the drug products that you manufacture on shared equipment, such as the various drugs for oral use discussed above. It is unacceptable as a matter of cGMP to continue manufacturing drugs using the same equipment you use to manufacture nonpharmaceutical products.

非药用产品中的原辅料可能会污染你公司在共享设备上生产的药品，如上面讨论的各种口服药品。从 cGMP 的角度来看，继续使用生产非药用产品的同一设备来生产药品是不可接受的。

In your response, you state each "follow up batch" is tested for microbial analysis, pH, taste, and other attributes prior to the filling process, and that it is not standard for a manufacturer to have a tank for every product and every flavor. You also state you have purchased a swab kit and a luminometer to assess the cleanliness of surfaces.

在回复中，你公司指出每个"后续批次"在灌装过程之前都经过微生物分析、pH、口味和其他属性检验，同时指出生产商为每种产品和每种口味配备一个罐并不是标准的做法。你公司还声称购买了拭子试剂盒和光度计，来评估表面的清洁度。

In response to this letter, discontinue manufacturing drugs on shared equipment in your facility, and if you intend to continue to manufacture both pharmaceutical and nonpharmaceutical products at your facility provide a plan to show how you will separate the areas in which you will maintain dedicated manufacturing equipment for your pharmaceutical manufacturing and nonpharmaceutical product manufacturing operations.

作为对本函的回应，请停止在你公司的设施中使用共享设备生产药品和非药用产品，如果你公司打算继续在你们的设施生产药品和非药品产品，请提供一份计划，说明如何分隔区域，确保专用设备用于药品生产，非药用产品制造操作则采用其他设备。

Also provide a risk assessment for all drugs you have previously produced on equipment shared with nonpharmaceutical products. For each product, assess the risk of potential contamination due to the shared equipment, and provide your plans for addressing the product quality and patient safety risks for any product still in distribution, including potential recalls

53

or market withdrawals.

此外，请对你公司先前在与非药用产品共用设备上生产的所有药品进行风险评估。对于每种药品，评估因共享设备而造成的潜在污染风险，并提供解决仍在流通的任何产品的产品质量和患者安全风险的计划，包括潜在的召回或市场撤回。

物料检验

2. Your firm failed to test samples of each component for conformity with all appropriate written specifications for purity, strength, and quality（21 CFR 211.84（d）（2））.

2. 你公司未能检验每种原辅料的样品，来确认其是否符合所有适当的纯度、规格和质量的书面质量标准［21 CFR 211.84（d）（2）］。

You relied on certificates of analysis（COA）for incoming components from your suppliers without establishing the reliability of your suppliers' test results. Additionally, a representative COA noted the use of nonpharmaceutical grade potassium nitrate in your drug product manufacturing. As a manufacturer, you have a responsibility to sample, test, and examine drug components before use in production to ensure acceptable quality parameters are met.

你公司依赖供应商的进场物料的分析证书（COA），但没有确定供应商检验结果的可靠性。此外，一份代表性的 COA 表明你公司药品生产中使用了非药品级硝酸钾。作为生产商，在生产使用之前，有责任对药物原辅料进行取样、检验和检查，以确保满足可接受的质量参数。

You also lacked appropriate testing of components used in the manufacture of your drug products. For example, you lacked a specific identity test to detect diethylene glycol（DEG）and ethylene glycol（EG）in all shipments, containers, and lots of glycerin before use in the manufacturing of drug products. Some of your firm's glycerin-containing products are intended for oral use in pediatric populations. The use of glycerin contaminated with diethylene glycol（DEG）has resulted in various lethal poisoning incidents in humans worldwide.

对于药品生产中使用的原辅料，你公司还缺乏进行适当的检验。例如，在用于药品生产之前，缺乏专属鉴别检验，来检测用于生产药品的所有货物、容器和批次的甘油中的二甘醇（DEG）和乙二醇（EG）。你公司的一些含甘油产品供儿童口服使用。在全球范围内，使用受二甘醇（DEG）污染的甘油已导致多起人类致命中毒事件。

In your response, you note you follow USP monographs for your raw materials, and you provided an additional nonpharmaceutical grade potassium nitrate COA. You state you "perform ID testing and/or review COAs for all incoming raw materials" at the time of delivery, and note you have a new logbook to document your raw material evaluations. You also state glycerin is tested for diethylene glycol (DEG) by a contract laboratory.

在回复中，你公司指出你们的原料遵循 USP 专论，并且提供了另外的非药品级硝酸钾 COA。你公司声明在收货时"对所有入厂原材料进行 ID 检验和（或）审查 COA"，并指出你公司有一个新的台账来记录原料评估。你公司还指出，甘油由委托实验室进行了二甘醇（DEG）检验。

Your response is inadequate. You do not address your use of a nonpharmaceutical grade component. You also fail to provide sufficient evidence showing you performed adequate testing on all containers of all lots of glycerin prior to its use in the manufacture of drug products. Additionally, you do not provide scientific evidence demonstrating that you have established the reliability of your suppliers' test results.

你公司的回应不够充分。你们没有阐明对非药品级原辅料的使用问题。也未能提供充分的证据来表明在将甘油用于药品生产之前对所有批次的所有容器进行充分的检验。此外，没有提供科学证据，来证明你公司已确定供应商检验结果的可靠性。

In response to this letter, provide:

在回复本函时，请提供：

● A comprehensive, independent review of your material system to determine whether all suppliers of components, containers, and closures are each qualified and the materials are assigned appropriate expiration or retest dates. The review should also determine whether incoming material controls are adequate to prevent use of unsuitable components, containers, and closures.

● 对物料系统进行全面、独立审查，以确定所有物料、容器和密封件的供应商是否均有资质，并为物料指定适当的有效期或复验期。审查还应确定进场物料控制是否足以防止使用不适当的物料、容器和密封件。

● The chemical and microbiological quality control specifications you use to test and release each incoming lot of components for use in manufacturing.

● 针对每批用于生产目的的进场物料，用于检验和放行的化学和微生物质控标准。

● A description of how you will test each component lot for conformity with all appropriate specifications for identity, strength, quality, and purity. If you intend to accept any results from your supplier's COA instead of testing each component lot for strength, quality, and purity, specify how you will robustly establish the reliability of your supplier's results through initial validation as well as periodic revalidation. In addition, include a commitment to always conduct at least one specific identity test for each incoming component batch.

● 说明如何检验每个批次，确定是否符合有关鉴别、规格、质量和纯度质量标准。如果你公司打算接受供应商 COA 的结果，而不是检验每个物料批次的规格、质量和纯度，请说明如何进行初始验证和定期再验证，从而稳健地确定供应商结果的可靠性。此外，还应承诺对于每个进场原辅料批次，至少进行一个专属鉴别检验。

● A summary of results obtained from testing all components to evaluate the reliability of the COA from each component manufacturer. Include your SOP that describes this COA validation program.

● 一份从所有物料检验获得的结果汇总，以评估每个物料生产商的 COA 可靠性。包括描述此 COA 验证计划的程序。

● A summary of your program for qualifying and overseeing contract facilities that test the drug products you manufacture.

● 对于检验你公司生产药品的外包设施，进行资质审查和监督计划的汇总。

● Results of tests for diethylene glycol（DEG）and ethylene glycol（EG）in retain samples of all containers for all lots of glycerin used to manufacture your drug products.

● 对用于生产的所有批次甘油的容器留样，提供二甘醇（DEG）和乙二醇（EG）的检验结果。

● A full risk assessment for drug products that contain glycerin and are within expiry in the U.S. market. Take prompt corrective actions and preventive actions, and detail your future actions to ensure appropriate selection of your suppliers, ongoing scrutiny of their supply chain, and appropriate incoming lot controls.

● 针对美国市场上含甘油且在有效期内的药品进行全面的风险评估。立即采取纠正和预防措施，并详细说明你公司将来的措施，以确保正确选择供应商、持续审查其供应链以及适当的进场批次控制。

See FDA's guidance document *Testing of Glycerin for Diethylene Glycol* to help you meet the cGMP requirements when manufacturing drugs containing glycerin at https://www.fda.gov/media/71029/download.

请参阅 FDA 指南，甘油中二甘醇检验，以帮助你公司在生产含有甘油的药品时满足 cGMP 要求，网址（略，见上）。

工艺验证

3. Your firm failed to establish written procedures for production and process control designed to assure that the drug products you manufacture have the identity, strength, quality, and purity they purport or are represented to possess(21 CFR 211.100(a)).

3. 你公司未建立用于生产和过程控制的书面程序，以确保所生产药品具有其声称或代表拥有的鉴别、规格、质量和纯度［21 CFR 211.100(a)］。

▣ Lack of Process Validation ｜ 缺乏工艺验证

You failed to provide data to demonstrate you have validated the manufacturing processes for all your drug products. During the inspection, when asked for validation documents for your manufacturing processes, you stated that you did not have any validation information.

你公司未能提供数据来证明已验证所有药品的生产工艺。在检查过程中，当被要求提供生产工艺的验证文件时，你公司表示没有任何验证信息。

In your response, you explain your equipment manufacturer validates the equipment's function with the same packaging components you use before delivery to your facility. You also state you will document this compatibility testing in each equipment logbook.

在回复中，你公司解释说，设备生产商在交付设施之前，使用和你公司相同包装材料验证了设备的功能。你公司还声明将在每个设备台账中记录此兼容性检测。

Your response is inadequate. You fail to demonstrate that the commercial manufacturing process performs as expected using your actual facility, utilities, equipment, personnel, controls, and other variables unique to your operation. In addition, your response does not address or otherwise include a risk assessment for any marketed drug products manufactured and distributed with unvalidated processes. Failure to perform adequate process validation can result in product quality attribute failure.

你公司的回应不够充分。你们未能使用实际设施、公用系统、设备、人员、控制和其他特定的操作变量，来证明商业生产工艺按预期执行。此外，针对任何未经验证的工艺生产和流通的市售药品，你公司的回复并未涉及或包括相应的风险。未能进行充分的工艺验证可能会导致产品质量属性不合格。

Successful process qualification studies are necessary before commercial distribution. Thereafter, ongoing vigilant oversight of process performance and product quality is necessary to ensure you maintain a stable manufacturing operation throughout the product lifecycle.

在商业流通之前，必须进行成功的工艺确认研究。此后，有必要对工艺性能和产品质量进行持续的警戒性监控，以确保你公司在整个产品生命周期内保持稳定的生产操作。

See FDA's guidance document *Process Validation*: *General Principles and Practices* for general principles and approaches that FDA considers appropriate elements of process validation at https://www.fda.gov/files/drugs/published/Process-Validation--General-Principles-and-Practices.pdf.

有关 FDA 认为适当的工艺验证要素的一般原则和方法，请参阅 FDA 指南，工艺验证：一般原则和实践，网址（略，见上）。

■ Inadequate Equipment Maintenance ｜设备维护不充分

You failed to adequately maintain equipment used in the manufacture of your drug products. For example, motorized mixing equipment located in your liquid manufacturing area was observed in a poor state of repair, with rust and paint chipping.

你公司未能充分维护药品生产中使用的设备。例如，位于液体生产区域的电动混合设备被发现维修状况不佳，出现生锈和油漆剥落的情况。

In your response, you state the motorized equipment has been refurbished, and the active ingredient is corrosive by nature. You also state you perform regular cleaning and wipe down the motors before use.

在回复中，你公司说电动设备已经翻新，原料药具有腐蚀性。你们还声明在使用前定期清洁并擦拭电机。

Your response is inadequate. You do not provide an assessment of your manufacturing equipment's material of construction to ensure compatibility with the products you manufacture. You also fail to provide evidence of your investigation into the scope of your equipment maintenance issues to determine if other equipment was in need of maintenance. Further, you do not provide a corrective action and preventive action (CAPA) plan to prevent equipment maintenance deficiencies in the future.

你公司的回应不够充分。你们未提供对生产设备结构物料的评估，以确保与所生产产品的兼容性，也未能提供证据，来证明对设备维护问题的范围进行了调查，以确定其他设备是否需要维护。此外，你公司没有提供纠正和预防措施（CAPA）计划，来防止未来出现设备维护缺陷。

In response to this letter, provide:

在回复本函时，请提供：

● A detailed summary of your validation program for ensuring a state of control throughout the product lifecycle, along with associated procedures. Describe your program for process performance qualification, and ongoing monitoring of both intra-batch and inter-batch variation to ensure a continuing state of control.

● 有关确保整个产品生命周期中控制状态的验证项目的详细汇总,以及相关程序。描述你公司的程序,以进行工艺性能确认,并持续监控批内和批间变化,以确保持续的控制状态。此外,还需包括设备和设施的确认计划。

● summary of your validation program for ensuring a state A timeline for performing process performance qualification (PPQ) for each of your marketed drug products.

● 对每种上市药品执行工艺性能确认(PPQ)的时间表。

● Include your process performance protocol (s), and written procedures for qualification of equipment and facilities.

● 包括你公司的工艺性能方案,以及设备和设施确认的书面程序。

● Provide a detailed program for designing, validating, maintaining, controlling and monitoring each of your manufacturing processes that includes vigilant monitoring of intra-batch and inter-batch variation to ensure an ongoing state of control. Also, include your program for qualification of your equipment and facility.

● 提供用于设计、验证、维护、控制和监测每个生产工艺的详细计划,包括对批内和批间变化进行警戒性的监测,以确保持续的控制状态。另外,请包含设备和设施确认计划。

● An assessment of each drug product process to ensure that there is a data-driven and scientifically sound program that identifies and controls all sources of variability, such that your production processes, and will consistently meet appropriate specifications and manufacturing standards. This includes, but is not limited to, evaluating suitability of equipment for its intended use, sufficiency of detectability in your monitoring and testing systems, quality of input materials, and reliability of each manufacturing process step and control.

● 对每个药品工艺的评估,以确保有一个以数据为依据的、科学合理的程序,该程序可以识别和控制所有可变性来源,并始终符合相应的质量标准和生产标准。这包括但不限于评估设备的预期用途适用性、监视和检验系统中可检验性的充分性、输入物料的质量以及每个生产工艺步骤和控制的可靠性。

● Timelines for completed process performance qualification (PPQ) for marketed drug products.

● 对于已完成的上市药品工艺性能确认（PPQ），提供时间表。

● Your CAPA plan to implement routine, vigilant operations management oversight of facilities and equipment. This plan should ensure, among other things, prompt detection of equipment/facilities performance issues, effective execution of repairs, adherence to appropriate preventive maintenance schedules, timely technological upgrades to the equipment/facility infrastructure, and improved systems for ongoing management review.

● 你公司的 CAPA 计划，以便对设施和设备实施常规的、警戒性的运营管理监督。该计划应确保及时发现设备 / 设施性能问题，有效执行维修，遵守适当的预防性维护计划，及时对设备 / 设施基础设施进行技术升级，并不断完善持续管理评审系统。

质量部门

4. Your firm failed to establish an adequate quality control unit with the responsibility and authority to approve or reject all components, drug product containers, closures, in-process materials, packaging materials, labeling, and drug products (21 CFR 211.22 (a)).

4. 你公司未能建立胜任的质量控制部门，负责批准或拒绝所有原辅料、药品容器、密封件、中间物料、包装材料、标签和药品 ［ 21 CFR 211.22 (a) ］。

You failed to provide adequate oversight of finished product testing, and other quality functions. For example, your Quality Unit (QU) failed to initiate and document an investigation into out-of-specification (OOS) results. During the inspection, our investigator observed your analyst obtained OOS finished drug product assay results. You stated the results would be discarded, and the tests would be reperformed by a different analyst.

你公司未能对成品检验和其他质量职能提供充分的监督。例如，质量部门（QU）未能启动并记录对不合格（OOS）结果的调查。在检查过程中，我们的调查员观察到，分析人员得到了成品制剂的 OOS 检验结果。你公司表示结果将被废弃，检验将由不同的分析人员重新进行。

In your response, you state you have no unexplained discrepancies. You provided your "Yield Deviation Report" and indicated it would be used if a test result was outside the appropriate range.

在回复中，你公司声明没有无法解释的偏差。你们提供了"偏差报告"，并表示如果检验结果超出适当范围，将使用该报告。

Your response is inadequate. Your investigation did not include sufficient detail as to the possible scope and probable root cause for the OOS results observed during the inspection.

For example, you failed to investigate the impact of the root cause on other batches you manufactured and distributed. You also failed to provide a retrospective review to ensure you have fully identified and thoroughly investigated all OOS results. Additionally, you failed to implement appropriate CAPAs to mitigate and prevent recurrence.

你公司的回应不够充分。针对检查期间观察到的 OOS 结果的可能范围和可能的根本原因，你们的调查没有详细说明。例如，未能调查根本原因对所生产和流通的其他批次的影响；也未能提供回顾性审查，以确保你公司已充分识别并彻底调查所有 OOS 结果。此外，你们未能实施适当的 CAPA，来缓解和防止再次发生。

In addition, we identified you did not perform stability testing at the intervals required by your procedure. Our inspection also noted you did not perform periodic evaluations of your drug products. You also lack an adequate change management system.

此外，我们发现你公司没有按照程序要求的时间间隔执行稳定性检验。检查还发现，你公司没有对药品进行定期评审。你们还缺乏适当的变更管理系统。

Your firm's quality systems are inadequate. See FDA's guidance document *Quality Systems Approach to Pharmaceutical cGMP Regulations* for help implementing quality systems and risk management approaches to meet the requirements of cGMP regulations 21 CFR, parts 210 and 211 at https://www.fda.gov/media/71023/download.

你公司的质量体系不完善。请参阅 FDA 的指南，药品 cGMP 法规质量体系方法，以帮助实施质量体系和风险管理方法，满足 cGMP 法规 21 CFR 第 210 和 211 部分的要求，网址（略，见上）。

In response to this letter, provide：

在回复本函时，请提供：

● A comprehensive independent assessment and remediation plan to ensure your QU is given the authority and resources to effectively function. The assessment should also include, but not be limited to：

● 全面的独立评估和整改计划，以确保你公司的 QU 获得有效运行的权力和资源。评估还应包括但不限于：

○ A determination of whether procedures used by your firm are robust and appropriate

○ 确定你公司使用的程序是否可靠和适当。

○ Provisions for QU oversight throughout your operations to evaluate adherence to appropriate practices

61

○ 在整个运营过程中 QU 进行监督的规定，以评估对相应规范的遵守情况。

○ A complete and final review of each batch and its related information before the QU disposition decision

○ 在 QU 决定处置之前，对每批产品及其相关信息进行完整和最终审查。

○ Oversight and approval of investigations and discharging of all other QU duties to ensure identity, strength, quality, and purity of all products

○ 监督和批准调查以及履行所有其他 QU 职责，以确保所有产品的鉴别、规格、质量和纯度。

● A comprehensive, independent assessment of your overall system for investigating deviations, discrepancies, complaints, OOS results, and failures. Provide a detailed action plan to remediate this system. Your action plan should include, but not be limited to, significant improvements in investigation competencies, scope determination, root cause evaluation, CAPA effectiveness, quality unit oversight, and written procedures. Address how your firm will ensure all phases of investigations are appropriately conducted.

● 对整个系统进行全面、独立的评估，以调查偏差、差异、投诉、OOS 结果和不合格。提供详细的行动计划，以整改此系统。行动计划应包括但不限于：调查能力、范围确定、根本原因评估、CAPA 有效性、质量部门监督和书面程序方面的显著提高。说明你公司将如何确保调查的所有阶段都得到适当实施。

● A retrospective, independent review of all invalidated OOS（including in-process and release/stability testing）results for U.S. products currently in the U.S. market and within expiry as of the date of this letter and a report summarizing the findings of the analysis, including the following for each OOS：

● 对目前在美国市场和截至本函日期到期的产品的所有无效 OOS（包括中控和放行 / 稳定性检验）结果进行回顾性独立审查，以及总结分析结果的报告，包括每个 OOS 的以下内容：

○ Determine whether the scientific justification and evidence relating to the invalidated OOS result conclusively or inconclusively demonstrates causative laboratory error.

○ 对于与无效 OOS 结果相关的科学论证和证据，确定其是否确凿或不确凿地证明了实验室相关的错误。

○ For investigations that conclusively establish laboratory root cause, provide rationale and ensure that all other laboratory methods vulnerable to the same or similar root cause are identified for remediation.

○ 对于最终确定实验室为根本原因的调查，提供论证，并确定所有其他易受相同或类似根本原因影响的实验室方法，以进行整改。

○ For all OOS results found by the retrospective review to have an inconclusive or no root cause identified in the laboratory, include a thorough review of production (e.g., batch manufacturing records, adequacy of the manufacturing steps, suitability of equipment/ facilities, variability of raw materials, process capability, deviation history, complaint history, batch failure history). Provide a summary of potential manufacturing root causes for each investigation, and any manufacturing operation improvements.

○ 在回顾性评估中，对于发现 OOS 结果在实验室中没有确定的根本原因，或没有根本原因的情况，应包括对生产的全面检查（例如，批生产记录、生产步骤是否适当、设备 / 设施的适用性、原料的可变性、工艺能力、偏差历史、投诉历史和批次不合格历史）。就每次调查的潜在生产根本原因，以及任何生产操作改进，提供总结。

● A comprehensive review and remediation plan for your OOS result investigation systems. The CAPA should include but not be limited to addressing the following:

● 针对你公司 OOS 结果调查系统的全面审查和整改计划。CAPA 应包括但不限于解决以下问题：

○ Quality unit oversight of laboratory investigations

○ 质量部门对实验室调查的监督

○ Identification of adverse laboratory control trends

○ 实验室控制异常趋势的识别

○ Resolution of causes of laboratory variation

○ 解决实验室波动的原因

○ Initiation of thorough investigations of potential manufacturing causes whenever a laboratory cause cannot be conclusively identified

○ 在无法最终确定实验室原因时，就应对潜在的生产原因进行彻底调查

○ Adequately scoping of each investigation and its CAPA

○ 充分探究每个调查及其 CAPA 的范围

○ Revised OOS investigation procedures with these and other remediations

○ 通过这些和其他整改措施修订 OOS 调查程序

● A comprehensive, independent assessment of your stability program and CAPA plan to ensure the adequacy of your stability program. Your remediated program should include, but not be limited to:

● 就稳定性计划进行全面、独立的评估和 CAPA 计划，以确保稳定性计划是充分的。你公司的整改计划应包括但不限于：

○ Stability indicating methods

○ 稳定性指示方法

○ Stability studies for each drug product in its marketed container-closure system before distribution is permitted

○ 在流通之前，对市售容器密闭系统中的每种药品进行稳定性研究

○ An ongoing program in which representative batches of each product are added each year to the program to determine if the shelf-life claim remains valid

○ 持续进行的计划，每年将每种产品的代表性批次添加到其中，以确定有效期声明是否仍然有效

○ Detailed definition of the specific attributes to be tested at each station (timepoint)

○ 每个点（时间点）要检验的特定属性的详细定义

● All procedures that describe these and other elements of your remediated stability program.

● 针对稳定性整改计划的这些以及其他元素，其所有相关的描述性程序。

● An assessment of manufacturing and quality data associated with each drug product you manufacture. Include remediated procedures and retrospective trending to identify any adverse findings and determine the need for changes to manufacturing processes or equipment, controls, or specifications.

● 对与你公司生产的每种药品相关的生产和质量数据进行评估。包括整改程序和回顾趋势，以识别任何不利结果，并确定是否需要变更生产工艺或设备、控制或质量标准。

● Describe how you intend to implement your annual product review (APR) program and how you intend to monitor effectiveness.

● 描述你公司打算如何实施年度产品回顾（APR）计划以及打算如何监控有效性。

● A comprehensive, independent assessment of your change management system.

This assessment should include, but not be limited to, your procedure to ensure changes are justified, reviewed, and approved by your quality unit. Your change management program should also include provisions for determining change effectiveness.

● 对你公司的变更管理系统进行全面、独立的评估。该评估应包括但不限于确保变更合理、经过质量部门审查和批准的程序。变更管理计划还应包括确定变更有效性的规定。

实验室控制措施

5. Your firm failed to establish laboratory controls that include scientifically sound and appropriate specifications, standards, sampling plans, and test procedures designed to assure that components, drug product containers, closures, in-process materials, labeling, and drug products conform to appropriate standards of identity, strength, quality, and purity (21 CFR 211.160(b)).

5. 你公司未能建立实验室控制措施，其中包括科学合理且相应的规范、标准、取样计划和检验程序，以确保物料、药品容器、密封件、中间体、标签和药品符合相关规定，即鉴别、规格、质量和纯度的标准〔21 CFR 211.160(b)〕。

You have inadequate laboratory controls. For example:

你公司的实验室控制措施不充分。例如：

● You failed to demonstrate your water system can consistently meet the minimum United States Pharmacopeia (USP) monograph specifications suitable for drug manufacturing. Specifically, you do not perform chemical analysis of your water, and you lack data to support your water system consistently produces water adhering to appropriate microbial limits (total counts, objectionable microbes). Furthermore, you stated you test your water system (b)(4), but you failed to test your water in 2021. This frequency does not provide meaningful information about the quality of the water used to manufacture your products throughout the year. Additionally, your system contains a dead leg with no recirculation loop. Inadequate control of water used as an ingredient in oral rinse products increases the risk of contaminated drug products reaching consumers, including pediatric patients.

● 你公司未能证明水系统能够始终满足适合药品生产的《美国药典》（USP）专论的最低质量标准。具体来说，你公司没有对水进行化学分析，并且缺乏数据来支持水系统持续生产符合适当微生物限度（总计数、有害微生物）的水。此外，你公司声称你们检验了水系统，基于（b）(4)的频率，但在2021年未能对水进行检验。就全年用于生产产品的水质量，该频率并不能提供有关有意义的信息。此外，你公司的系统包含一个没有再循环回路的死角。对口腔冲洗产品原辅料用水控制不力，这会增加消费者（包括儿科患者）受到药品污染的风险。

● You failed to establish adequate finished product testing procedures. You send finished product samples to a contract laboratory for microbial analysis. However, you have not adequately evaluated the suitability of the laboratory's test methods for use with your drug products. In addition, you use an（b）（4）to quantify fluoride content as part of your finished drug products' in-house testing. However, you lack sufficient evidence showing your method is equivalent or better than applicable USP compendial methods.

● 你公司未能建立充分的成品检验程序。你们将成品样品发送到委托实验室进行微生物分析。然而，你们没有充分评估实验室检验方法对药品的适用性。此外，你们使用（b）（4）来量化氟化物含量，以作为成品制剂内部检验的一部分。但是，缺乏充分的证据表明你公司的方法相当于或优于适用的药典方法。

For further information regarding the significance of Burkholderia cepacia complex and other objectionable contamination of non-sterile, water-based drug products, see FDA's advisory notice posted on July 7, 2021, at https://www.fda.gov/Drugs/DrugSafety/ucm559508.htm.

有关洋葱伯克霍尔德菌复合体和其他非无菌、水基药品污染显著性的更多信息，请参阅 FDA 于 2021 年 7 月 7 日发布的咨询通知，网址（见上，略）。

In your response, you state your water system's "quality light" assures the system is sufficient, and it is an "effective form of validation of system function." You also state you send your water to a third-party lab for microbial analysis, and you perform（b）（4）testing. In addition, you indicate you are considering incorporating（b）（4）and testing for "（b）（4）."

在回复中，你公司表示水系统中的"质量指示灯"可确保系统的充分性，并且它是"验证系统功能的有效形式"。你们还声明将水送到第三方实验室进行微生物分析，并进行（b）（4）检验。此外，你们表示正在考虑合并（b）（4），并检验"（b）（4）。"

Your response is inadequate. You lack adequate evidence that your water system meets the minimum USP monograph specifications suitable for drug manufacturing, and you fail to adequately address the deficiencies of your water system's design. In addition, you do not provide evidence that your proposed corrective actions would address the quality of your water system. Furthermore, your response regarding finished product testing fails to provide an adequate evaluation of your contract laboratory's microbial test methods.

你公司的回应不够充分。你们缺乏充分的证据，来证明水系统符合适合药品生产的最低 USP 专论质量标准，并且未能充分解决水系统设计的缺陷。此外，你们没有提供证据来证明纠正措施可以解决水系统的质量问题。此外，就委托实验室的微生物检验方法，你公司对成品检验的回复未能进行充分的评估。

In response to this letter, provide:

在回复本函时，请提供:

- A comprehensive, independent assessment of your water system design, control, and maintenance.

- 对水系统设计、控制和维护进行全面、独立的评估。包括对水系统中可能停滞的所有区域的描述。

- A thorough remediation plan to install and operate a suitable water system. Include a robust ongoing control, maintenance, and monitoring program to ensure the remediated system design consistently produces water adhering to (b)(4) Water, USP monograph specifications and appropriate microbial limits.

- 对于安装和运行适当的水系统，提供彻底整改计划。包括可靠的持续控制、维护和监测计划，以确保整改后的系统设计始终如一地生产符合（b）（4）、USP 专论质量标准和适当微生物限度要求的水。

- Regarding the latter, ensure that your total microbial count limit for water is appropriate in view of the intended use of the products produced by your firm.

- 关于后者，请确保你公司水的微生物总计数限度适合所生产产品的预期用途。

- A detailed risk assessment addressing the potential effects of the water system on the quality of all drug product lots currently within expiry. Specify actions that you will take in response to the risk assessment, such as customer notifications and product recalls.

- 详细的风险评估，阐明水系统对目前到期的所有药品批次质量的潜在影响。界定你公司将针对风险评估采取的措施，例如，客户通知和产品召回。

- A procedure for your water system monitoring that specifies routine microbial testing of water to ensure its acceptability for use in each batch of drug products produced by your firm.

- 你公司的水系统监测程序，规定了水的常规微生物检验，以确保其在生产的每批药品中的使用可接受性。

- The current action/alert limits for total counts and objectionable organisms used for your (b)(4) Water system. Ensure that the total count limits for your (b)(4) water are appropriately stringent in view of the intended use of each of the products produced by your firm.

● 用于水系统的总计数和有害微生物的当前行动／警戒限。鉴于你公司生产的每种产品的预期用途，确保（b）(4）水的总计数限度适当严格。

● A procedure governing your program for ongoing control, maintenance, and monitoring that ensures the remediated system consistently produces water that meets（b）(4）Water, USP monograph specifications and appropriate microbial limits.

● 一项用于监管持续控制、维护和监测计划的程序，以确保整改后的系统可以持续生产符合（b）(4）、USP 专论质量标准和适当微生物限度要求的水。

● A comprehensive, independent assessment of your laboratory practices, procedures, methods, equipment, documentation, and analyst competencies. Based on this review, provide a detailed plan to remediate and evaluate the effectiveness of your laboratory system.

● 对你公司的实验室实践、程序、方法、设备、文件和分析人员能力进行全面、独立的评估。在此审查的基础上，提供一个详细的计划来整改和评估你们的实验室系统的有效性。

● A list of chemical and microbial specifications, including test methods, used to analyze each lot of your drug products before a lot disposition decision.

● 在做出批处置决定之前，用于分析每批药品的化学和微生物质量标准（包括检验方法）清单。

○ An action plan and timelines for conducting full chemical and microbiological testing of retain samples to determine the quality of all batches of drug product distributed to the United States that are within expiry as of the date of this letter.

○ 行动计划和时间表：对留样进行全面的化学和微生物检验，对于流通给美国的所有效期内（本函发出之日计）药品批次，确定其质量。

○ A summary of all results obtained from testing retain samples from each batch. If such testing reveals substandard quality drug products, take rapid corrective actions, such as notifying customers and product recalls.

○ 所有批次的留样检验汇总。如果此类检验表明药品质量不合格，请迅速采取整改措施，例如，通知客户和产品召回。

● If any of the assessments performed to address the violations listed in this letter indicate substandard quality of drug product you manufacture, specify actions that you will take in response to the assessments, such as customer notifications and product recalls.

● 如果为解决本警告信中列出的违规情况而进行的任何评估表明你公司生产的药品质量不合格，请具体说明你们将针对评估采取的行动，例如，客户通知和产品召回。

Use of Contract Manufacturers | 使用合同生产商

Drugs must be manufactured in conformance with cGMP. FDA is aware that many drug manufacturers use independent contractors such as production facilities, testing laboratories, packagers, and labelers. FDA regards contractors as extensions of the manufacturer.

药品的生产必须符合 cGMP。FDA 意识到很多药品生产商使用独立合同商，例如生产设施、检验实验室、包装商和贴标商。FDA 将合同商视为生产商的延伸。

You are responsible for the quality of your drugs regardless of agreements in place with your contract facilities. You are required to ensure that drugs are made in accordance with section 501 (a)(2)(B) of the FD&C Act to ensure safety, identity, strength, quality, and purity. See FDA's guidance document *Contract Manufacturing Arrangements for Drugs : Quality Agreements* at https://www.fda.gov/media/86193/download.

无论与委托机构签订了何种协议，你公司都应对药品质量负责。你们需要确保根据 FD&C 法案第 501 (a)(2)(B) 条生产药品，以确保安全性、鉴别、规格、质量和纯度。请参阅 FDA 的指南，药品合同生产安排：质量协议，网址（略，见上）。

Data Integrity Remediation | 数据可靠性整改

Your quality system does not adequately ensure the accuracy and integrity of data to support the safety, effectiveness, and quality of the drugs you test. See FDA's guidance document *Data Integrity and Compliance with Drug cGMP* for guidance on establishing and following cGMP compliant data integrity practices at https://www.fda.gov/media/119267/download.

你公司的质量体系没有充分确保数据的准确性和可靠性，以支持检验药品的安全性、有效性和质量。有关建立和遵循 cGMP 合规数据可靠性实践的指南，请参阅 FDA 的指南，数据可靠性和药品 cGMP 合规性，网址（略，见上）。

A. A comprehensive investigation into the extent of the inaccuracies in data records and reporting, including results of the data review for drugs distributed to the United States. Include a detailed description of the scope and root causes of your data integrity lapses.

A. 对数据记录和报告的不准确程度进行全面调查，包括流通到美国的药品的数据审查结果。包括对数据可靠性失效的范围和根本原因的详细描述。

B. A current risk assessment of the potential effects of the observed failures on the quality of your drugs. Your assessment should include analyses of the risks to patients caused by the release of drugs affected by a lapse of data integrity, and analyses of the risks posed by ongoing operations.

B. 就观察到的失效对你公司药品质量的潜在影响，进行的当前风险评估。评估应包括：就因数据可靠性失效而影响的药品放行，分析其对患者造成的风险，以及分析对当前持续运营带来的风险。

C. A management strategy for your firm that includes the details of your global corrective action and preventive action plan. The detailed corrective action plan should describe how you intend to ensure the reliability and completeness of all data generated by your firm, including microbiological and analytical data, manufacturing records, and all data submitted to FDA.

C. 你公司的管理战略，包括整体纠正和预防措施计划的详细信息。详细的纠正措施计划应描述：你公司打算如何确保所有数据的可靠性和完整性，包括微生物和分析数据、实验室记录以及提交给 FDA 的所有数据。

4 原辅料鉴别方面存在疏漏

警告信编号： MARCS-CMS 644745-M

签发时间： 2023-3-1；**公示时间：** 2023-3-14

签发机构： 药品质量业务四处（Division of Pharmaceutical Quality Operations IV）

公　　司： Formology Lab Inc.

所在国家／地区： 美国

主　　题： cGMP/成品制剂/掺假（cGMP/Finished Pharmaceuticals/ Adulterated）

简　　介： 2022 年 8 月至 9 月，FDA 对该加利福尼亚州药品生产设施进行检查。令人遗憾的是，检查发现该公司在确认药物原辅料鉴别方面存在疏漏——在生产药品之前未对原料药（API）进行检验。FDA 指出，物料检验是药品质量的基础。FDA 要求公司说明每个批次的检验流程，并确保符合鉴别、规格、质量和纯度标准。如果接受供应商 COA 结果而非检验每批物料，请提供初始验证和定期再验证的方法，确保供应商结果可靠；同时，对每个进场物料批次至少进行一次鉴别检验。

本警告信以下部分与本书此前其他警告信内容类似，故略去：前言、作为合同商的责任（Responsibilities as a Contractor）、结论（Conclusion）。

物料鉴别

1. Your firm failed to conduct at least one test to verify the identity of each component of a drug product（21 CFR 211.84（d）（1））.

1. 你公司未能进行至少一项检验，来确认药品中每个原辅料均被鉴别［21 CFR 211.84（d）（1）］。

Your firm failed to test Active Pharmaceutical Ingredients（API）prior to use in manufacturing drug products. Specifically, at least（b）（4）drug product batches were manufactured and subsequently released, before identity testing was performed. Component testing is fundamental to drug product quality. Without adequate testing, you do not have scientific evidence that your incoming components conform to appropriate specifications before use in the manufacture of drug products.

在用于药品生产之前，你公司未能检验原料药（API）。具体而言，在进行鉴别检验之前，至少生产了（b）（4）个药品批次并随后放行。原辅料检验是药品质量的基础。如果没有充分的检验，就没有科学证据，来证明你公司的进场原辅料在用于药品生产之前符合相应的质量标准。

In your response, you indicate that your firm is currently developing, reviewing, and updating all quality management system procedures and processes and assessing the roles and responsibilities of all personnel. You also indicate that procedures around testing and receiving of components will be enhanced.

在回复中，你公司表明目前正在开发、审查和更新所有质量管理体系程序和流程，并评估人员角色和职责。你们还表示将加强有关物料检验和接收的程序。

Your response is inadequate. The revision of the procedure for receiving and testing components lacks details such as timelines for implementation of revised procedures and specific testing to be performed. The use of components and release of the drug products containing these components prior to conducting identity testing, and the qualification of suppliers was not addressed. An impact assessment or investigation into this practice is not provided, nor is there any evaluation if other components were inappropriately utilized.

你公司的回应不够充分。接收和检验物料程序的修订缺乏细节，例如实施修订程序的时间表和要执行的具体检验。没有阐明如何解决以下问题：在进行鉴别检验之前使用物料、放行含这些物料的药品，以及供应商的资质确认。没有提供对此实践的影响评估或调查，也没有对其他物料使用不当进行任何评估。

In response to this letter, provide：

在回复本函时，请提供：

● A comprehensive review of your material system to determine whether all suppliers of components, containers, and closures, are each qualified and the materials are assigned appropriate expiration or retest dates. The review should also determine whether incoming material controls are adequate to prevent use of unsuitable components, containers, and closures.

● 对你公司物料系统进行全面审查，以确定所有物料、容器和密封件的供应商是否均合格，并为物料指定适当的有效期或复验日期。审查还应确定进场物料控制是否足以防止使用不合适的物料、容器和密封件。

● A description of how you will test each component lot for conformity with all appropriate specifications for identity, strength, quality, and purity. If you intend to accept any results from your supplier's Certificates of Analysis(COA) instead of testing each component lot for strength, quality, and purity, specify how you will robustly establish the reliability of your supplier's results through initial validation as well as periodic revalidation. In addition, include a commitment to always conduct at least one specific identity test for each incoming component lot.

● 说明如何检验每个批次，确定是否符合有关鉴别、规格、质量和纯度质量标准。如果你公司计划接受供应商的 COA 结果，而不是检验每个物料批次的规格、质量和纯度，请说明如何进行初始验证和定期再验证，从而稳健地确定供应商结果的可靠性。此外，还应承诺对于每个进场原辅料批次，至少进行一个专属鉴别检验。

工艺验证

2. Your firm failed to establish written procedures for production and process control designed to assure that the drug products you manufacture have the identity, strength, quality, and purity they purport or are represented to possess(21 CFR 211.100(a)).

2. 未能建立书面的生产和过程控制程序，以确保药品具有其声称或声称拥有的鉴别、规格、质量和纯度［21 CFR 211.100(a)］。

Your firm lacked an adequate ongoing program for monitoring process controls to ensure stable manufacturing operations and consistent drug quality. Specifically, you did not provide documentation to show that the manufacturing processes for your over-the-counter(OTC) sunscreen drug products have been validated.

你公司缺乏充分的持续计划来监控过程控制，以确保稳定的生产操作和一致的药品质量。具体来说，你公司没有提供文件，来证明非处方（OTC）防晒药品的生产工艺已经过验证。

See the FDA's guidance document *Process Validation：General Principles and Practices* for general principles and approaches that the FDA considers appropriate elements of process validation at https://www.fda.gov/media/71021/download.

有关 FDA 认为适当的工艺验证要素的一般原则和方法，请参阅 FDA 指南，工艺验证：一般原则和实践，网址（略，见上）。

In addition, your firm could not provide data to demonstrate that the water used to manufacture drug products met the United States Pharmacopeia（USP）monograph for（b）（4）water and was fit for pharmaceutical use. Specifically, conductivity and total organic carbon （TOC）testing was not performed.

此外，你公司无法提供数据，来证明用于生产药品的水符合 USP（b）（4）水的专论，适合制药用途。具体来说，没有进行电导率和总有机碳（TOC）检验。

In your response, you provide a Master Validation Plan. Additionally, your firm commits （b）（4）.

在回复中，你公司提供了主验证计划。此外，你们承诺（b）（4）。

Your response is inadequate because it lacks sufficient information on your planned validation activities, including timelines for completion. Also, your response does not discuss TOC and conductivity testing.

你公司的回复不充分，因为其缺乏有关你们计划的验证活动的足够信息，包括完成时间表。此外，你们的回复没有讨论 TOC 和电导率检验。

In response to this letter, provide：

在回复本函时，请提供：

● A detailed summary of your validation program for ensuring a state of control throughout the product lifecycle, along with associated procedures, for each of your manufacturing processes. Describe your program for process performance qualification and ongoing monitoring of both intra-batch and inter-batch variation to ensure a continuing state of control.

● 有关确保整个产品生命周期中控制状态的验证项目的详细汇总，以及相关程序。描述你公司的程序，以进行工艺设计、工艺性能确认，并持续监控批内和批间变化，以确保持续的控制状态。

● A timeline for performing process performance qualification（PPQ）for each of your marketed drug products.

● 对每种上市药品执行工艺性能确认（PPQ）的时间表。

● Include your process performance protocol（s）, and written procedures for qualification of equipment and facilities.

● 包括工艺性能方案，以及设备和设施确认的书面程序。

● A comprehensive assessment of your water system design, control, and maintenance.

● 对你公司的水系统设计、控制和维护的全面评估。

● A thorough remediation plan to install and operate a suitable water system. Include a robust ongoing control, maintenance, and monitoring program to ensure the（b）（4）system consistently produces water adhering to（b）（4）Water, USP monograph specifications and appropriate microbial limits.

● 对于安装和运行适当的水系统，提供彻底整改计划。包括可靠的持续控制、维护和监测计划，以确保整改后的系统设计始终如一地生产符合（b）（4）、USP 专论质量标准和适当微生物限度要求的水。

● Regarding the latter, ensure that your total microbial count limit for water is appropriate in view of the intended use of the products produced by your firm.

● 关于后者，请确保水的微生物总计数限度适合你公司产品的预期用途。

● A detailed risk assessment addressing the potential effects of the observed water system deficiencies on the quality of all drug product lots currently in U.S. distribution or within expiry. Specify actions that you will take in response to the risk assessment, such as customer notifications and product recalls.

● 详细的风险评估，以阐明观察到的水系统缺陷对目前在美国上市或有效期内的所有药品批次质量的潜在影响。指定你公司为回应风险评估将采取的操作，例如，客户通知和产品召回。

质量部门未能履责

3. Your firm failed to establish an adequate quality unit and the responsibilities and procedures applicable to the quality control unit are not in writing and fully followed（21 CFR 211.22（a）and（d））.

3. 你公司未能建立适当的质量部门，适用于质量部门的责任和程序未以书面形式呈现，且未得到完全遵守［21 CFR 211.22（a）和（d）］。

Specifically, your quality unit（QU）failed to establish procedures describing critical oversight responsibilities including but not limited to, the following: investigations, management of changes, customer complaints, training, corrective actions and preventive actions（CAPAs）, deviations, annual product reviews, and written procedures for quality unit operations.

具体来说，你公司质量部门（QU）未能建立描述关键监督责任的程序，包括但不限于以下内容：调查、变更管理、客户投诉、培训、纠正和预防措施（CAPA）、偏差、年度产品回顾，以及质量部门运行的书面程序。

Furthermore, you did not have appropriate stability data to demonstrate that the chemical and microbiological properties of your drug products met established specifications and remain acceptable throughout their assigned shelf-life. For example, your firm did not place an appropriate number of batches of each drug product formulation on stability. Additionally, out-of-specification (OOS) viscosity results were obtained for your (b)(4) and (b)(4) formula stability samples. You failed to conduct an adequate investigation for the OOS viscosity results.

此外，你公司没有适当的稳定性数据，来证明药品的化学和微生物特性符合既定质量标准，并且在指定的有效期内保持可接受的状态。例如，你公司没有对每种药品处方的稳定性进行适当数量的批次的检验。此外，还获得了（b）（4）及（b）（4）处方稳定性的不合格（OOS）黏度结果。你公司未能对 OOS 黏度结果进行充分的调查。

In your response, you state that you are currently developing, or reviewing and updating all quality management system procedures and processes. You plan to provide training for all applicable personnel as procedures are implemented and include documented evidence in subsequent response updates. Your firm also provides information on how viscosity impacts your product and may shift during stability testing. You commit to continuing to evaluate your viscosity specifications and OOS investigations are initiated for the failures.

在回复中，你公司声明目前正在开发或审查和更新所有质量管理体系程序和流程。你公司计划在实施程序时为所有适用人员提供培训，并在后续回应更新中包含书面证据。你公司还提供了有关黏度如何影响产品，以及在稳定性检验期间可能发生变化的信息。你们承诺继续评估黏度质量标准，并针对不合格启动 OOS 调查。

Your response is inadequate. You do not provide target completion dates for the updated procedures. In addition, it is not appropriate to train personnel without a training procedure in place.

你公司的回应不够充分。你们没有提供更新程序的目标完成日期。此外，在没有适当培训程序的情况下培训人员是不合适的。

In response to this letter, provide:

在回复本函时，请提供：

● A comprehensive independent assessment and remediation plan to ensure your QU is given the authority and resources to effectively function. The assessment should also include, but not be limited to:

● 全面的独立评估和整改计划，以确保你公司的 QU 获得有效运行的权力和资源。

评估还应包括但不限于：

○ A determination of whether procedures used by your firm are robust and appropriate

○ 确定你公司使用的程序是否可靠和适当。

○ Provisions for QU oversight throughout your operations to evaluate adherence to appropriate practices

○ 在整个运营过程中 QU 进行监督的规定，以评估对相应规范的遵守情况。

○ A complete and final review of each batch and its related information before the QU disposition decision

○ 在 QU 决定处置之前，对每批产品及其相关信息进行完整和最终审查。

○ Oversight and approval of investigations and discharging of all other QU duties to ensure identity, strength, quality, and purity of all products

○ 监督和批准调查以及履行所有其他 QU 职责，以确保所有产品的鉴别、规格、质量和纯度。

● A comprehensive assessment and CAPA plan to ensure the adequacy of your stability program. Your remediated program should include, but not be limited to:

● 进行全面、独立的评估和 CAPA 计划，以确保你公司的稳定性计划是充分的。整改计划应包括但不限于：

○ Stability indicating methods

○ 稳定性指示方法

○ Stability studies for each drug product in its marketed container-closure system before distribution is permitted

○ 在流通之前，对市售容器密闭系统中的每种药品进行稳定性研究

○ An ongoing program in which representative batches of each product are added each year to the program to determine if the shelf-life claim remains valid

○ 持续进行的计划，每年将每种产品的代表性批次添加到其中，以确定有效期声明是否仍然有效

○ Detailed definition of the specific attributes to be tested at each station（timepoint）

○ 每个点（时间点）要检验的特定属性的详细定义

- All procedures that describe these and other elements of your remediated stability program.

- 针对稳定性整改计划的这些以及其他元素，其所有相关的描述性程序。

5 水系统未经充分设计与监控

警告信编号： MARCS-CMS 645558

签发时间： 2023-3-10；**公示时间：** 2023-3-21

签发机构： 药品质量业务四处（Division of Pharmaceutical Quality Operations IV）

公　　司： Cosmetic Science Laboratories LLC

所在国家 / 地区： 美国

主　　题： cGMP/ 成品制剂 / 掺假（cGMP/Finished Pharmaceuticals/ Adulterated）

简　　介： FDA 于 2022 年 9 月对位于美国加利福尼亚的药品生产设施进行了审查。FDA 指出该公司在生产药品时使用水作为原辅料使用，然而公司并未能确保其水系统经过充分设计、控制、维护和监控，以持续提供适合其预期用途的水质。作为回应，FDA 要求该公司制定水系统监测程序，并规定了水的常规微生物检验，以确保每批公司生产的药品的使用安全性。此外，还要求该公司提供水系统的总微生物计数和有害微生物的当前行动 / 警戒限。鉴于该公司生产的每种产品的预期用途，这些措施需要确保其水系统的总微生物计数限度达到适当严格的标准。

本警告信以下部分与本书此前其他警告信内容类似，故略去：前言、结论（Conclusion）。

入厂物料鉴别问题

1. Your firm failed to conduct at least one test to verify the identity of each component of a drug product. Your firm also failed to validate and establish the reliability of your component supplier's test analyses at appropriate intervals（21 CFR 211.84（d）（1）and 211.84（d）（2））.

1. 你公司未进行至少一项检验来确认药品中每种原辅料都被鉴别。也未能在适当的时间间隔内验证和确定供应商检验结果的可靠性［21 CFR 211.84（d）（1）和 211.84（d）（2）］。

You failed to test your incoming active pharmaceutical ingredients（APIs）for identity prior to manufacturing your bulk over-the-counter（OTC）drug products，including SPF-50（b）（4）Sunscreen. Additionally，you relied on certificates of analysis（COAs）from your suppliers to use incoming APIs without establishing the reliability of the specifications and characteristics of each supplier's COAs.

在生产包括 SPF-50（b）（4）防晒霜在内的半成品非处方（OTC）药品之前，你公司未能对进场原料药（API）进行鉴别检验。此外，你们依赖供应商的分析证书（COA）来使用进场 API，而没有确定每个供应商 COA 的质量标准和特征的可靠性。

Your response is inadequate.

你公司的回应不够充分。

Identity testing for each component lot used in drug product manufacturing is required，and you may only rely on certificates of analysis（COAs）for other component attributes by validating the suppliers' test results at appropriate intervals.

需要对药品生产中使用的每个原辅料批次进行鉴别检验。只有通过定期验证供应商的检验结果，你公司才能依赖分析证书（COA）确认原辅料属性。

In response to this letter，provide the following：

在回复本函时，请提供以下信息：

（略）

此处与 FDA 发给 Dunagin Pharmaceuticals Inc. dba Massco Dental 的警告信（编号：MARCS-CMS 644335，即"3 与非药用产品的共线生产问题"）的要求类似，故略去。

验证

2. Your firm failed to establish adequate written procedures for production and process control designed to assure that the drug products you manufacture have the identity，strength，quality，and purity they purport or are represented to possess. Your firm also failed to prepare batch production and control records with complete information relating to the production and control of each batch of drug product produced（21 CFR 211.100（a）and 21 CFR 211.188）.

你公司未建立用于生产和过程控制充分的书面程序，以确保所生产药品具有其声称或代表拥有的鉴别、规格、质量和纯度。你公司也未能准备批生产和控制记录，其中包含与所生产的每批药品的生产和控制相关的完整信息［21 CFR 211.100（a）和 21 CFR 211.188］。

Process Validation ｜ 工艺验证

Your firm did not provide process validation documents for your contract manufactured over-the-counter（OTC）bulk drug products. During the inspection, you failed to provide your protocols, reports, or data to support that each OTC drug product met predetermined quality requirements consistently and reliably.

针对你公司委托生产的非处方（OTC）原料药产品，你们未能提供工艺验证文件。在检查过程中，你公司未能提供方案、报告或数据，来支持每种非处方药产品一致且可靠地满足预定的质量要求。

You also failed to provide detailed process performance qualification（PPQ）protocols for the validation of your different OTC drug product manufacturing processes.

你公司还未能提供详细的工艺性能确认（PPQ）方案，来验证不同的 OTC 药品生产工艺。

（略）

此处与 FDA 发给 Profounda, Inc. 的警告信（编号：MARCS-CMS 642595，即"2 未能提供生产工艺的验证数据"）中有关工艺验证的重要性部分的内容类似，故略去。

Batch Production Records ｜ 批生产记录

Your firm lacked adequate batch records. You did not include specific information such as equipment identification and process parameters that demonstrate control in the manufacture of your bulk drug products.

你公司缺乏充分的批记录。你们没有提供具体信息，例如，设备标识和工艺参数，以证明对原料药生产的控制。

Cleaning Validation ｜ 清洁验证

During the inspection, your firm could not provide investigators with evidence that you have performed cleaning validation and equipment qualification.

在检查过程中，你公司无法向调查员提供已进行清洁验证和设备确认的证据。

You manufacture drug products using the same equipment that you use to manufacture nonpharmaceutical products such as cosmetics. Chemical and microbiological residues on equipment from previous manufacturing activities can adversely impact the purity, quality, and safety of drug products also manufactured on that equipment.

你公司生产药品所使用的设备与生产非药用产品（例如化妆品）所用的设备相同。设备上可能残留有先前生产活动中的化学成分和微生物，这些残留物可能对在该设备上生产的药品的纯度、质量和安全性产生不利影响。

Additionally, you lacked cleaning logs and usage logs for kettles and mixers used in compounding your bulk drug products.

此外，你公司缺乏用于配制产品半成品的罐子和混合器的清洁台账和使用台账。

■ （b）（4）Water System ｜（b）（4）水系统

Your firm uses（b）（4）Water as a component to manufacture your drug products that are released for distribution to U.S. consumers. You did not establish that the（b）（4）Water system you use to manufacture your drug product is adequately designed, controlled, maintained, and monitored to ensure that it consistently produces water suitable for its intended use.

你公司使用（b）（4）水作为生产药品的原辅料，然后向美国消费者销售。你们没有确定用于生产药品的（b）（4）水系统经过充分设计、控制、维护和监控，以确保其持续生产适合其预期用途的水。

（b）（4）water must be suitable for its intended use and routinely tested to ensure ongoing conformance with appropriate chemical and microbiological attributes.

（b）（4）水必须适合其预期用途并定期进行检验，以确保持续符合适当的化学和微生物特性。

Your response is inadequate.

你公司的回应不够充分。

In response to this letter, provide the following：

在回复本函时，请提供以下信息：

（略）

此处为工艺验证观察项对应的回应要求，与 FDA 发给 Dunagin Pharmaceuticals Inc. dba Massco Dental 的警告信（编号：MARCS-CMS 644335，即 "3 与非药用产品的共线生产问题"）中有关工艺验证的回应要求部分的内容类似，故略去。

- Your master production and control records for your drug products, to demonstrate that they fully document each significant and validated manufacturing step.

- 你公司药品的主要生产和控制记录，以证明它们完整记录了每个重要且已验证生产步骤。

- A complete assessment of documentation systems used throughout your manufacturing operations, to determine where documentation practices are insufficient. Include a detailed corrective action and preventive action (CAPA) plan that comprehensively remediates your firm's documentation practices, to ensure you retain attributable, legible, complete, original, accurate, and contemporaneous records throughout your operation.

- 对整个生产操作中使用的文档系统进行全面评估，以确定记录实践的不足之处。包括详细的 CAPA 计划，以全面整改公司的记录规范，以确保你公司在整个运营过程中保存可追溯的、清晰的、完整的、原始的、准确的和同步的记录。

- Appropriate improvements to your cleaning validation program, with special emphasis on incorporating conditions identified as worst-case in your drug manufacturing operation. This should include but not be limited to identification and evaluation of all worst-case：

- 对你公司的清洁验证程序进行适当的改进，特别强调在药品生产操作中纳入被确定为最差情况的条件。这应包括但不限于所有最差情况的识别和评估：

  ○ drugs with higher toxicities

  ○ 毒性较高的药物

  ○ drugs with higher drug potencies

  ○ 药效较高的药物

  ○ drugs of lower solubility in their cleaning solvents

  ○ 在其清洁溶剂中溶解度较低的药物

  ○ drugs with characteristics that make them difficult to clean

  ○ 具有难以清洁特征的药物

  ○ swabbing locations for areas that are most difficult to clean

  ○ 最难以清洁区域的擦拭位置

  ○ maximum hold times before cleaning

    ○ 清洁前的最长存放时间

● A summary of updated SOPs that ensure an appropriate program is in place for verification and validation of cleaning procedures for products, processes, and equipment.

● 更新的 SOP 的汇总，以确保制定适当的程序，来确认和验证产品、工艺和设备的清洁程序。

● A procedure for your water system monitoring that specifies routine microbial testing of water to ensure its acceptability for use in each batch of drug products produced by your firm.

● 你公司水系统监测程序，规定了水的常规微生物检验，以确保其在生产的每批药品中使用的可接受性。

● The current action/alert limits for total counts and objectionable organisms used for your (b)(4) water system. Ensure that the total count limits for your (b)(4) water are appropriately stringent in view of the intended use of each of the products produced by your firm.

● 用于水系统的总计数和有害微生物的当前行动 / 警戒限。鉴于你公司生产的每种产品的预期用途，确保（b）(4) 水的总计数限度适当严格。

● A procedure governing your program for ongoing control, maintenance, and monitoring that ensures the remediated system consistently produces water that meets (b)(4) water, USP monograph specifications and appropriate microbial limits.

● 一项用于监管持续控制、维护和监测计划的程序，以确保整改后的系统可以持续生产符合（b）(4)、USP 专论质量标准和适当微生物限度要求的水。

质量部门

3. Your firm's quality control unit failed to exercise its responsibility to ensure drug products manufactured are in compliance with cGMP, and meet established specifications for identity, strength, quality, and purity (21 CFR211.22).

3. 你公司质量控制部门未能履行职责，以确保所生产的药品符合 cGMP 要求，并符合有关鉴别、规格、质量和纯度的既定质量标准（21 CFR 211.22）。

Your quality unit (QU) did not provide adequate oversight for the manufacture of your OTC drug products. In an affidavit dated September 20, 2022, you stated that you could not provide documents related to several cGMP activities such as, out-of-specification (OOS) results, non-conformances, deviations and investigations, annual product review, and cGMP training.

你公司质量部门（QU）没有对 OTC 药品的生产提供充分的监督。在 2022 年 9 月 20 日的宣誓书中，你公司表示无法提供与多项 cGMP 活动相关的文件，例如不合格（OOS）结果、不合格项、偏差和调查、年度产品回顾和 cGMP 培训。

In addition, you used（b）（4）hold-time studies to support a（b）（4）expiration date for bulk drug products, such as your SPF-30 Daily Protect Sunscreen. These（b）（4）hold-time studies do not support a（b）（4）hold time for bulk drug products. You have not determined the impact these inadequate hold-time studies may have had on the stability and quality attributes of your bulk drug products. Additionally, customers may rely on these claims to establish（b）（4）expiration dates on finished drug products.

此外，你公司还使用（b）（4）存放时间研究，来支持半成品制剂（例如 SPF-30 每日防护防晒霜）的（b）（4）有效期。这些（b）（4）存放时间研究不支持半成品制剂的（b）（4）存放时间。这些不充分的放置时间研究可能对半成品制剂的稳定性和质量属性产生的影响，对此你公司尚未确定。此外，客户可以依靠这些声明来确定成品的（b）（4）有效期。

An adequate QU overseeing all manufacturing operations is necessary to consistently ensure drug quality. Your firm's quality systems are inadequate. See FDA's guidance document *Quality Systems Approach to Pharmaceutical cGMP Regulations* for help in implementing quality systems and risk management approaches to meet the requirements of cGMP regulations 21 CFR parts 210 and 211, at https://www.fda.gov/media/71023/download.

需要有充分的 QU 来监督所有生产操作，以始终如一地确保药品质量。请参阅 FDA 指南，药品 cGMP 法规的质量体系方法，帮助实施质量体系和风险管理方法，以满足 cGMP 法规 21 CFR 第 210 和 211 部分的要求，网址（略，见上）。

Your response is inadequate.

你公司的回应不够充分。

In response to this letter, provide：

在回复本函时，请提供：

● A comprehensive assessment and remediation plan to ensure your QU is given the authority and resources to effectively function. The assessment should also include, but not be limited to：

● 全面的评估和整改计划，以确保你公司 QU 获得有效运作的权限和资源。评估还应包括但不限于：

○ A determination of whether procedures used by your firm are robust and appropriate.

○ 确定你公司使用的程序是否可靠和适当。

○ Provisions for QU oversight throughout your operations to evaluate adherence to appropriate practices.

○ 在整个运营过程中 QU 进行监督的规定，以评估对相应规范的遵守情况。

○ A complete and final review of each batch and its related information before the QU disposition decision.

○ 在 QU 决定处置之前，对每批产品及其相关信息进行完整和最终审查。

○ Oversight and approval of investigations and discharging of all other QU duties to ensure identity, strength, quality, and purity of all products

○ 监督和批准调查以及履行所有其他 QU 职责，以确保所有产品的鉴别、规格、质量和纯度。

6 未能进行充分的放行检验

警告信编号： MARCS-CMS 645821

签发时间： 2023-3-13；**公示时间：** 2023-3-28

签发机构： 药品质量业务四处（Division of Pharmaceutical Quality Operations IV）

公　　司： NuGeneration Technologies LLC

所在国家 / 地区： 美国

主　　题： cGMP/ 成品制剂 / 掺假（cGMP/Finished Pharmaceuticals/ Adulterated）

简　　介： FDA 于 2022 年 9 月对位于加利福尼亚州的药品生产设施进行了检查。该公司专注于生产手部消毒药品，这在新冠肺炎疫情期间显得尤为重要且供不应求。在检查中，FDA 指出该公司依赖未经确认的乙醇供应商提供的 COA，而乙醇是手部消毒剂的关键原料药。根据 cGMP 的要求，药品生产中每一批次的原辅料都必须至少进行了鉴别检验。更为重要的是，公司只有通过定期验证供应商所提供的检验结果，才能依赖分析证书来确认其他质量属性。FDA 特别强调了该公司对于乙醇中甲醇杂质检验不足的问题。全球范围内已发生多起由使用受甲醇污染乙醇引发的人类致命中毒事件。因此，该公司需要高度重视这一问题，并立即采取相应措施，以确保产品的安全性和合规性。

本警告信以下部分与本书此前其他警告信内容类似，故略去：前言、cGMP 顾问推荐（cGMP Consultant Recommended）、使用合同生产商（Use of Contract Manufacturers）、结论（Conclusion）。

产品检验

1. Your firm failed to have, for each batch of drug product, appropriate laboratory

determination of satisfactory conformance to final specifications for the drug product, including the identity and strength of each active ingredient, prior to release.（21 CFR 211.165（a））.

1. 你公司没有对每批药品进行适当的实验室确认，以在放行之前确定其是否符合最终产品的质量标准要求，包括每种原料药的鉴别和规格［21 CFR 211.165（a）］。

Your firm failed to conduct adequate release testing of your NuRinse Hand Sanitizer drug product. You only conducted（b）（4）, and（b）（4）testing prior to release. Full release testing, which includes strength and identity testing of the active ingredient（e.g., ethanol）, and appropriate impurity and microbiological testing, must be performed before drug product release and distribution. Without adequate testing, you do not have adequate scientific evidence to assure that your drug products conform to appropriate specifications before release.

你公司未能对 NuRinse 手部消毒药品进行充分的放行检验。在放行前，仅对（b）（4）和（b）（4）进行检验。在药品放行和流通之前，必须进行全面放行检验，包括原料药（例如乙醇）的规格和鉴别检验，以及适当的杂质和微生物检验。如果没有充分的检验就没有充分的科学证据，来确保你公司的药品在放行前符合相应的质量标准。

In response to this letter, provide：

在回复本函时，请提供：

● A list of chemical and microbial test methods and specifications used to analyze each lot of your drug product before making a lot disposition decision, and the associated written procedures.

● 在做出批处置决定之前，用于分析每批药品的化学和微生物检验方法和质量标准的清单，以及相关的书面程序。

● A comprehensive, independent assessment of your laboratory practices, procedures, methods, equipment, documentation, and analyst competencies. Based on this review, provide a detailed plan to remediate and evaluate the effectiveness of your laboratory system.

● 对实验室操作、程序、方法、设备、文件和分析人员的能力，进行全面的独立评估。在此审查的基础上，提供详细计划，以整改和评估实验室系统的有效性。

物料检验

2. Your firm failed to test samples of each component for identity and conformity with all appropriate written specifications for purity, strength, and quality. Your firm also failed to validate and establish the reliability of your component supplier's test analyses at appropriate

intervals（21 CFR 211.84（d）（1）and 211.84（d）（2）).

2. 你公司未进行至少一项检验来确认药品中每种原辅料都被鉴别，并使其符合所有适当的纯度、规格和质量的书面质量标准。你公司也未能在适当的时间间隔内，验证和确定物料供应商检验分析的可靠性［21 CFR 211.84（d）（1）和 211.84（d）（2）]。

Your firm failed to test incoming active pharmaceutical ingredients（API）（e.g., ethanol）and other components（e.g., deionized（DI）water）used to manufacture over-the-counter drug products to determine their identity, purity, strength, and other appropriate quality attributes. Additionally, you have not shown that your water system can consistently produce water suitable for drug manufacturing, and, at a minimum, meets the USP monograph for Purified Water and appropriate microbial limits.

针对用于生产非处方药品的进场原料药（API）（例如乙醇）和其他原辅料［例如去离子（DI）水］，你公司未能检验，以确定其鉴别、纯度、规格和其他原辅料适当的质量属性。此外，还没有证明你公司的水系统，确保其能够持续生产适合药品生产的水，并且至少符合 USP 专论的纯化水和适当的微生物限度要求。

■ Inadequate API Testing ｜原料药检验不充分

Your firm relied on the COA from unqualified suppliers of ethanol. This component is used as an active ingredient in the manufacture of your NuRinse Hand Sanitizer drug product. cGMP requires identity testing for each component lot used in drug product manufacturing, and you can only rely on the COA for other component attributes by appropriately validating the supplier's test results at appropriate intervals. You also failed to appropriately test your incoming ethanol, used as an active ingredient, for methanol.

你公司依赖于未经确认的乙醇供应商提供的分析证书（COA）。该原辅料用作 NuRinse 手部消毒药品生产中的原料药。cGMP 要求对药品生产中使用的每个原辅料批次进行鉴别检验，且只有通过定期验证供应商的检验结果，才能依赖 COA 确认其他原辅料属性。针对进场原料药乙醇中的甲醇杂质，你公司也能进行适当的检验。

The use of ethanol contaminated with methanol has resulted in various lethal poisoning incidents in humans worldwide. See FDA's guidance document *Policy for Testing of Alcohol（Ethanol）and Isopropyl Alcohol for Methanol, Including During the Public Health Emergency（COVID-19）* to help you meet the cGMP requirements when manufacturing drugs containing ethanol at https://www.fda.gov/media/145262/download.

在全球范围内，使用被甲醇污染的乙醇已导致多起人类致命中毒事件。请参阅 FDA 指南，酒精（乙醇）和异丙醇检验政策——包括在公共卫生紧急事件（COVID-19）期间的要求，网址（见上，略）。

▨ Inadequate Component Water｜水作为物料存在问题

Your firm has not shown that your DI water is suitable for aqueous-based dosage form drug product manufacturing, and, at a minimum, meets the USP Purified Water monograph and appropriate microbials limits. Your firm lacked sufficient testing of your DI water system. For example, you failed to appropriately test for total organic carbon or microbial organisms, and you failed to ensure that your conductivity results are accurate and recorded.

你公司尚未证明去离子水适合水基剂型药品的生产，并且至少符合 USP 纯化水专论和适当的微生物限度。你公司缺乏对去离子水系统的充分检验。例如，未能正确检验总有机碳或微生物，也未能确保电导率结果准确并记录。

Without routine water monitoring of an appropriately designed system, you cannot ensure that your water meets minimum microbiological and chemical standards suitable for the manufacture of your drug products.

如果没有对适当设计的系统进行常规水监测，就无法确保你公司的水符合适合药品生产的最低微生物和化学标准。

In response to this letter, provide：

在回复本函时，请提供：

● A comprehensive, independent review of your material system to determine whether all suppliers of components, containers, and closures, are each qualified and the materials are assigned appropriate expiration or retest dates. The review should also determine whether incoming material controls are adequate to prevent use of unsuitable components, containers, and closures.

● 对你公司的物料系统进行全面、独立审查，以确定所有物料、容器和密封件的供应商是否均有资质，并为物料指定了适当的有效期或复验期。审查还应确定进场物料控制是否足以防止使用不适当的物料、容器和密封件。

● The chemical and microbiological quality control specifications you use to test and release each incoming lot of component for use in manufacturing.

● 针对每批用于生产目的的进场物料，用于检验和放行的化学和微生物质控标准。

● A description of how you will test each component lot for conformity with all appropriate specifications for identity, strength, quality, and purity. If you intend to accept any results from your supplier's COA instead of testing each component lot for strength, quality, and purity, specify how you will robustly establish the reliability of your supplier's results through initial validation as well as periodic re-validation. In addition, include a commitment to always conduct at least one specific identity test for each incoming component lot.

● 说明如何检验每个批次，确定是否符合有关鉴别、规格、质量和纯度质量标准。如果你公司打算接受供应商 COA 的结果，而不是检验每个物料批次的规格、质量和纯度，请说明如何进行初始验证和定期再验证，从而稳健地确定供应商结果的可靠性。此外，还应承诺对于每个进场原辅料批次，至少进行一个专属鉴别检验。

● A thorough remediation plan to install and operate a suitable water system. Include a robust ongoing control, maintenance, and monitoring program to ensure the remediated system consistently produces water adhering to Purified Water, USP monograph specifications and appropriate microbial limits.

● 对于安装和运行适当的水系统，提供彻底整改计划。包括可靠的持续控制、维护和监测计划，以确保整改后的系统设计始终如一地生产符合纯化水、USP 专论质量标准和适当微生物限度要求的水。

● Regarding the latter, ensure that your total microbial count limit for water is appropriate in view of the intended use of the products produced by your firm.

● 关于后者，请确保水的微生物总计数限度适合你公司所生产产品的预期用途。

● A detailed risk assessment addressing the potential effects of the observed water system failures on the quality of all drug product lots currently in U.S. distribution or within expiry. Specify actions that you will take in response to the risk assessment, such as customer notifications and product recalls.

● 详细的风险评估，以阐明观察到的水系统缺陷对目前在美国上市或有效期内的所有药品批次质量的潜在影响。指定你公司为回应风险评估将采取的操作，例如，客户通知和产品召回。

稳定性研究

3. Your firm failed to establish and follow an adequate written testing program designed to assess the stability characteristics of drug products and to use results of stability testing to determine appropriate storage conditions and expiration dates（21 CFR 211.166（a））.

3. 你公司未能建立并遵循适当的书面检验程序，以评估药品的稳定性特征；未能使用稳定性检验结果，来确定适当的储存条件和有效期［21 CFR 211.166（a）］。

Your firm lacked stability data to support the expiration dates for your NuRinse Hand Sanitizer drug product currently in distribution. Without an adequate stability program, you cannot confirm that your drug product will meet established specifications and all predetermined quality criteria throughout their shelf life.

你公司缺乏稳定性数据，来支持目前正在销售的 NuRinse 手部消毒药品的有效期。如果没有充分的稳定性计划，就无法确认你公司的药品在整个有效期内符合既定的规格和所有预先确定的质量标准。

In response to this letter, provide：

在回复本函时，请提供：

● A comprehensive independent assessment and corrective action and preventive action（CAPA）plan to ensure the adequacy of your stability program. Your remediated program should include，but not be limited to：

● 全面、独立的评估和 CAPA 计划，以确保你公司的稳定性计划是充分的。整改计划应包括但不限于：

○ Stability indicating methods

○ 稳定性指示方法

○ Stability studies for each drug product in its marketed container-closure system before distribution is permitted

○ 在流通之前，对市售容器密闭系统中的每种药品进行稳定性研究

○ An ongoing program in which representative batches of each product are added each year to the program to determine if the shelf-life claim remains valid

○ 持续进行的计划，每年将每种产品的代表性批次添加到其中，以确定有效期声明是否仍然有效

○ Detailed definition of the specific attributes to be tested at each station（timepoint）

○ 每个点（时间点）要检验的特定属性的详细定义

● All procedures that describe these and other elements of your remediated stability program.

● 针对稳定性整改计划的这些以及其他元素，其所有相关的描述性程序。

工艺验证

4. Your firm failed to establish written procedures for production and process control

designed to assure that the drug products you manufacture have the identity, strength, quality, and purity they purport or are represented to possess (21 CFR 211.100 (a)).

4. 未能建立书面的生产和过程控制程序，以确保药品具有其声称或声称拥有的鉴别、规格、质量和纯度［21 CFR 211.100 (a)］。

Your firm failed to validate the manufacturing process for NuRinse Hand Sanitizer drug product currently in distribution.

你公司未能验证目前正在销售的 NuRinse 手部消毒药品的生产工艺。

（略）

此处与 FDA 发给 Profounda, Inc. 的警告信（编号：MARCS-CMS 642595，即"2 未能提供生产工艺的验证数据"）中有关工艺验证的重要性部分的内容类似，故略去。

In response to this letter, provide:

在回复本函时，请提供：

（略）

此处与 FDA 发给 Dunagin Pharmaceuticals Inc. dba Massco Dental 的警告信（编号：MARCS-CMS 644335，"3 与非药用产品的共线生产问题"）中有关工艺验证的回应要求类似，故略去。

Quality Systems | 质量体系

Your firm's quality systems are inadequate. See FDA's guidance document *Quality Systems Approach to Pharmaceutical cGMP Regulations* for help implementing quality systems and risk management approaches to meet the requirements of cGMP regulations 21 CFR, parts 210 and 211 at https://www.fda.gov/regulatory-information/search-fda-guidance-documents/quality-systems-approach-pharmaceutical-current-good-manufacturing-practice-regulations.

你公司的质量体系不完善。请参阅 FDA 指南，药品 cGMP 法规质量体系方法，以帮助实施质量体系和风险管理方法，满足 cGMP 法规 21 CFR 第 210 和 211 部分的要求，网址（略，见上）。

7 建议聘请顾问，对公司进行全面审计

警告信编号： MARCS-CMS 649122

签发时间： 2023-3-20；**公示时间：** 2023-4-11

签发机构： 药品质量业务一处（Division of Pharmaceutical Quality Operations I ）

公　　司： Omega Packaging Corp

所在国家／地区： 美国

主　　题： cGMP／成品制剂／掺假（cGMP/Finished Pharmaceuticals/ Adulterated ）

简　　介： FDA 于 2022 年 10 月至 11 月对位于新泽西州的药品生产设施进行了全面检查。该公司也是手部消毒药品的生产商。在检查中，FDA 指出该公司未能适当检验进场原料药中是否存在甲醇等杂质，并且其程序没有确保检验甘油中是否存在二甘醇。此外，FDA 还注意到，该公司用于生产药品的 API 的 COA 声明称"该物料不被视为，且不作为原料药出售"。最后，FDA 强调根据其在公司发现的违规情况的性质，公司应聘请有资格的顾问，协助公司满足 cGMP 要求。根据 FDA 指南——药品 cGMP 法规质量体系方法，有资格的顾问应对公司的整个运营进行全面的六大系统审计，包括质量系统、设施和设备系统、物料系统、生产系统、包装和贴标系统，以及实验室控制系统。在该公司与 FDA 寻求解决合规状态之前，顾问应评估所有 CAPA 的完成情况和有效性。

本警告信以下部分与本书此前其他警告信内容类似，故略去：前言、作为合同商的责任（Responsibilities as a Contractor）、结论（Conclusion）。

物料检验

1. Your firm failed to test samples of each component for identity and conformity with all

appropriate written specifications for purity, strength, and quality (21 CFR 211.84 (d) (1) and 211.84 (d) (2)).

你公司未能检验每种原辅料的样品，以确定其纯度、规格和质量符合相应的书面质量标准 [21 CFR 211.84 (d) (1) 和 211.84 (d) (2)]。

■ Inadequate API Testing ｜原料药检验不充分

Your firm contract manufactures ethanol-based over-the-counter (OTC) hand rub drug products (also referred to as consumer hand sanitizer). You failed to adequately test your incoming components for identity before using the components to manufacture your OTC drug products, and you relied on certificates of analysis (COAs) from unqualified suppliers. Specifically, you failed to appropriately test your incoming (b) (4) active pharmaceutical ingredient (API) for impurities such as methanol, and your procedures did not ensure that you test glycerin for presence of diethylene glycol (DEG). We also note that the COA for the (b) (4) API you used to manufacture your drug products states that "this material is not considered to be, and is not sold as, an Active Pharmaceutical Ingredient."

你公司合同生产乙醇基非处方（OTC）手部消毒药品（也称为消费者手部消毒剂）。在使用这些物料来生产非处方药品之前，针对收到的物料，你公司未能充分检验鉴别项，并且依赖于未经确认的供应商分析证书（COA）。具体来说，对于进场（b）（4）原料药（API）中是否存在甲醇等杂质，你公司未能进行适当的检验，并且你们没有确保甘油中是否存在二甘醇（DEG）的检验程序。我们还注意到，你公司用于生产药品的（b）（4）API 的 COA 声明"该物料不被视为，且不作为原料药出售。"

You manufacture multiple drugs that contain ethanol. The use of ethanol contaminated with methanol has resulted in various lethal poisoning incidents in humans worldwide.

你公司生产多种含有乙醇的药品。在全球范围内，使用被甲醇污染的乙醇已导致多起人类致命中毒事件。

See FDA's guidance document *Policy for Testing of Alcohol (Ethanol) and Isopropyl Alcohol for Methanol, Including During the Public Health Emergency (COVID-19)* to help you meet the cGMP requirements when manufacturing drugs containing ethanol at https://www.fda.gov/regulatory-information/search-fda-guidance-documents/policy-testing-alcohol-ethanol-and-isopropyl-alcohol-methanol-including-during-public-health.

请参阅 FDA 指南，酒精（乙醇）和异丙醇检验政策——包括在公共卫生紧急事件（COVID-19）期间的要求，以帮助你们在生产含有乙醇的药物时满足 cGMP 要求，网址（略，见上）。

You manufacture products that contain glycerin. The use of glycerin contaminated with

DEG has resulted in various lethal poisoning incidents in humans worldwide.

你公司生产含有甘油的产品。在全球范围内，使用受 DEG 污染的甘油已导致多起人类致命中毒事件。

See FDA's guidance document *Testing of Glycerin for Diethylene Glycol* to help you meet the cGMP requirements when manufacturing drugs containing glycerin at https://www.fda.gov/regulatory–information/search–fda–guidance–documents/testing–glycerin–diethylene–glycol.

请参阅 FDA 指南，甘油中二甘醇检验，以帮助你公司在生产含有甘油的药品时满足 cGMP 要求，网址（略，见上）。

■ Inadequate Component Water Testing ｜水的检验不充分

You use water as a component in your drug products. You failed to provide data supporting the frequency of the testing of your water system for resistivity and microbiological growth. Pharmaceutical water must be suitable for its intended use, and routinely and adequately tested to ensure ongoing conformance with appropriate chemical and microbiological attributes.

你公司使用水作为药品的原辅料。你们未能提供支持水系统电阻率和微生物生长检验频率的数据。制药用水必须适合其预期用途，并定期进行充分检验，以确保持续符合适当的化学和微生物属性。

验证问题

2. Your firm failed to establish written procedures for production and process control designed to assure that the drug products you manufacture have the identity, strength, quality, and purity they purport or are represented to possess（21 CFR 211.100（a））.

2. 未能建立书面的生产和过程控制程序，以确保药品具有其声称或声称拥有的鉴别、规格、质量和纯度［21 CFR 211.100（a）］。

■ Production Process Validation ｜生产工艺验证

You failed to validate the processes used to manufacture your drug products.

你公司未能验证用于生产药品的工艺。

（略）

此处与 FDA 发给 Profounda, Inc. 的警告信（编号：MARCS-CMS 642595，即"2 未能提供生产工艺的验证数据"）中有关工艺验证的重要性部分的内容类似，故略去。

■ Water System Design and Validation ｜水系统设计和验证

You failed to validate your water system and you lacked written procedures for the validation of the water system. Your firm lacked evidence to demonstrate that you could effectively control, maintain, sanitize, and monitor the system, so it consistently produces pharmaceutical grade water that, at a minimum, meets the Purified Water USP monograph and appropriately stringent microbiological limits. You must design and control your water system to reproducibly yield suitable water for use in production operations.

你公司未能验证水系统，并且缺乏验证水系统的书面程序。你公司缺乏证据，来证明可以有效地控制、维护、消毒和监控该系统，使其始终生产出制药用水，至少符合纯化水 USP 专论和适当严格的微生物限度的要求。你公司必须设计和控制水系统，以可重现地产生适合生产操作的水。

质量部门

3. Your firm's quality control unit failed to exercise its responsibility to ensure drug products manufactured are in compliance with cGMP, and meet established specifications for identity, strength, quality, and purity（21 CFR211.22）.

3. 质量控制部门未能履行职责，以确保所生产的药品符合 cGMP 要求，并符合有关鉴别、规格、质量和纯度的既定质量标准（21 CFR 211.22）

Your quality unit（QU）did not provide adequate oversight for the manufacture of your drug products. For example, your QU failed to ensure the following：

你公司质量部门（QU）没有对药品生产提供充分的监督。例如，未能确保以下事项：

● Establishment of an adequate cleaning validation program for your non-dedicated equipment（21 CFR 211.67（b））.

　● 针对你公司的非专用设备，建立适当的清洁验证计划［21 CFR 211.67（b）］。

● Establishment of an adequate ongoing stability program（21 CFR 211.166（a））.

　● 建立充分的持续稳定计划［21 CFR 211.166（a）］。

● Establishment of appropriate data integrity controls（21 CFR 211.68（b））.

● 建立适当的数据可靠性控制［21 CFR 211.68（b）］。

● Adequate batch control and production records for your hand sanitizer drug products（21 CFR 211.188）.

● 充分的手部消毒药品批次控制和生产记录（21 CFR 211.188）。

● Appropriate quality-related procedures were written and approved, such as for finished product release, master batch record review, annual product reviews, recalls, and change control（21 CFR 211.22（d））.

● 制定并批准了适当的质量相关程序，例如成品放行、工艺规程审查、年度产品回顾、召回和变更控制［21 CFR 211.22（d）］。

An adequate QU overseeing all manufacturing operations is necessary to consistently ensure drug quality. Your firm's quality systems are inadequate. See FDA's guidance document *Quality Systems Approach to Pharmaceutical cGMP Regulations* for help in implementing quality systems and risk management approaches to meet the requirements of cGMP regulations 21 CFR parts 210 and 211, at https://www.fda.gov/media/71023/download.

需要有充分的 QU 来监督所有生产操作，以始终如一地确保药品质量。你公司的质量体系不完善。请参阅 FDA 指南，药品 cGMP 法规的质量体系方法，帮助实施质量体系和风险管理方法，以满足 cGMP 法规 21 CFR 第 210 和 211 部分的要求，网址（略，见上）。

Your quality system does not adequately ensure the accuracy and integrity of data to support the safety, effectiveness, and quality of the drugs you manufacture. See FDA's guidance document *Data Integrity and Compliance with Drug cGMP* for guidance on establishing and following cGMP compliant data integrity practices at https://www.fda.gov/regulatory-information/search-fda-guidance-documents/data-integrity-and-compliance-drug-cGMP-questions-and-answers.

你公司的质量体系没有充分确保数据的准确性和可靠性，以支持检验药品的安全性、有效性和质量。有关建立和遵循 cGMP 合规数据可靠性实践的指南，请参阅 FDA 指南，数据可靠性和药品 cGMP 合规性，网址（略，见上）。

In response to this letter, provide：

在回复本函时，请提供:

（略）

此处与 FDA 发给 Dunagin Pharmaceuticals Inc. dba Massco Dental 的警告信（编号：MARCS-CMS 644335，即"3 与非药用产品的共线生产问题"）中数据可靠性整改部分的回应内容类似，故略去。

Systemic Remediation | 系统性整改

In response to this letter, confirm whether you intend to continue manufacturing any drugs at this facility or any other facility in the future. If you plan to continue cGMP activities, you are responsible for resolving all deficiencies and systemic flaws to ensure your firm is capable of ongoing cGMP compliance.

在回复本函时，请确认你公司将来是否打算继续在该设施或任何其他设施生产任何药品。如果计划继续 cGMP 活动，你公司有责任解决所有缺陷和系统性问题，以确保有能力持续遵守 cGMP。

Based upon the nature of the violations we identified at your firm, you should engage a consultant qualified as set forth in 21 CFR 211.34 to assist your firm in meeting cGMP requirements. The qualified consultant should also perform a comprehensive six-system audit of your entire operation for cGMP compliance and evaluate the completion and efficacy of all CAPAs before you pursue resolution of your firm's compliance status (i.e., Quality System, Facilities & Equipment System, Materials System, Production System, Packaging & Labeling System, and Laboratory Control System) per FDA's guidance document *Quality Systems Approach to Pharmaceutical cGMP Regulations*.

根据我们在你公司发现的违规情况的性质，你们应该聘请符合 21 CFR 211.34 规定的有资质的顾问，来协助你公司满足 cGMP 要求。基于 FDA 指南，药品 cGMP 法规质量体系方法，有资质的顾问还应对你公司整个运营进行全面的六大系统审计（即质量系统、设施和设备系统、物料系统、生产系统、包装和贴标系统，以及实验室控制系统），以确保 cGMP 合规性，并在你们寻求解决公司合规状态之前，评估所有 CAPA 的完成情况和有效性。

8 未验证药品微生物检验方法

警告信编号： MARCS-CMS 646619

签发时间： 2023-3-24；**公示时间：** 2023-5-23

签发机构： 药品质量业务一处（Division of Pharmaceutical Quality Operations I）

公　　司： Sure-Biochem Laboratories, LLC

所在国家/地区： 美国

主　　题： cGMP/成品制剂/掺假（cGMP/Finished Pharmaceuticals/ Adulterated）

简　　介： FDA于2022年9月至10月对这家委托检验实验室进行了检查，该实验室开展药品的微生物委托检验业务。在检查中，FDA发现该实验室未验证用于药品检验的替代微生物方法，以确保这些方法与USP方法一致或优于USP方法。FDA强调，客户依赖该实验室的数据来获取关于药品质量的关键信息。因此，确保检验方法经过正确的确认或验证，并使用适当的检验方法，对于客户做出正确决策至关重要。使用未经确认或验证的方法产生的结果可能会误导客户，并可能使消费者面临风险。为此，FDA要求对先前检验进行追溯性评估，以确保过去4年检验方法的"适用性"，并承诺在发现任何缺陷时通知客户。此外，FDA指出，包括委托检验实验室在内的所有实验室都必须保存所有与cGMP相关的数据，以便质量部门和客户能够进行适当的评估和决策。

本警告信以下部分与本书此前其他警告信内容类似，故略去：前言、cGMP顾问推荐（cGMP Consultant Recommended）、数据可靠性整改（Data Integrity Remediation）、结论（Conclusion）。

实验室控制

1. Your firm failed to follow required laboratory control mechanisms and to establish

laboratory controls that include scientifically sound and appropriate specifications, standards, sampling plans, and test procedures designed to assure that components, drug product containers, closures, in-process materials, labeling, and drug products conform to appropriate standards of identity, strength, quality, and purity (21 CFR 211.160 (a) and 211.160 (b)).

1. 你公司未能遵循所需的实验室控制机制，并建立实验室控制，其中包括科学合理且相应的规范、标准、取样计划和检验程序，以确保原辅料、药品容器、密封件、在制品、标签和药品符合适当的鉴别、规格、质量和纯度标准［21 CFR 211.160 (a) 和211.160 (b)］。

You failed to adequately establish and follow procedures for growth promotion testing of your microbiological media to assure suitability before use, including failing to establish appropriate challenge conditions and acceptance criteria to ensure the media could support appropriate growth. For example, your growth promotion testing conducted on July 13, 2022, for Salmonella media lot number (b)(4), identified light and moderate growth for the challenge organisms including Escherichia coli. You accepted the lot for use without noting the deviation as required by your established procedure that specifies the growth of Escherichia coli should be inhibited. Further, you also failed to conduct growth promotion for each lot of media received.

你公司未能充分建立并遵循微生物培养基的生长促进检验程序，以确保使用前的适用性，包括未能建立适当的挑战条件和可接受标准，以确保培养基能够支持适当的生长。例如，你公司于 2022 年 7 月 13 日针对沙门菌培养基批号（b)(4)，确定了挑战微生物（包括大肠埃希菌）的轻度和中度生长。你公司接受并使用了该批次，但没有启动偏差，即既定程序要求应抑制大肠埃希菌的生长。此外，你公司也未能对收到的每批培养基进行促生长。

Additionally, you did not validate your alternative microbial methods used to test drug products to assure the methods were equivalent to or better than USP methods. Specifically, you failed to adequately establish that your microbiological testing methods can reliably detect objectionable microorganisms. For example, Lab Numbers (b)(4) and (b)(4) were samples of (b)(4) drug products marketed for pre- and post-surgical oral care and intended for use with patients who are particularly susceptible to infection.

此外，你公司没有验证用于检验药品的替代微生物方法，以确保这些方法相当于或优于 USP 方法。具体来说，你们未能充分证明你们的微生物检测方法能够可靠地检测出有害微生物。例如，实验室编号（b)(4) 和（b)(4) 是（b)(4) 药品的样品，用于手术前和术后口腔护理，用于特别容易受到感染影响的患者。

Your microbial method failed to detect *Burkholderia cepacia complex* (*Bcc*), and you reported "Not Detected" to your client. Subsequently, you sent microbial subcultures from these samples to another external laboratory that detected *Burkholderia contaminans* in both

101

samples, a species that is part of *Bcc*. The ability of microbial testing methods to detect objectionable microorganisms in the presence of each drug product to be tested must be established and validated.

你公司的微生物方法未能检测到洋葱伯克霍尔德菌复合体（Bcc），并向客户报告了"未检测到"。随后，你公司将这些样品的微生物传代培养物发送到另一个外部实验室，该实验室在两个样本中检测到了伯克霍尔德菌污染，这是 Bcc 的一部分。必须建立并验证微生物检验方法，确保其具有在每种药品中可以检测到有害微生物的能力。

In your response, you commit to performing growth promotion for every lot of purchased media and revising your growth promotion procedure to ensure media can support acceptable growth. You also acknowledge that your alternative method used to test drug products was insufficient to detect *Bcc*, and state that you will develop a procedure for the USP <60> test method. However, your response is inadequate because it does not address how you will review the validity of previous results using your alternative methods, or how you will communicate with your clients about these potentially noncompliant analyses. You also state that you will perform method suitability verifications for each type of product, but do not detail the actions you would take if suitability verifications are found inadequate.

在回复中，你公司承诺对每批购买的培养基进行促生长，并修订促生长程序，以确保培养基能够支持可接受的生长。你们还承认用于检验药品的替代方法不足以检测 Bcc，并声明你们将制定符合 USP <60> 检验方法的程序。但是，回复是不充分的，因为没有说明你公司将如何审查先前结果（使用替代方法）的有效性；以及就这些可能不合规的分析结果，你们将如何与客户就进行沟通。你公司还声明将为每种类型的产品执行方法适用性验证，但没有就如发现适用性确认结果不能接受时，详细说明将采取的行动。

Your clients rely on your laboratory data for critical information about the quality of their drugs. Thus, it is important that your test methods are properly verified or validated, and that you use appropriate test methods to enable your clients to make proper decisions (e.g., lot disposition). Results generated using unverified or unvalidated methods can mislead customers and may put consumers at risk.

客户依靠你公司的实验室数据来获取有关其药品质量的关键信息。因此，重要的是你公司的检验方法经过正确的确认或验证，并且使用适当的检验方法，从而使客户能够做出正确的决策（例如批次处置）。使用未经确认或未经验证的方法生成的结果，这可能会误导客户，并可能使消费者面临风险。

In response to this letter, provide：

在回复本函时，请提供：

● A comprehensive, independent assessment of your laboratory practices, procedures, methods, equipment, documentation, and analyst competencies. Based on this review, provide a detailed plan to remediate and evaluate the effectiveness of your laboratory system.

● 对你公司实验室实践、程序、方法、设备、文件和分析员能力进行完整、全面、独立的评估。在此审查的基础上，提供详细的计划来整改和评估实验室系统的有效性。

● A retrospective assessment of prior testing to assure 'suitability' of your methods for the last (b)(4) years of testing, and a commitment to notify customers of any deficiencies. Include any revised testing results provided to your clients with incorrect enumeration calculations.

● 对先前检验的追溯性评估，以确保过去（b）(4）年检验中方法的"适用性"，并承诺在发现任何缺陷时通知客户。请纳入所有向客户提供的修订检验结果，其中包含不正确的计数计算。

● A comprehensive investigation into the extent of the inaccuracies in data, records, and reporting, including results of the data review for drugs tested. Include a detailed description of the scope and root causes of your data integrity lapses.

● 对数据记录和报告的不准确程度进行全面调查，包括流通到美国的药物数据审查结果。包括对数据可靠性失效的范围和根本原因的详细描述。

● A procedure to establish a quantitative, acceptance criteria rather than qualitative growth entries(e.g., (b)(4)) included in your growth promotion testing.

● 一个程序，以便在生长促进检验中建立一个定量的可接受标准，而不是仅包含定性生长记录［例如（b）(4）］。

● Raw data from inoculation studies of your drugs to ensure appropriate identification of objectionable microorganisms including, but not limited to Bcc.

● 提供药品接种研究的原始数据，以确保对有害微生物（包括但不限于 Bcc）进行适当的鉴别。

质量部门未能履责

2. Your firm failed to establish an adequate quality unit and the responsibilities and procedures applicable to the quality control unit are not in writing and fully followed(21 CFR 211.22(a)and 211.22(d)).

2. 你公司未能建立适当的质量部门，适用于质量部门的责任和程序未以书面形式呈现且未得到完全遵守［21 CFR 211.22（a）和 211.22（d）］。

Your quality unit（QU）lacked adequate control over your testing operations and failed to ensure that you had suitable procedures. For example, your QU failed:

你公司质量部门（QU）对检验操作缺乏充分的控制，并且未能确保你们有适当的程序。例如，你公司的 QU 未能：

● To adequately retain documentation for the review, approval, or rejection, of laboratory testing materials such as buffers, reagents, and media. There is a lack of assurance that testing materials used to conduct microbial testing meet all appropriate specifications before use of an incoming lot, and include evaluation of certificates of analysis（COA）.

● 对于实验室检验用物料（例如缓冲液、试剂和介质）的审查、批准或拒放，保存充分的记录。针对用于进行微生物检验用物料的进场批次，无法保证其在使用之前符合所有相应的质量标准，包括分析证书（COA）的评估。

● To ensure procedures were followed to document and retain records such as laboratory investigations, corrective action and preventive action plans（CAPA）, and change controls. You told our investigators that you were not following a number of your standard operating procedures（SOPs）.

● 确保遵循程序，对实验室调查、纠正和预防措施计划（CAPA）以及变更控制等记录进行文件化和保存文档。你公司告知我们调查员，你们没有遵守一些标准操作程序（SOP）。

● To establish an adequate cGMP training program. You lacked appropriate resources to perform QU related functions and our inspection revealed basic cGMP violations.

● 建立适当的 cGMP 培训计划。你公司缺乏适当的资源来执行 QU 相关职能，而我们的检查发现存在基本的 cGMP 违规情况。

In your response, you admit to not adhering to your SOPs and state that you will document receipt of all incoming testing materials and retain the associated documentation. You also committed to hiring a quality consultant to develop a cGMP training program and perform quality functions. However, your response is inadequate because you did not commit to conducting a retrospective review to ensure materials used for drug product testing were suitable for their intended use. In addition, you state that your lab technician will attend "21 CFR 820 training," which is applicable to medical devices, but does not address the lack of cGMP training for drugs.

在回复中，你公司承认没有遵守 SOP，并声明你们将记录收到的所有检验物料并保存相关文档。你公司还承诺聘请一名质量顾问，来制定 cGMP 培训计划并履行质量职能。然而，你们的回复是不充分的，因为没有承诺进行回顾性审查，以确保用于药品检验的物料适合其预期用途。此外，你公司还声明你们的实验室技术员将参加"21 CFR 820 培训"，该培训适用于医疗器械，但并未解决缺乏药品 cGMP 培训的问题。

Your firm's quality systems are inadequate. See FDA's guidance document *Quality Systems Approach to Pharmaceutical cGMP Regulations* for help implementing quality systems and risk management approaches to meet the requirements of cGMP regulations 21 CFR, parts 210 and 211 at https://www.fda.gov/downloads/Drugs/GuidanceComplianceRegul atoryInformation/Guidances/UCM070337.pdf .

你公司的质量体系不完善。请参阅 FDA 指南，药品 cGMP 法规的质量体系方法，帮助实施质量体系和风险管理方法，以满足 cGMP 法规 21 CFR 第 210 和 211 部分的要求，网址（略，见上）。

In response to this letter, provide：

在回复本函时，请提供：

● A retrospective review of records for testing using received materials to assure correct materials were used and acceptable.

● 针对收到并使用的物料，对其检验记录进行回顾性审查，以确保使用正确的物料并可接受。

（略）

此处与 FDA 发给 Dunagin Pharmaceuticals Inc. dba Massco Dental 的警告信（编号：MARCS-CMS 644335，"3 与非药用产品的共线生产问题"）中有关 QU 的回应要求部分的内容类似，故略去。

● A comprehensive, independent assessment of your change management system. This assessment should include, but not be limited to, your procedure（s）to ensure changes are justified, reviewed, and approved by your QU. Your change management program should also include provisions for determining change effectiveness.

● 对你公司的变更管理系统进行全面、独立的评估。该评估应包括但不限于确保变更合理、经过质量部门审查和批准的程序。你公司的变更管理计划还应包括确定变更有效性的规定。

● An independent summary of your retrospective review of records for（b）（4）years of testing using received materials to assure correct materials were used and acceptable.

● 针对收到并使用的物料，提供对其（b）（4）年检验记录回顾性审查的独立总结，以确保使用正确的物料并可接受。

数据可靠性

3. Your firm failed to ensure that laboratory records included complete data derived from all tests necessary to ensure compliance with established specifications and standards（21 CFR 211.194（a））.

3. 你公司未能确保实验室记录包含所有检验的完整数据，以确保符合既定质量标准和标准［21 CFR 211.194（a）］。

Your laboratory records do not include complete testing data to support the analysis performed. For example, your records lack a statement of methods used for testing, a statement of the results of tests and how they compare to the established specifications, a record of all critical equipment used, and confirmation of compliance with testing conditions. Furthermore, you were unable to provide raw data to support the suitability of your alternative methods for each drug tested.

你公司的实验室记录不包括支持所执行分析的完整检验数据。例如，你们的记录缺少检验方法的声明、检验结果的声明，以及检验结果与既定质量标准的比较情况、使用的所有关键设备的记录以及符合检验条件的确认。此外，你公司无法提供原始数据，来支持替代方法对每种检验药品的适用性。

All cGMP-related data must be retained by all laboratories, including contract testing laboratories, to enable appropriate assessments and decisions by the QU and customers, and to demonstrate ongoing control.

所有实验室（包括委托检验实验室）都必须保存所有 cGMP 相关数据，以便 QU 和客户能够进行适当的评估和决策，并证明持续的控制。

In your response, you state that you will revise your records to include the missing information. Your response is inadequate because you make no commitment to retrospectively review prior testing for completeness, validity, or for errors.

在回复中，你公司声明将修订你们的记录以包含缺失的信息。你公司的回应是不充分的，因为你们没有承诺回顾之前的检验的完整性、有效性或错误。

In response to this letter, provide：

在回复本函时，请提供：

● A comprehensive independent assessment of documentation practices used throughout your laboratory operations to determine where documentation is insufficient. Include a detailed CAPA plan that comprehensively remediates your firm's documentation practices to ensure you retain attributable, legible, complete, original, accurate, contemporaneous records throughout your operation.

● 对整个实验室运营过程中使用的文档记录实践进行全面的独立评估，以确定文档记录的不足之处。包括一份详细的 CAPA 计划，全面整改你公司的文件记录实践，以确保在整个运营过程中保存可追溯的、清晰的、完整的、原始的、准确的和同步的记录。

● An independent assessment that summarizes the potential impact on product quality of the inadequate documentation.

● 一项独立评估，总结了不充分的文档对产品质量的潜在影响。

Responsibilities of a Contract Testing Lab
委托检验实验室的职责

FDA considers contractors as extensions of the manufacturer's own facility. Your failure to comply with cGMP may affect the quality, safety, and efficacy of the drugs you test for your clients. It is essential that you understand your responsibility to operate in full compliance with cGMP when performing analytical work for your customers. Your laboratory role is critical to the pharmaceutical supply chain, and it is essential that you meet all cGMPs related to your function. As part of this responsibility, it is essential that you provide prompt, complete, and transparent analytical information to your customers (e.g., manufacturers) to enable them to handle their quality responsibilities related to batch evaluation and contractor oversight. This responsibility includes, but is not limited to, conveying to the customer any out-of-specification (OOS) investigations performed by your firm.

FDA 将合同方视为生产商自身设施的延伸。你公司未能遵守 cGMP 可能会影响你们为客户检验的药物的质量、安全性和有效性。在为客户执行分析工作时，你们必须了解自己有责任完全遵守 cGMP。你公司的实验室角色对于药品供应链至关重要，并且满足与你们职能相关的所有 cGMP 很有必要。作为此责任的一部分，你公司必须向客户（例如生产商）提供及时、完整和透明的分析信息，以使他们能够履行与批次评估和合同商监督相关的质量责任。此责任包括但不限于向客户传达你公司执行的任何不合格（OOS）调查。

For additional information refer to FDA guidance for *Industry Contract Manufacturing Arrangements for Drugs*: *Quality Agreements* (https://www.fda.gov/media/86193/download).

如需更多信息，请参阅 FDA 指南，药品合同生产安排：质量协议，网址（略，见上）

9 产品苯污染，未能充分调查

警告信编号： MARCS-CMS 643600

签发时间： 2023-4-20；**公示时间：** 2023-4-25

签发机构： 药品质量业务三处（Division of Pharmaceutical Quality Operations III）

公　　司： Accra-Pac, Inc. dba Voyant Beauty

所在国家／地区： 美国

主　　题： cGMP/ 成品制剂 / 掺假（cGMP/Finished Pharmaceuticals/ Adulterated）

简　　介： FDA 于 2022 年 8 月至 9 月对位于印第安纳的药品生产设施进行了检查。该公司使用共享设备为众多客户生产非处方外用气雾剂药品和化妆品。在检查中，FDA 发现该公司未能充分调查其药品中高达 13.3ppm 的苯污染。由于苯污染的根本原因未能得到充分调查，因此该公司产品的影响范围也未能得到充分确定。作为与其客户进行的联合调查的一部分，该公司和其客户选择性地检验了一部分成品制剂的留样。然而，他们未能充分检验其他留样，以确定是否所有药品批次都受到影响。在检查过程中，FDA 调查员特别采集了三种药品的样品。经 FDA 实验室检验，这些样品显示出杂质苯污染达到了不可接受的水平，表明质量保证未按照 cGMP 要求发挥作用。在 FDA 的要求下，产品持有方扩大了正在进行的全国自愿召回范围，受苯污染的多个批次也包括在内。

本警告信以下部分与本书此前其他警告信内容类似，故略去：前言、结论（Conclusion）。

偏差调查

1. Your firm failed to thoroughly investigate any unexplained discrepancy or failure of a

batch or any of its components to meet any of its specifications, whether or not the batch has already been distributed(21 CFR 211.192).

1. 无论批次是否已经流通，对于该批次或其原辅料不满足其质量标准、无法解释的偏差或不合格，你公司未能进行彻底调查（21 CFR 211.192）。

Your firm manufactures over-the-counter (OTC) topical aerosol drug products as well as cosmetic products for numerous customers using shared equipment. Your firm failed to perform adequate investigations into benzene contamination in your drug products as high as 13.3 parts per million (ppm). After obtaining information, including data from your customers, indicating that your finished drug products manufactured with isobutane propellants were contaminated with benzene, your propellant investigation was limited to isobutane propellants. However, you failed to expand your investigation to other propellants, such as dimethyl ether, when you received information from a customer that your cosmetic products using dimethyl ether as the propellant also contained unacceptable levels of benzene. We note that you also use dimethyl ether as a propellant in drug products. Your investigation, focused on isobutane's role in the benzene contamination, was therefore flawed because it failed to account for other potential root causes when unacceptable levels of benzene were found in your finished cosmetic products manufactured using a different propellant on equipment shared with your drug products.

你公司使用共享设备为众多客户生产非处方（OTC）外用气雾剂药品和化妆品。你公司未能对药品中高达 13.3ppm 的苯污染进行充分调查。在获得信息（包括来自你公司的客户数据）后，表明你们用异丁烷推进剂生产的成品制剂受到苯污染，推进剂调查仅限于异丁烷推进剂。然而，当从客户那里收到信息，称你公司使用二甲醚作为推进剂的化妆品也含有不可接受的苯含量时，你们未能将调查范围扩大到其他推进剂，例如二甲醚。我们注意到，你公司还在药品中使用二甲醚作为推进剂。因此，你们的调查重点关注异丁烷在苯污染中的作用，这存在缺陷，因为当发行在与你公司药品共用的设备上使用不同推进剂生产的化妆品成品中苯含量不可接受时，你们的调查未能包括其他潜在的根本原因。

Because the root cause of the benzene contamination is not well understood, the scope of your product impact investigation was also inadequate. As part of the joint investigation conducted by you and your customers, you and your customers selectively tested reserve samples of finished drug products with higher propellant concentrations but failed to adequately test other reserve samples to identify if all drug product batches were impacted.

由于苯污染的根本原因尚不清楚，因此你公司的产品影响调查范围也不充分。作为你公司和你公司客户联合调查的一部分，你们选择性地检验了推进剂浓度较高的成品制剂的留样，但未能充分检验其他留样，以确定是否所有药品批次都受到影响。

Your response is inadequate. Your sampling and testing approach for risk assessment is based on tracing propellant batches used in finished product batches. However, your ability to accurately trace propellant is undermined by your failures to test for benzene in each batch of the incoming propellants and to routinely test for benzene in your propellant storage tanks because you use non-dedicated tanks for hydrocarbon propellants. Therefore, your risk assessment may underestimate the numbers of impacted drug product batches. We acknowledge that you are now testing each batch of propellant prior to use. However, your response states, "the heels of each (propellent) blend that remained in the (storage) tanks were blended with propellant with a result of ≤ 1.0 ppm, then retested, assuring the final result met specification." Based on your response, it is unclear if your procedure allows you to blend non-conforming propellant with conforming propellant. The practice of blending non-conforming lots with other lots for the purpose of meeting specifications is not acceptable. Verify in response to this letter that no propellant containing benzene above a scientifically sound and appropriate specification is permitted to be blended with any other propellant for use on site.

你公司的回应不够充分。你公司用于风险评估的取样和检验方法是基于追踪成品批次中使用的推进剂批次。然而，由于使用非专用碳氢化合物推进剂储罐，你公司未能检验每批进场推进剂中的苯，也未能定期检验推进剂储罐中的苯，削弱了你们准确追踪推进剂的能力。这可能导致风险评估低估受影响药品批次的数量。我们知晓，目前你公司在使用前对每批推进剂进行检验。然而，你们的回复指出，"将（储）罐中的（推进剂）混合残留物与 ≤ 1.0ppm 的推进剂混合，然后复验，确保最终结果符合质量标准。"根据这一回复，尚不清楚你公司的程序是否允许将不合格推进剂与合格推进剂混合。将不合格批次与其他批次混合以满足质量标准的做法是不可接受的。在针对本函的回复中，对于含有超过科学合理和适当质量标准苯的推进剂，确认其不得与设施使用的任何其他推进剂混合。

In response to this letter, provide：

在回复本函时，请提供：

● A comprehensive assessment of your overall system for investigating deviations, discrepancies, complaints, OOS results, and failures. Provide a detailed action plan to remediate this system. Your action plan should include, but not be limited to, significant improvements in investigation competencies, scope determination, root cause evaluation, corrective action and preventive action (CAPA) effectiveness, quality unit oversight, and written procedures. Address how your firm will ensure all phases of investigations are appropriately conducted.

● 对调查偏差、差异、投诉、OOS 结果和不合格的整个系统进行全面、独立的评估。提供一个详细的行动计划来整改该系统。你公司的行动计划应包括但不限于在调查能力、范围确定、根本原因评估、纠正和预防措施（CAPA）有效性、质量部门监督和书面程序方面的显著提高。说明你公司将如何确保适当地进行所有阶段的调查。

● Test results of all reserve samples for finished products that were not subject to recall and are currently on the U.S. market within expiry, using a suitable method for testing for benzene in finished products.

● 使用适当的方法检测成品中苯的含量，对目前在美国市场上市的未召回成品的所有留样进行检验，提供检验结果。

● A detailed description of the method you establish to test for benzene in finished products prior to release, until you have demonstrated you have a comprehensive understanding of the root cause of the benzene contamination and have implemented adequate controls to prevent such contamination of your drug products.

● 详细描述在放行前为成品中的苯进行检验所建立的方法，直至证明你公司对苯污染的根本原因有全面的了解，并已实施适当的控制措施来防止药品受到此类污染。

● A report of periodic assessments of the implementation and effectiveness of CAPAs.

● CAPA 实施和有效性的定期评估报告。

● A detailed description of your current sampling and testing procedure of each batch of incoming propellants before or after it is transferred to your storage tanks.

● 每批进场推进剂在转移到储罐之前或之后的取样和检验程序的详细描述。

微生物检验

2. Your firm failed to conduct, for each batch of drug product, appropriate laboratory testing, as necessary, required to be free of objectionable microorganisms (21 CFR 211.165 (b)).

2. 你公司未能根据需要，对每批药品进行适当的实验室检验，以确保不含有害微生物［21 CFR 211.165（ b ）］。

You failed to test many of your topical drug products for critical microbiological attributes. Without testing each batch prior to release, you did not have scientific evidence that all drug product batches were free of microbial contamination that is objectionable in view of its intended use.

对于很多外用药品，你公司未能检验其关键微生物属性。如放行前未对每批产品进行检验，则无法获得科学证据，来证明所有药品批次均不含微生物污染，而鉴于其预期用途，微生物污染是有害的。

In your response, you note that you are a contract manufacturer, and that per your quality agreements, your customers determine the test plans and specifications. You also state that you would evaluate the water content of the products and conduct risk assessment for all your drug products that are not being evaluated for microbiological attributes.

在回复中，你公司指出你们是合同生产商，活动是基于质量协议，你公司的客户确定检验计划和质量标准。你们还声明，将评估产品的含水量，并对所有未进行微生物属性评估的药品进行风险分析。

Your response is inadequate. You are responsible for the quality of drugs you produce as a contract facility, regardless of agreements in place with product owners. In addition, the water activity, and not water content, of a product can provide useful information about the potential for a product to support microbial growth. It is also well established that many microorganisms are known to survive and persist even in drug products that typically have minimal water activity.

你公司的回应不够充分。无论与产品所有者达成何种协议，作为外包设施生产，你公司应对生产的药品质量负责。此外，产品的水活度，而非水含量，可以提供有关产品支持微生物生长潜力的有用信息。但众所周知，即使在具有最低水活度的药品中，通常也有很多微生物存活并持续存在。

In response to this letter, provide:

在回复本函时，请提供：

● A list of microbiological specifications (i.e., total counts, objectionable microorganisms), including test methods, used to analyze each lot of your drug products before a lot disposition decision.

● 微生物质量标准清单（即总计数、有害微生物），包括检验方法，其用于在做出批次处置决定之前检验每批药品。

● A summary of all results obtained from testing retain samples from each batch. If such testing reveals substandard quality drug products, take rapid corrective actions, such as notifying customers and product recalls.

● 所有批次的留样检验汇总。如果此类检验表明药品质量不合格，请迅速采取整改措施，例如通知客户和产品召回。

物料鉴别

3. Your firm failed to conduct at least one test to verify the identity of each component of

a drug product (21 CFR 211.84 (d)(1)).

3. 你公司未能进行至少一项检验，来确认药品每个原辅料都被鉴别［21 CFR 211.84（d）（1）］。

You failed to adequately test the incoming components used to manufacture your drug products. Specifically, your component identity testing does not include a limit test for diethylene glycol (DEG) and ethylene glycol (EG) on all lots of glycerin before use in the manufacture or preparation of drug products. You manufacture multiple drug products that contain glycerin.

你公司未能充分检验用于生产药品的原料。具体来说，在用于制备药品之前，原辅料鉴别检验未能包括对所有批次的甘油进行二甘醇（DEG）和乙二醇（EG）的限度检验。你公司生产多种含有甘油的药品。

In your response, you provided conforming DEG and EG test results of reserve samples for glycerin lots used to manufacture drug products. However, you did not test for DEG and EG in glycerin item(b)(4), which was used to manufacture sunscreen products for children, as it appears that your inventory for glycerin item (b)(4) is depleted. You also failed to provide a risk assessment for finished products on the market and within expiry manufactured with glycerin item(b)(4).

在回复中，你公司提供了用于生产药品的甘油批次留样符合要求的 DEG 和 EG 检验结果。然而，你公司没有检验用于生产儿童防晒产品的甘油（b）（4）中的 DEG 和 EG，因为其库存似乎已耗尽。就市场上和有效期内使用甘油项目（b）（4）生产的成品，你公司也未能提供风险评估。

In response to this letter, provide：

在回复本函时，请提供:

● A summary of test results for reserve samples of all finished product lots manufactured with glycerin item(b)(4).

● 对于使用甘油项目（b）（4）生产的所有成品批次留样，提供检验结果汇总。

● A description of how you will test each component lot for conformity with all appropriate specifications for identity, strength, quality, and purity. If you intend to accept any results from your supplier's Certificates of Analysis (COA) instead of testing each component lot for strength, quality, and purity, specify how you will robustly establish the reliability of your supplier's results through initial validation as well as periodic re-validation. In addition, include a commitment to always conduct at least one specific identity test for each incoming component lot. In the case of glycerin, we note that this includes the performance of parts A, B, and C of the United States Pharmacopeia (USP) monograph.

● 说明如何检验每个批次，确定是否符合有关鉴别、规格、质量和纯度质量标准。如果你公司打算接受供应商 COA 的结果，而不是检验每个物料批次的规格、质量和纯度，请说明如何进行初始验证和定期再验证，从而稳健地确定供应商结果的可靠性。此外，还应承诺对于每个进场原辅料批次，至少进行一个专属鉴别检验。就甘油而言，我们注意到这包括 USP 专论 A、B 和 C 部分的性能表现。

● A comprehensive review of the components used in your drug products to ensure appropriate identity tests are performed.

● 对药品中使用的原辅料进行全面审查，以确保进行适当的鉴别检验。

The use of glycerin contaminated with DEG has resulted in various lethal poisoning incidents in humans worldwide. For more information, see FDA's guidance document *Testing of Glycerin for Diethylene Glyco*l at https://www.fda.gov/media/71029/download

在全球范围内，使用受 DEG 污染的甘油已导致多起人类致命中毒事件。请参阅 FDA 指南，甘油中二甘醇检验，网址（略，见上）。

FDA Tested Drug Samples | FDA 检验的药品样品

During the inspection, FDA investigators collected samples of three drug products. FDA laboratory testing of these samples found the following:

在检查过程中，FDA 调查员采集了三种药品的样品。FDA 实验室对这些样品进行了检验，结果如下：

Product Name 产品名称	Customer Lot Number 客户批号	Expiration Date 截止日期	Benzene Test Results 苯检验结果（ppm）
(b)(4)	(b)(4)	(b)(4)	6
(b)(4)	(b)(4)	(b)(4)	3
(b)(4)	(b)(4)	(b)(4)	1

* Not distributed in the United States 未在美国流通

Manufacturers should not use benzene in the manufacture of drugs because it is a known human carcinogen that causes leukemia and other blood disorders. FDA has alerted all drug manufacturers to the known risk factors for contamination with benzene. For more information see https://www.fda.gov/drugs/pharmaceutical-quality-resources/fda-alerts-drug-manufacturers-risk-benzene-contamination-certain-drugs

生产商不应在药品生产中使用苯，因为它是一种已知的人类致癌物，会导致白血病和其他血液疾病。FDA 已提醒所有药品生产商注意已知的苯污染风险因素。了解更多信息，请参阅（网址略，见上）

On（b）（4），FDA recommended your customer，（b）（4），consider removing the adulterated batch of（b）（4）drug product from the U.S. market.

在（b）（4）日，FDA 建议你公司客户（b）（4）考虑从美国市场上移除掺假批次的（b）（4）药品。

On（b）（4），（b）（4）expanded an ongoing voluntary nationwide recall to include the contaminated batch of（b）（4）due to the presence of benzene above 2 ppm.

在（b）（4）日，（b）（4）扩大了正在进行的全国自愿召回范围，将受污染批次（b）（4）包括在内，因为苯含量超过 2ppm。

The contamination with benzene in a drug product manufactured in your facility, in addition to the significant violations documented in the inspection, demonstrate that the quality assurance within your facility is not functioning in accordance with cGMP requirements under section 501（a）（2）（B）of the FD&C Act.

除了检查中记录的重大违规情况外，你公司设施生产的药品中存在苯污染，这表明设施内的质量保证未按照 FD&C 法案第 501（a）（2）（B）条下的 cGMP 要求发挥作用。

Quality Agreement | 质量协议

Drugs must be manufactured in conformance with cGMP. FDA is aware that many drug manufacturers use independent contractors such as production facilities, testing laboratories, packagers, and labelers. FDA regards contractors as extensions of the manufacturer.

药品必须按照 cGMP 要求 生产。FDA 意识到很多药品生产商使用独立合同商，例如生产设施、检验实验室、包装商和贴标商。FDA 将合同商视为生产商的延伸。

You are responsible for the quality of drugs you produce as a contract facility, regardless of agreements in place with product owners. You are required to ensure that drugs are made in accordance with section 501（a）（2）（B）of the FD&C Act for safety, identity, strength, quality, and purity. For more information, see FDA's guidance document *Contract Manufacturing Arrangements for Drugs*: *Quality Agreements* at https://www.fda.gov/downloads/drugs/guidances/ucm353925.pdf.

无论与产品所有者达成何种协议，作为外包设施生产，你公司应对生产的药品质量负责。你们需要确保按照 FD&C 法案第 501（a）（2）（B）条的规定生产药品，以确保安全性、鉴别、规格、质量和纯度。请参阅 FDA 指南，药品合同生产安排：质量协议，网址（略，见上）。

SULFATRIM™ PEDIATRIC SUSPENSION Production Ceased
SULFATRIM™ 小儿混悬剂停止生产

We acknowledge your commitment to cease production of SULFATRIMTM PEDIATRIC SUSPENSION at this facility. In response to this letter, clarify whether you intend to resume manufacturing this drug at this facility in the future.

我们知晓，你公司承诺停止在该设施生产 SULFATRIM™ 小儿混悬剂。在回复本函时，请澄清你公司是否打算将来在该设施恢复生产该药品。

Cosmetic Products | 化妆品

In addition, we note that some of the products you manufacture may be regulated as cosmetics, as defined in section 201（i）of the FD&C Act. A cosmetic is adulterated under section 601（a）of the FD&C Act, 21 U.S.C. 361（a）, if it bears or contains any poisonous or deleterious substance, such as benzene, which may render it injurious to users under the conditions of use prescribed in the labeling thereof, or, under such conditions of use as are customary or usual. Some of the practices that cause the OTC drug products you manufacture to be contaminated with benzene may also cause the cosmetic products you manufacture to be contaminated with benzene. We note that under section 301（a）of the FD&C Act, 21 U.S.C. 331（a）, it is a prohibited act to introduce or deliver for introduction into interstate commerce a cosmetic product that is adulterated.

此外，我们注意到，按照 FD&C 法案第 201（i）条的定义，你公司生产的某些产品可能会作为化妆品进行监管。根据 FD&C 法案第 601（a）条、21 U.S.C. 361（a），如果化妆品带有或含有任何有毒或有害物质，例如苯，在规定的使用条件下可能对使用者造成伤害，则该化妆品属于掺假。一些导致你公司生产的非处方药品受到苯污染的实践也可能导致生产的化妆品受到苯污染。我们注意到，根据 FD&C 法案第 301（a）条、21 U.S.C. 331（a），引入或交付掺假化妆品进入州际贸易属于禁止行为。

10 未能建立有胜任力的质量部门

警告信编号： MARCS-CMS 652756

签发时间： 2023-7-17；**公示时间：** 2023-8-1

签发机构： 药 品 质 量 业 务 三 处（Division of Pharmaceutical Quality Operations III）

公　　　司： LXR Biotech, LLC

所在国家 / 地区： 美国

主　　　题： cGMP/ 成 品 制 剂 / 掺 假（cGMP/Finished Pharmaceuticals/Adulterated）

简　　　介： 2023 年 1 月，FDA 对该药品生产设施进行了检查。该公司未能建立一个胜任的质量部门（Quality Unit, QU），用以监督药品的生产。具体而言，未能确保建立完善的投诉处理程序、遵守全面的稳定性计划、保持一致且完整的批记录，以及对不符合事件进行充分调查等。FDA 强调，即使质量部门只是由一人或少数几人组成，这些人员仍然需要负责监督所有系统和程序的持续有效性，并审查生产结果，以确保控制状态并遵守所有质量标准。

本警告信以下部分与本书此前其他警告信内容类似，故略去：前言、作为合同商的责任（Responsibilities as a Contractor）、结论（Conclusion）。

物料检验

1. Your firm failed to test samples of each component for identity and conformity with all appropriate written specifications for purity，strength，and quality. Your firm also failed to validate and establish the reliability of your component supplier's test analyses at appropriate

117

intervals（21 CFR 211.84（d）（1）and 211.84（d）（2）).

1. 你公司未进行至少一项检验来确认药品中每种原辅料都被鉴别，并使其符合所有适当的纯度、规格和质量的书面质量标准。你公司也未能在适当的时间间隔内，验证和确定物料供应商检验分析的可靠性［21 CFR 211.84（d）（1）和 211.84（d）（2）]。

Your firm contract manufactured an over–the–counter（OTC）（b）（4）drug product（e.g.,（b）（4）). You failed to conduct adequate testing on components used to manufacture this drug product. Additionally, your firm accepted components from suppliers without establishing the reliability of suppliers' test analyses. You also did not routinely obtain or review the suppliers' certificate of analysis（COA）for components（e.g., the active ingredient（b）（4）). For instance, you provided only a certificate of conformance for your（b）（4）component.

你公司合同生产了一种非处方药（OTC）（b）（4）药品［例如，（b）（4）]。你们未能对用于生产该药品的原辅料进行充分的检验。此外，你公司在没有确定供应商检验分析可靠性的情况下，接受了供应商的物料。你们也没有定期获取或审查供应商的原辅料分析证书（COA）［例如原料药（b）（4）]。例如，你公司仅提供了（b）（4）物料的符合性证书。

Without adequate testing, you do not have appropriate assurance that the components conform to appropriate specifications prior to use in the drug products you manufacture.

如果没有充分的检验，你公司就无法保证这些原辅料在用于生产药品之前符合相应的质量标准。

产品检验

2. Your firm failed to have, for each batch of drug product, appropriate laboratory determination of satisfactory conformance to final specifications for the drug product, including the identity and strength of each active ingredient, prior to release.（21 CFR 211.165（a）).

2. 你公司没有对每批药品进行适当的实验室确认，以在放行之前确定其是否符合最终产品的质量标准要求，包括每种原料药的鉴别和规格［21 CFR 211.165（a）]。

Your firm failed to conduct adequate release testing of（b）（4）drug product. You only conducted heavy metals and microbiological testing prior to batch release.

你公司未能对（b）（4）药品进行充分的放行检验。你们仅在批放行前进行了重金属和微生物检验。

Full release testing, which includes strength and identity testing of the active ingredient (e.g., (b)(4)), must be performed before drug product batch release and distribution. Without adequate testing, you do not have adequate scientific evidence to assure that drug product batches conform to appropriate specifications before release.

全面放行检验，包括原料药的规格和鉴别检验［如（b）(4)]，需要在药品批放行和流通之前进行。如果没有充分的检验，你公司就没有充分的科学证据，来确保药品批次在放行前符合相应的质量标准。

工艺验证

3. Your firm failed to establish adequate written procedures for production and process control designed to assure that the drug products you manufacture have the identity, strength, quality, and purity they purport or are represented to possess (21 CFR 211.100 (a)).

3. 你公司未充分建立用于生产和过程控制的书面程序，以确保所生产的药品具有其声称或声称拥有的鉴别、规格、质量和纯度［21 CFR 211.100 (a)]。

Your firm failed to adequately qualify the equipment and validate the processes used to manufacture (b)(4) drug product. You have not performed process performance qualification (PPQ) studies, nor do you have a meaningful ongoing program for monitoring process control, to ensure stable manufacturing operations and consistent drug quality.

对于用于生产（b）(4）药品的设备和工艺，你公司未能充分验证。你们尚未进行工艺性能确认（PPQ）研究，也没有有意义的持续监控工艺控制的计划，以确保稳定的生产操作和一致的药品质量。

（略）

此处与 FDA 发给 Profounda, Inc. 的警告信（编号：MARCS–CMS 642595，即 "2 未能提供生产工艺的验证数据"）中有关工艺验证的重要性部分的内容类似，故略去。

质量部门

4. Your firm's quality control unit failed to exercise its responsibility to ensure drug products manufactured are in compliance with cGMP, and meet established specifications for identity, strength, quality, and purity (21 CFR 211.22).

4. 质量控制部门未能履行职责，以确保所生产的药品符合 cGMP 要求，并符合有

关鉴别、规格、质量和纯度的既定质量标准（21 CFR 211.22）

Your firm failed to establish an adequate quality unit（QU）with the responsibilities and authority to oversee the manufacture of drug products. For example，you failed to ensure：

你公司未能建立一个胜任的质量部门（QU）来负责监督药品的生产。例如，你公司未能确保：

● An adequate complaint handling process（21 CFR 211.198）.

● 充分的投诉处理流程（21 CFR 211.198）。

● Adherence to an adequate stability program（21 CFR 211.166（a））.

● 遵守充分的稳定性计划［21 CFR 211.166（a）］。

● Consistent and complete batch records（21 CFR 211.188）.

● 一致且完整的批记录（21 CFR 211.188）。

● Adequate investigations into non-conformances（21 CFR 211.192）.

● 对不符合事件进行充分调查（21 CFR 211.192）。

● Appropriate examination of labeling and packaging materials for correctness，including but not limited to sufficiently accounting for all ingredients used in manufacturing，prior to packaging operations（21 CFR 211.130（d））.

● 对标签和包装材料的正确性进行适当检查，包括但不限于在包装操作之前充分考虑生产中使用的所有物料［21 CFR 211.130（d）］。

There was a fundamental failure of production management to effectively oversee the procedures，practices，and suitability of the manufacturing operations. In addition，even when a QU consists of one or only a few，those persons are still accountable for overseeing ongoing effectiveness of all systems and procedures，and review of the results of manufacture to ensure state of control and adherence to all quality standards.

在根本上，生产管理未能有效监督生产操作的程序、实践和适用性，有着根本性的失效。此外，即使 QU 由一人或少数几人组成，这些人员仍然负责监督所有系统和程序的持续有效性，并审查生产结果，以确保控制状态并遵守所有质量标准。

Drug Production | 药品生产

We acknowledge your commitment to cease production of drugs at this facility. Please verify you no longer manufacture drugs and provide us with a detailed list of the name and NDC numbers for those products. Additionally, respond to this letter by informing FDA if you are currently the manufacturer of any (b)(4) or (b)(4) products for (b)(4).

你公司承诺停止在该设施生产药品。请确认你们不再生产药品，并向我们提供这些产品的名称和 NDC 编号的详细清单。此外，如果你公司目前是（b）（4）的任何（b）（4）或（b）（4）产品的生产商，请回复本函时告知 FDA.

If you plan to resume any operations regulated under the FD&C Act, notify this office prior to resuming your drug manufacturing operations. If you resume cGMP activities at this or another facility, you are responsible for resolving all deficiencies and systemic flaws to ensure your firm is capable of ongoing cGMP compliance. In your notification to the agency, provide a summary of your remediations to demonstrate that you have appropriately completed all CAPAs.

如果你公司计划恢复 FD&C 法案规定的任何运营，请在恢复药品生产运营之前通知本办公室。如果在此或其他设施恢复 cGMP 活动，你公司有责任解决所有缺陷和系统性问题，以确保你们有能力持续遵守 cGMP。在你公司向 FDA 发出的通知中，请提供你们的整改措施汇总，以证明已正确完成所有 CAPA.

If you resume cGMP activities, you should engage a consultant qualified as set forth in 21 CFR 211.34 to assist your firm in meeting cGMP requirements. The qualified consultant should also perform a comprehensive six-system audit of your entire operation for cGMP compliance and evaluate the completion and efficacy of all CAPAs before you pursue resolution of your firm's compliance status with FDA.

如果你公司恢复 cGMP 活动，你们应该聘请符合 21 CFR 211.34 规定的有资质的顾问，来协助你公司满足 cGMP 要求。有资质的顾问还应对你们的整个运营进行全面的六大系统审计，以确保 cGMP 合规性，并在你公司寻求解决公司合规状态之前，评估所有 CAPA 的完成情况和有效性。

11 机械润滑剂的污染问题

警告信编号： MARCS-CMS 654226

签发时间： 2023-7-26；**公示时间：** 2023-8-15

签发机构： 药品质量业务一处（Division of Pharmaceutical Quality Operations I）

公　　司： Denison Pharmaceuticals, LLC

所在国家/地区： 美国

主　　题： cGMP/成品制剂/掺假（cGMP/Finished Pharmaceuticals/Adulterated）

简　　介： FDA 于 2023 年 1 月对该药品生产设施进行了检查。该生产设施受托生产的药品包括标有"新生儿安全"标签的婴儿和儿童药品。然而，该公司未能对所有可能受到机械润滑剂污染影响的批次进行充分调查，且没有扩大范围进行调查。此外，对于多起臭味投诉的调查也未充分展开。该公司确定造成臭味的微生物为表皮葡萄球菌，其调查进一步表明，该微生物"是一种兼性厌氧细菌，在口服液体中不会对顾客造成健康风险"，并且"该批次仍然适合使用"。然而，FDA 并不认可此结论，认为该公司未能充分评估微生物污染情况。作为整改要求，该公司需要对整个系统进行全面、独立的评估，以调查偏差、差异、投诉、OOS 结果和不合格。此外，该公司需提供详细的行动计划，以整改该系统的情况。

本警告信以下部分与本书此前其他警告信内容类似，故略去：前言、未经批准的新药（Unapproved New Drugs）、作为合同商的责任（Responsibilities as a Contractor）、cGMP 顾问推荐（cGMP Consultant Recommended）、结论（Conclusion）。

偏差调查

1. Your firm failed to thoroughly investigate any unexplained discrepancy or failure of a batch or any of its components to meet any of its specifications, whether or not the batch has already been distributed (21 CFR 211.192).

1. 无论批次是否已经流通，对于该批次或其原辅料不满足其质量标准、无法解释的偏差或不合格，你公司未能进行彻底调查（21 CFR 211.192）。

You contract manufacture homeopathic and over-the-counter (OTC) drug products including those intended for infants and children and labeled "safe for newborn."

你公司受委托生产顺势疗法和非处方（OTC）药品，包括用于婴儿和儿童并标有"新生儿安全"的药品。

■ Lubricant Contamination ｜润滑剂污染

You failed to perform adequate investigations and expand investigations to all batches and drug products that may have been impacted from contamination by machinery lubricant. For example, your investigation into the contamination of (b) (4) with (b) (4) lubricant, a non-food grade lubricant not intended for ingestion, concluded that only Lot (b) (4) was impacted and was rejected. However, your investigation did not consider other potentially affected drug products manufactured in the same mixing tank, and indicated that no corrective action and preventive action (CAPA) was required. The lubricant was used for manufacturing equipment for approximately (b) (4) previous months, during which more than (b) (4) batches of drug products were manufactured, including products for infants. The safety data sheet (SDS) from the manufacturer of (b) (4) lubricant lists health hazards such as skin and respiratory irritation, genetic defects, and cancer. The (b) (4) lubricant is unsuitable for pharmaceutical purposes.

对于可能受到机械润滑剂污染影响的所有批次和药品，你公司未能进行充分的调查并扩大调查范围。例如，你们对（b）(4）润滑剂（一种不适合摄入的非食品级润滑剂）污染调查的结论是，只有批次（b）(4）受到影响并被拒收。然而，调查没有考虑在同一混合罐中生产的其他可能受影响的药品，并表明不需要采取纠正和预防措施（CAPA）。该润滑剂在过去大约（b）(4）个月内用于生产设备，在此期间生产了超过（b）(4）批次的药品，其中包括婴儿产品。（b）(4）润滑剂制造商的安全数据表（SDS）列出了健康危害，例如皮肤和呼吸道刺激、遗传缺陷和癌症。（b）(4）润滑剂不适合制药用途。

It is necessary to conduct a thorough investigation to evaluate all potentially affected batches and implement a timely and effective CAPA.

有必要进行彻底调查，评估所有可能受影响的批次，并实施及时有效的 CAPA。

Odor Complaints ｜气味投诉

You failed to adequately investigate multiple foul odor complaints for（b）（4）. For complaints COMP 20–161 and COMP 20–162, you tested retains of（b）（4）, Berry, Lot（b）（4）, which failed microbiological testing due to too numerous to count（TNTC）results for total count of yeast and mold（TCYM）. Your investigation noted "there was a trend for foul odor complaints for lot（b）（4）. The organism which caused of［sic］the odor in this lot was determined to be *Staphylococcus epidermis*." Your investigation further stated that the organism "is a facultative anaerobic bacteria and poses no health risk to the customer in an oral dose liquid" and "the lot remains fit for use." You failed to adequately assess the microbiological contamination and extend the investigation to additional batches manufactured after Lot（b）（4）that may also have been impacted. The TNTC microbiological testing results for your（b）（4）posed an unacceptable risk to public health, yet you failed to take any market action.

你公司未能充分调查针对（b）（4）的多起臭味投诉。对于 COMP 20–161 和 COMP 20–162 的投诉，你们检验了（b）（4）浆果口味、批次（b）（4），由于酵母菌和霉菌总计数（TCYM）多不可计（TNTC），其未能通过微生物检验。你公司的调查指出，"批次（b）（4）有臭味投诉的趋势。经确定，造成该批次气味的微生物为表皮葡萄球菌"。你公司进一步调查指出，该微生物 "是一种兼性厌氧细菌，在口服液体中不会对顾客造成健康风险"，并且 "该批次仍然适合使用"。你公司未能充分评估微生物污染，也未能将调查范围扩大到批次（b）（4）之后生产的其他批次，这些批次可能也受到影响。TNTC 微生物检测结果对你公司的（b）（4）造成了不可接受的公共健康风险，但你们未能采取任何市场行动。

Microbiological contamination may not be uniformly distributed, and a sample may not be representative of the type or level of contamination that may exist in other individual units of a batch.

微生物污染可能不均匀分布，并且样品可能不能代表批次中其他单元中可能存在的污染类型或水平。

Water System Excursions ｜水系统异常

You failed to initiate investigations for multiple microbiological excursions for your purified water system used to manufacture aqueous drug products. For example, you did not investigate several testing results for your water system that indicated the bacteria were too numerous to count (TNTC), and above your total aerobic microbial count action limit of (b)(4) cfu/mL. You also failed to consider how flaws in design, control, and maintenance of your water system contribute to these excessive microbial counts. Furthermore, your procedure for sampling and testing of the water system lacks a mechanism to trigger an investigation in response to severe microbiological excursions from water testing.

你公司未能对用于生产含水药品的纯化水系统的多次微生物异常启动调查。例如，没有调查水系统的多项检验结果，这些结果表明细菌数量多不可计（TNTC），超出了需氧微生物总计数行动限（b）（4）cfu/ml。对于水系统的设计、控制和维护方面的缺陷是如何导致微生物多不可计，你公司也未能进行考量。此外，针对水检验中的严重微生物偏差，缺乏触发水系统取样和检验程序的调查机制。

In addition, your investigation INV-21-051 was inadequate because you failed to identify the microbial species in the water samples and did not extend the impact assessment to other potentially affected products manufactured using the same water system. Indeed, your procedure does not specify the need for microbial identification of water system sample isolates and the level of identification required (e.g., genus or species).

此外，你公司对INV-21-051的调查是不充分的，因为未能鉴别水样中的微生物种类，也没有将影响评估扩展到使用同一水系统生产的其他可能受影响的产品。事实上，对于水系统样品分离物，你公司程序没有规定进行微生物鉴别的必要性，以及所需的鉴别水平（例如属或种）。

Notably, you use water as a component in your aqueous based products, which is the prominent ingredient in your (b)(4) indicated for infants.

值得注意的是，你公司使用水作为含水产品的原辅料，这是（b）（4）产品中的主要原辅料，该产品适用于婴儿。

In your response, you state you are revising your procedures and conducting additional investigations. However, your response is inadequate because your investigations are limited in scope and lack comprehensive review for potentially affected products and root cause determination. You also did not provide any supporting documentation, including details of your corrective actions with your initial 483 response.

在回复中，你公司声明正在修订程序并进行额外的调查。然而，你公司的回应并不充分，因为你们的调查范围有限，缺乏对潜在受影响产品的全面审查和根本原因确定。你公司也没有提供任何支持文档，包括最初的483表格回复中整改措施的详细信息。

Well documented, thorough, scientifically sound investigations are necessary to identify the root cause and implement the appropriate CAPA.

为了查明根本原因并实施适当的 CAPA，必须进行有据可查、彻底、科学合理的调查。

In response to this letter, provide：

在回复本函时，请提供：

● A comprehensive, independent assessment of your overall system for investigating deviations, discrepancies, complaints, out-of-specification（OOS）results, and failures. Provide a detailed action plan to remediate this system. Your action plan should include, but not be limited to, significant improvements in investigation competencies, scope determination, root cause evaluation, CAPA effectiveness, quality unit（QU）oversight, and written procedures. Address how your firm will ensure all phases of investigations are appropriately conducted.

● 对整个系统进行全面、独立的评估，以调查偏差、差异、投诉、OOS 结果和不合格。提供详细的行动计划，以整改此系统。行动计划应包括但不限于：调查能力、范围确定、根本原因评估、CAPA 有效性、质量部门监督和书面程序方面的显著提高。说明你公司将如何确保：调查的所有阶段都得到适当实施。

● An independent assessment and remediation plan for your CAPA program. Provide a report that evaluates whether the program includes effective root cause analysis, ensures CAPA effectiveness, analyzes investigations trends, improves the CAPA program when needed, implements final QU decisions, and is fully supported by executive management.

● 针对你公司 CAPA 计划的独立评估和整改计划。提供一份报告，评估是否有效地进行了根本原因分析，确保 CAPA 的有效性，分析调查趋势，在需要时对 CAPA 计划进行了改进，确保了适当的 QU 决策权，并得到了高级管理层的全面支持。

● A comprehensive, independent assessment of your water system design, control, and maintenance.

● 对你公司的水系统设计、控制和维护进行全面、独立的评估。

● A thorough remediation plan to install and operate a suitable water system. Include a robust ongoing control, maintenance, and monitoring program to ensure the remediated system design consistently produces water adhering to Purified Water, United States Pharmacopeia（USP）monograph specifications and appropriate microbial limits（total counts, objectionable microbes）.

● 对于安装和运行适当的水系统，提供彻底整改计划。包括可靠的持续控制、维护和监测计划，以确保整改后的系统设计始终如一地生产符合纯化水、USP 专论质量标准和适当微生物限度要求的水。

● A procedure for your water system monitoring that specifies routine microbial testing of water to ensure its acceptability for use in each batch of drug products produced by your firm.

● 你公司的水系统监测程序，规定了水的常规微生物检验，以确保其在所生产的每批药品中的使用可接受性。

● A procedure governing your program for ongoing control and monitoring that ensures the system consistently produces water that meets Purified Water, United States Pharmacopeia（USP）monograph specifications and appropriate microbial limits.

● 管理你公司的持续控制和监测计划的程序，确保系统持续生产符合纯化水、USP 专论质量标准和适当微生物限度的水。

物料鉴别

2. Your firm failed to conduct at least one test to verify the identity of each component of a drug product（21 CFR 211.84（d）（1））.

2. 你公司未能进行至少一项检验，来确认药品每个原辅料都被鉴别［21 CFR 211.84（d）（1）］。

You lacked testing for each shipment of each lot of components at high risk of diethylene glycol（DEG）and ethylene glycol（EG）contamination, used in the manufacture of your drug products. For example, you lacked a specific identity test to detect DEG and EG in all lots of glycerin and propylene glycol, prior to determining acceptability for use in manufacturing drug products. The identity testing of glycerin and propylene glycol includes a limit test per the USP to ensure that the component meets the relevant safety limits for the levels of DEG or EG. We note that both glycerin and propylene glycol are ingredients used in your（b）（4）and （b）（4）drug products. As a drug manufacturer, you are responsible for performing specific identity tests for all incoming shipments of component lots prior to determining suitability for release for use in manufacturing.

针对每批用于生产药品的二甘醇（DEG）和乙二醇（EG）高风险污染物料，你公司缺乏相应检验程序。例如，在确定用于生产药品的可接受性之前，你们缺乏专属鉴别检验来检测所有批次的甘油和丙二醇中的 DEG 和 EG。甘油和丙二醇的鉴别检验包括根据 USP 进行的限度检验，以确保该原辅料符合 DEG 或 EG 水平的相关安全限度。我们注意到，（b）（4）和（b）（4）中使用了甘油和丙二醇两种原辅料。作为药品生产商，你公司有责任在确定是否适合放行用于生产之前，对所有进场原辅料批次进行专属鉴别检验。

In your response, you state that you performed DEG and EG testing for 3 lots of glycerin and 4 lots of propylene glycol. In response to the FDA teleconference held with you on April 19, 2023, you indicate that testing of all additional lots of retain samples of glycerin and propylene glycol was initiated. However, your response did not indicate whether you intend to perform a risk assessment for other components at high-risk for DEG or EG contamination.

在回复中，你公司声明你们对 3 批甘油和 4 批丙二醇进行了 DEG 和 EG 检验。为了回应 FDA 于 2023 年 4 月 19 日与你们举行的电话会议，你们表示已开始对所有额外批次的甘油和丙二醇留样进行检验。然而，回复并未表明你公司是否打算对其他 DEG 或 EG 高风险污染原辅料进行风险评估。

Without appropriate testing of components and ingredients, you cannot ensure the quality and safety of your drug products.

如果不对物料和原辅料进行适当的检验，你公司就无法确保药品的质量和安全性。

The use of ingredients contaminated with DEG or EG has resulted in various lethal poisoning incidents in humans worldwide. See FDA's guidance document *Testing of Glycerin, Propylene Glycol, Maltitol Solution, Hydrogenated Starch Hydrolysate, Sorbitol Solution, and Other High-Risk Drug Components for Diethylene Glycol and Ethylene Glycol* to help you meet the cGMP requirements when manufacturing drugs containing ingredients at risk for DEG or EG contamination, at https://www.fda.gov/media/167974/download.

在全球范围内，使用受 DEG 或 EG 污染的原辅料已导致多起人类致命中毒事件。请参阅 FDA 指南，甘油、丙二醇、麦芽糖醇溶液、氢化淀粉水解物、山梨醇溶液和其他高风险药品原辅料中二甘醇和乙二醇的检验，以帮助你公司在生产含有 DEG 或 EG 污染风险原辅料的药品时满足 cGMP 要求，请访问（网址略，见上）。

In response to this letter, provide a full risk assessment for drug products that are within expiry which contain any ingredient at risk for DEG or EG contamination (including, but not limited to, glycerin). Take prompt and appropriate actions to determine the safety of all lots of the component(s) and any related drug product that could contain DEG or EG, including customer notifications and product recalls for any contaminated lots. Identify additional appropriate CAPA that secure supply chains in the future including, but not limited to, ensuring that all incoming raw material lots are from fully qualified manufacturers and free from unsafe impurities. Detail these actions in your response to this letter.

作为对本函的回应，就含有任何 DEG 或 EG 污染风险的原辅料（包括但不限于甘油），且在效期内的药品，提供全面的风险评估。立即采取适当的措施，就任何可能含有 DEG 或 EG 的原辅料或相关药品批次，确定其安全性，包括通知客户和召回任何受污染批次的产品。确定其他适当的 CAPA，以确保未来的供应链安全，包括但不限于：

确保所有进场原料批次均来自有充分资质的生产商，且不含不安全的杂质。在你公司对本函的回复中详细说明这些行动。

检验方法

3. Your firm failed to establish and document the accuracy, sensitivity, specificity, and reproducibility of its test methods(21 CFR 211.165(e)).

3. 你公司未能建立和记录其检验方法的精确度、灵敏度、专属性和重现性〔21 CFR 211.165(e)〕。

You failed to adequately validate your alternative rapid microbiological test methods, demonstrate they were equivalent to, or better than USP compendial methods, and suitable for their intended use.

你公司未能充分验证替代的快速微生物检验方法，未能证明它们相当于或优于 USP 药典方法，并且适合其预期用途。

For example, our investigators observed the(b)(4)system used for rapid microbiological release testing(total counts, objectionable microorganisms)of(b)(4) and(b)(4)drug products was not validated, and that your investigation of OOS results concluded the system should be reassessed before future use. You failed to demonstrate that the(b)(4)system is appropriate for total count testing or detection of objectionable microorganisms, such as *Burkholderia cepacia* complex, in your drug products.

例如，我们的调查员观察到：针对（b）(4）和（b）(4）药品（总计数、有害微生物）的快速微生物放行检验，其（b）(4）系统未经验证，且你公司对 OOS 结果的调查得出结论，在将来使用该系统之前应对其重新评估。你公司未能证明（b）(4）系统适合进行总计数检验或有害微生物（例如，药品中的洋葱伯克霍尔德菌复合体）检测。

Notably, microbiological testing for(b)(4)lots(b)(4)for total count and objectionable microorganisms revealed failing results using the(b)(4)system. Objectionable microbes detected by(b)(4)included *Pseudomonas aeruginosa* and *Staphylococcus aureus*. Retesting confirmed the failures.

值得注意的是，（b）(4）批次的微生物检验（b）(4）使用（b）(4）系统对总计数和有害微生物显示不合格结果。对于（b）(4）检出有害微生物包括铜绿假单胞菌及金黄色葡萄球菌，复验结果确认了其不合格。

However, your firm invalidated these failing total count and objectionable microorganism findings based on limited retest using traditional compendial methods(USP <60>, <61>, and < 62>). The investigation speculated that the failures could be due to interferences from analytes and extra incubation time, but lacked data to support any root cause (s). Although you lacked sufficient investigation, scientific justification, and data to establish a root cause, you released (b)(4) lots. You did not adequately investigate manufacturing operations, including but not limited to review of process state of control and testing microbial quality of units from other parts of the batch, as contamination is not a uniform attribute.

但是，你公司基于使用传统药典方法（USP <60><61> 和 <62>）进行的有限复验，使这些不合格的总计数和有害微生物结果判定为无效。调查推测，不合格可能是由于分析物的干扰和额外的培养时间造成的，但缺乏支持根本原因的数据。尽管你公司缺乏充分的调查、科学论证和数据来确定根本原因，但还是放行了（b）（4）批次。你们没有充分调查生产操作，包括但不限于：审查过程控制状态、检验批次其他部分的微生物质量，这是考虑到污染不是一种统一的属性。

The investigation ultimately concluded in June 2021 that a reassessment of the suitability of the (b)(4) system was required prior to any future use, and stated "all future testing to be done using compendial methods."

调查最终于 2021 年 6 月得出结论，在未来使用之前，需要重新评估（b）（4）系统的适用性，并指出"所有未来的检验都将使用药典方法进行。"

But your firm decided not to undertake this CAPA, despite the lack of methods validation and your investigation conclusion that the method was unreliable. Instead of reassessing the (b)(4) method due to your lack of confidence in its validity, you continued to use the method for (b)(4) from June 2021 through March 2023, per your response.

但是，尽管缺乏方法验证且调查结论表明该方法不可靠，但你公司决定不执行此 CAPA。根据回复，你公司对（b）（4）方法的有效性缺乏信心，但未因此有重新评估该方法，而是在 2021 年 6 月到 2023 年 3 月期间继续使用该方法（b）（4）。

In your response, you state that you have now suspended the use of the (b)(4) testing system until validation is performed. Your response is inadequate because it does not adequately address how you intend to validate your alternative method for its intended use.

在回复中，你公司声明现已暂停使用（b）（4）检验系统，直至执行验证。你公司的回复不充分，因为它没有充分说明你们打算如何验证替代方法的预期用途。

Test methods must be validated to show they are suitable for their intended use, and equivalent or better than applicable USP compendial methods. The reproducibility of your test methods is essential to determine if your drug products meet established specifications for microbial attributes.

检验方法必须经过验证，以表明它们适合其预期用途，且等同于或优于适当的USP 药典方法。对于确定你公司药品是否符合微生物属性的既定质量标准来说，检验方法的重现性至关重要。

In response to this letter, provide：

在回复本函时，请提供：

● A comprehensive, independent assessment of your laboratory practices, procedures, methods, equipment, documentation, supervision, and analyst competencies. Based on this review, provide a detailed plan to remediate and evaluate the effectiveness of your laboratory system.

● 对你公司实验室实践、程序、方法、设备、文件和分析员能力进行完整、全面、独立的评估。在此审查的基础上，提供详细的计划来整改和评估实验室系统的有效性。

● Comprehensively evaluate your method and fully address its inadequacies, including but not limited to those cited in this letter. Once this full evaluation is complete, provide all findings, data, and deviations encountered.

● 全面评估你公司的方法并充分解决其不足之处，包括但不限于本警告信所述的不足之处。完整评估完成后，提供所有发现、数据和遇到的偏差。

● Updated validation protocols and final reports for each product that include specificity, limit of detection, robustness, ruggedness, and repeatability. Where non-compendial methods are used, provide studies evaluating equivalence or superiority of the method to the USP method.

● 更新每种产品的验证方案和最终报告，包括特异性、检测限、稳健性、耐用性和重现性。如果使用非药典方法，请提供评估该方法与 USP 方法的等效性或优越性研究。

● A retrospective, independent review of all invalidated OOS（including in-process and release/stability testing）results for US products currently in the U.S. market and within expiry as of the date of this letter and a report summarizing the findings of the analysis, including the following for each OOS：

● 对目前在美国市场和截至本函日期到期产品的所有无效 OOS（包括中控和放行/稳定性检验）结果进行回顾性独立审查，以及总结分析结果的报告，包括每个 OOS 的以下内容：

（略）

此处与 FDA 发给 Dunagin Pharmaceuticals Inc. dba Massco Dental 的警告信（编号：

MARCS–CMS 644335，即 "3 与非药用产品的共线生产问题"）中的 OOS 调查要求类似，故略去。

● A more detailed investigation into the failure of(b)(4) lots (b)(4).

● 对不合格的（b）（4）批次（b）（4），进行更详细的调查。

○ Include details regarding the apparent over-incubation of the starting samples that specifies how much longer the plates were allowed to incubate than established by your procedures(or USP <61> and <62>), and what day the plates were read after incubation.

○ 包括有关起始样品明显过度培养的详细信息，说明培养皿允许培养的时间如何比你公司程序（或 USP <61> 和 <62>）确定的时间长，以及培养后对培养皿进行读数发生在哪一天。

○ Specify what interferences were postulated to be present in the samples that caused the failing results and what actions you took to prevent repeat failures.

○ 指定假设样品中存在哪些干扰导致结果不合格，以及你公司采取了哪些措施来防止重复不合格。

○ Provide all accompanying raw data from the analysis of the(b)(4) lots (b)(4).

○ 提供（b）（4）批次分析中的所有附带原始数据（b）（4）。

○ Evaluate your manufacturing operations to determine what variables may have led to contamination in portions of the batch.

○ 评估你公司的生产操作，以确定哪些变量可能导致部分批次的污染。

Recall | 召回

In your March 2, 2023 response, you indicated you were conducting an investigation and considering recalling drug products.

在 2023 年 3 月 2 日的回复中，你公司表示正在开展调查并考虑召回药品。

On April 19, 2023, FDA held a teleconference with you. We recommended you remove any batches of drug products currently in distribution from the U.S. market that were manufactured between April 2020, and December 2020, when you used the non-food grade (b)(4) lubricant for the(b)(4) mixing vessel.

2023 年 4 月 19 日，FDA 与你公司召开了电话会议。我们建议你们下架目前在美国市场上市且在 2020 年 4 月至 2020 年 12 月期间生产的所有批次药品，当时，在（b）（4）

混合容器中，你公司使用了非食品级（b）（4）润滑剂。

On May 3, 2023, you issued a voluntary nationwide recall of the following four products: Safe tussin DM, DAY TIME Cough Relief; Safe tussin PM, NIGHT TIME Cough Relief; Colic Calm, Colic, Gas & Reflux, Homeopathic Medicine; and Pin–Away PYRENTAL PAMOATE (Pyrantel base 50mg / mL) Pinworm Treatment.

2023 年 5 月 3 日，你公司在全国范围内自愿召回以下四种产品：(名称略，见上)。

Ineffective Quality Systems | 质量体系失效

Significant findings in this letter demonstrate that your firm does not operate an effective quality system in accord with cGMP. In addition to the lack of effective production operations oversight to ensure reliable facilities and equipment, we found that your QU is not enabled to exercise proper authority and/or has insufficiently implemented its responsibilities. You should immediately and comprehensively assess your company's global manufacturing operations to ensure that systems, processes, and the products manufactured conform to FDA requirements.

本函中的重要调查结果表明，你公司没有按照 cGMP 运行有效的质量体系。除了缺乏有效的生产操作监督来确保设施和设备可靠之外，我们还发现你公司的 QU 无法行使适当的权力和（或）没有充分履行其职责。你公司应该立即全面评估整体生产操作，以确保系统、工艺和生产的产品符合 FDA 的要求。

12 批生产记录存在倒记问题

警告信编号： MARCS-CMS 657682

签发时间： 2023-8-11；**公示时间：** 2023-8-29

签发机构： 药物审评与研究中心 | CDER（Center for Drug Evaluation and Research | CDER）

公　　司： Cosmobeauti Laboratories & Manufacturing Inc.

所在国家 / 地区： 美国

主　　题： cGMP/ 成 品 制 剂 / 掺 假（cGMP/Finished Pharmaceuticals/Adulterated）

简　　介： FDA 于 2023 年 3 月对位于加利福尼亚州的该药品生产设施进行了检查。FDA 指出质量控制部门未能履行职责。具体来说，对其生产的非处方防晒药品，其质量部门（QU）未能提供充分监督。例如，其 QU（包括其法规顾问）未能确保批生产记录审核步骤记录的同步性。在检查过程中，其法规顾问告诉 FDA 调查员，在 OTC 药品批生产记录的审核步骤中，都进行了倒记。FDA 指出，cGMP 活动必须在执行时记录，批生产记录存在非同步文件的问题，这引起了对整个公司生产记录的有效性和可靠性的质疑。因此，FDA 要求公司对整个生产操作中使用的文档系统进行全面评估，以确定记录规范的不足之处。此外，要求提供详细的 CAPA 计划，以全面整改公司的记录规范，以确保其在整个运营过程中保持可追溯、清晰、完整、原始、准确和同步的记录。

本警告信以下部分与本书此前其他警告信内容类似，故略去：前言、作为合同商的责任（Responsibilities as a Contractor）、cGMP 顾问推荐（cGMP Consultant Recommended）、质量体系（Quality Systems）、数据可靠性整改（Data Integrity Remediation）、结论（Conclusion）。

质量部门

1. Your firm's quality control unit failed to exercise its responsibility to ensure drug products manufactured are in compliance with cGMP, and meet established specifications for identity, strength, quality, and purity (21 CFR211.22).

1. 质量控制部门未能履行职责，以确保所生产的药品符合 cGMP 要求，并符合有关鉴别、规格、质量和纯度的既定质量标准（21 CFR 211.22）

Your quality unit (QU) did not provide adequate oversight for the manufacture of your over-the-counter (OTC) sun protection factor (SPF) sunscreen drug products. For example, your QU, which includes you and your regulatory consultant, failed to ensure that the review of batch production record steps was contemporaneously recorded. During the inspection, your regulatory consultant told FDA investigators that you both backdated review steps on batch production records for your OTC drug products.

对你公司的非处方（OTC）防晒系数（SPF）防晒药品的生产，你公司质量部门（QU）没有提供充分的监督。例如，QU（包括你们和你们的法规顾问）未能确保批生产记录审核步骤记录上的同步性。在检查过程中，你公司法规顾问告诉 FDA 调查员，在 OTC 药品批生产记录的审核步骤时间上，你们都进行了倒记。

cGMP activities must be documented at the time of performance. Non-contemporaneous documentation on batch production records raises concerns about the validity and integrity of your firm's production records.

cGMP 活动必须在执行时同步记录。批生产记录存在非同步文件这一问题，引起了对公司生产记录有效性和可靠性的质疑。

In response to this letter, provide：

在回复本函时，请提供：

● A complete assessment of documentation systems used throughout your manufacturing and laboratory operations to determine where documentation practices are insufficient. Include a detailed corrective action and preventive action (CAPA) plan that comprehensively remediates your firm's documentation practices to ensure you retain attributable, legible, complete, original, accurate, contemporaneous records throughout your operation.

● 对整个生产操作中使用的文档系统进行全面评估，以确定记录规范的不足之处。包括详细的 CAPA 计划，以全面整改公司的记录规范，以确保你公司在整个运营过程中保存可追溯的、清晰的、完整的、原始的、准确的和同步的记录。

● A comprehensive assessment and remediation plan to ensure your QU is given the authority and resources to effectively function. The assessment should also include, but not be limited to：

● 全面的评估和整改计划，以确保你公司 QU 获得有效运作的权限和资源。评估还应包括但不限于：

○ A determination of whether procedures used by your firm are robust and appropriate.

○ 确定你公司使用的程序是否可靠和适当。

○ Provisions for QU oversight throughout your operations to evaluate adherence to appropriate practices.

○ 在整个运营过程中 QU 进行监督的规定，以评估对相应规范的遵守情况。

○ A complete and final review of each batch and its related information before the QU disposition decision.

○ 在 QU 决定处置之前，对每批产品及其相关信息进行完整和最终审查。

○ Oversight and approval of investigations and discharging of all other QU duties to ensure identity, strength, quality, and purity of all products

○ 监督和批准调查以及履行所有其他 QU 职责，以确保所有产品的鉴别、规格、质量和纯度。

○ Also describe how top management supports quality assurance and reliable operations, including but not limited to timely provision of resources to proactively address emerging manufacturing/quality issues and to assure a continuing state of control.

○ 还应说明高层管理人员如何支持质量保证和可靠运营，包括但不限于及时提供资源以主动解决新出现的生产 / 质量问题，并确保持续的控制状态。

稳定性研究

2. Your firm failed to conduct, for each batch of drug product, appropriate laboratory testing, as necessary, required to be free of objectionable organisms. Your firm also failed to test an adequate number of batches of each drug product to determine an appropriate expiration date.（21 CFR 211.165（b）and 21 CFR 211.166（b）).

2. 你公司未能根据需要，对每批药品进行适当的实验室检验，以确保其不含有害微生物。你公司也未能对每种药品进行足够批次的检验，以确定适当的有效期［21

CFR 211.165（b）和 21 CFR 211.166（b）]。

You failed to perform microbiological testing on each batch of your finished drug products. In addition, you lacked sufficient stability data to support the assigned shelf-life for your OTC drug products.

你公司未能对每批成品进行微生物检验。此外，你们缺乏充分的稳定性数据来支持非处方药的指定有效期。

Testing is an essential part of ensuring that the drug products you manufacture conform to all pre-determined quality attributes and are appropriate for their intended use, including microbiological specifications.

对于确保你公司生产的药品符合所有预先确定的质量属性，并适合其预期用途（包括微生物质量标准），检验是重要组成部分。

In response to this letter, provide:

在回复本函时，请提供：

● A comprehensive, independent assessment and CAPA plan to ensure the adequacy of your stability program. Your remediated program should include, but not be limited to:

● 全面、独立的评估和 CAPA 计划，以确保你公司的稳定性计划是充分的。整改计划应包括但不限于：

○ Stability indicating methods

○ 稳定性指示方法

○ Stability studies for each drug product in its marketed container-closure system before distribution is permitted

○ 在许可流通之前，对市售容器密闭系统中的每种药品进行稳定性研究

○ An ongoing program in which representative batches of each product are added each year to the program to determine if the shelf-life claim remains valid

○ 持续进行的计划，每年将每种产品的代表性批次添加到其中，以确定有效期声明是否仍然有效

○ Detailed definition of the specific attributes to be tested at each station（timepoint）

○ 每个点（时间点）要检验的特定属性的详细定义

● All procedures that describe these and other elements of your remediated stability program.

● 针对稳定性整改计划的这些以及其他元素，其所有相关的描述性程序。

● A list of chemical and microbiological test methods and specifications used to analyze each batch of your drug products before making a batch disposition decision, and the associated written procedures.

● 用于在做出批次处置决定之前，分析每批药品的化学和微生物检验方法和质量标准清单，以及相关的书面程序。

● A comprehensive, independent assessment of your laboratory practices, procedures, methods, equipment, documentation, and analyst competencies. Based on this review, provide a detailed plan to remediate and evaluate the effectiveness of your laboratory system.

● 对你公司的实验室实践、程序、方法、设备、文件和分析员能力进行完整、全面、独立的评估。在此审查的基础上，提供详细的计划来整改和评估实验室系统的有效性。

工艺验证

3. Your firm failed to establish adequate written procedures for production and process control designed to assure that the drug products you manufacture have the identity, strength, quality, and purity they purport or are represented to possess. Your firm also failed to prepare batch production and control records with complete information relating to the production and control of each batch of drug product produced（21 CFR 211.100（a）and 21 CFR 211.188）.

3. 你公司未充分建立用于生产和过程控制的书面程序，以确保所生产的药品具有其声称或声称拥有的鉴别、规格、质量和纯度。你公司也未能准备批生产和控制记录，其中包含与每批药品的生产和控制相关的完整信息［21 CFR 211.100（a）和 21 CFR 211.188］。

Batch Production Records and Process Validation
批生产记录和工艺验证

Your batch production records for your sunscreen drug products do not include adequate production details, including but not limited to, identification of major manufacturing equipment and critical steps in your manufacturing processes such as critical parameters（e.g., mixing speed and mixing times）. Additionally, numerous steps were not recorded on your batch production records for the sunscreen drug products. Complete and accurate batch production and control records are necessary to ensure that manufacturing processes are consistently followed and reproducible. Additionally, incomplete manufacturing records deprive you of the ability to adequately investigate deviations and batch failures, and to perform process validation.

你公司防晒药品批生产记录不包括充分的生产细节，包括但不限于主要生产设备的识别和生产工艺中的关键步骤，例如关键参数（混合速度和混合时间）。此外，防晒药品批生产记录中没有记录很多步骤。对于确保生产工艺得到一致遵循和重现性，完整而准确的批生产和控制记录是必要的。此外，不完整的生产记录使你公司无法充分调查偏差和批次不合格，以及执行工艺验证。

■ Water System Validation and Cleaning Validation 水系统验证和清洁验证

You lack adequate validation for your (b)(4) water system. You use water from your (b) (4) water system to rinse your non-dedicated drug manufacturing equipment.

你公司的（b）（4）水系统缺乏充分的验证。你们使用（b）（4）水系统中的水来冲洗非专用药品生产设备。

You also failed to perform cleaning validation for your non-dedicated drug manufacturing equipment. You must demonstrate that your cleaning processes for equipment prevents cross-contamination between the products manufactured at your facility.

你公司还未能对非专用药品生产设备进行清洁验证。你们必须证明设备清洁工艺可以防止你公司设施生产的产品之间发生交叉污染。

In response to this letter, provide:

在回复本函时，请提供：

（略）

此处与 FDA 发给 Dunagin Pharmaceuticals Inc. dba Massco Dental 的警告信（编号：MARCS-CMS 644335，即 "3 与非药用产品的共线生产问题"）中有关验证回应要求类似，故略去。

● A comprehensive remediation plan for the design, control, and maintenance of the water system.

● 针对水系统的设计、控制和维护的全面整改计划。

○ A (b)(4) water system validation report. Also include the summary of any improvements made to system design and to the program for ongoing control and maintenance.

○（b）（4）水系统验证报告。还包括对系统设计以及持续控制和维护程序所做的任何改进的汇总。

● A procedure for your water system monitoring that specifies routine microbial testing of water to ensure its acceptability for use in each batch of drug products produced by your firm.

● 水系统监测程序，规定了水的常规微生物检验，以确保其在你公司生产的每批药品中的使用是可以接受的。

● The current action/alert limits for total counts and objectionable organisms used for your（b）（4）water system. Ensure that the total count limits for your（b）（4）water are appropriately stringent in view of the intended use of each of the products produced by your firm.

● 用于水系统的总计数和有害微生物的当前行动 / 警戒限。鉴于你公司生产的每种产品的预期用途，确保你们（b）（4）水的总计数限度是相应严格符合的。

● A procedure governing your program for ongoing control, maintenance, and monitoring that ensures the remediated system consistently produces water that meets（b）（4）Water, USP monograph specifications and appropriate microbial limits.

● 一项用于监管持续控制、维护和监测计划的程序，以确保整改后的系统可以持续生产符合（b）（4）水、USP 专论质量标准和适当微生物限度要求的水。

（略）

此处与 FDA 发给 Cosmetic Science Laboratories LLC 的警告信（编号：MARCS–CMS 645558，即"5 水系统未经充分设计与监控"）中有关清洁验证的回应要求部分的内容类似，故略去。

● In addition, describe the steps that must be taken in your change management system before introduction of new manufacturing equipment or a new product.

● 另外，描述在引入新的生产设备或新产品之前，变更管理系统必须采取的步骤。

○ A summary of updated standard operating procedures（SOPs）that ensure an appropriate program is in place for verification and validation of cleaning procedures for products, processes, and equipment.

○ 更新的 SOP 汇总，以确保制定适当的程序，来确认和验证产品、工艺和设备的清洁程序。

Repeat Observations at Facility | 在设施中重复观察

In a previous inspection, dated November 14 to November 17, 2017, the FDA cited similar cGMP observations. You proposed specific remediation for these observations in your response. Repeated failures demonstrate that executive management oversight and control over the manufacture of drugs is inadequate.

在 2017 年 11 月 14 日至 17 日的前次检查中，FDA 引用了类似的 cGMP 观察结果。你公司在回复中针对这些观察项提出了具体的整改措施。屡次不合格表明高级管理层对药品生产的监督和控制不够。

13 实验室设备缺乏权限控制

警告信编号： MARCS-CMS 656056

签发时间： 2023-8-17；**公示时间：** 2023-9-5

签发机构： 药品质量业务二处（Division of Pharmaceutical Quality Operations Ⅱ）

公　　司： Lex Inc.

所在国家 / 地区： 美国

主　　题： cGMP/ 成 品 制 剂 / 掺 假（cGMP/Finished Pharmaceuticals/Adulterated）

简　　介： 2023 年 2 月，FDA 对该药品生产设施进行了检查。在检查中，FDA 指出，该公司对用于生成放行检验分析数据的实验室设备缺乏限制访问和充分的控制。具体来说，某些实验室工作人员拥有管理员权限，这可能导致未受控制的访问，从而可能删除或修改 HPLC 色谱文件。与此同时，公司没有充分维护实验室设备的数据备份。在其回复中，该公司承认了其在 HPLC 软件使用方面的知识缺乏。对此，FDA 认为该公司需要在确保数据可靠性方面做出改进，包括加强管理监督和提高人员的胜任力。此外，该公司回复中没有涵盖关于回顾性审查和 CAPA 等方面的内容，以确保数据的准确性和可靠性，从而支持其生产药品的安全性、有效性和质量。

本警告信以下部分与本书此前其他警告信内容类似，故略去：前言、质量体系失效（Ineffective Quality System）、cGMP 顾问推荐（cGMP Consultant Recommended）、作为合同商的责任（Responsibilities as a Contractor）、结论（Conclusion）。

质量部门

1. Your firm's quality control unit failed to exercise its responsibility to ensure drug products manufactured are in compliance with cGMP, and meet established specifications for identity, strength, quality, and purity (21 CFR211.22).

1. 你公司质量控制部门未能履行职责，以确保所生产的药品符合 cGMP 要求，并符合有关鉴别、规格、质量和纯度的既定质量标准（21 CFR 211.22）

Your firm's quality system was inadequate. Your quality unit (QU) did not provide adequate oversight for the manufacture of your over the counter (OTC) drug products. For example, your QU failed to ensure：

你公司的质量体系不够完善。质量部门（QU）没有对非处方（OTC）药品的生产提供充分的监督。例如，你公司 QU 未能确保：

- Adequate oversight, including but not limited to authority and responsibility for：

- 充分的监督，包括但不限于以下方面的权力和责任：

○ Written procedures for QU roles and responsibilities.

○ QU 角色和职责的书面程序。

○ Approval or rejection of all components and drug products.

○ 批准或拒放所有原辅料和药品。

○ Review of production and control records to assure completeness and no errors that need investigation.

○ 审查生产和控制记录，确保完整性且没有需要进行调查的错误。

○ Approval or rejection of all procedures or specifications impacting the identity, strength, quality, and purity of drug products.

○ 批准或拒绝所有影响药品鉴别、规格、质量和纯度的程序或质量标准。

○ Each lot of components, drug product containers, and closures was withheld from use until the lot was sampled, tested, or examined, as appropriate, and released for use.

○ 每批次的物料、药品容器和密封件均不得使用，直至该批次酌情进行取样、检验或检查并放行使用。

In your response, you state that you intend to establish and implement new procedures to comply with cGMP. However, you do not provide detailed corrective actions and preventive actions（CAPA）, updated procedures for change management, annual product reviews, well-defined QU roles, and timeframes for implementation. You also do not indicate how your QU will provide oversight of your operations to ensure all requirements are met and that errors are identified prior to the release of batches.

在回复中，你公司声明你们打算建立并实施新的程序以遵守 cGMP。但是，没有提供详细的纠正和预防措施（CAPA）、更新的变更管理程序、年度产品回顾、明确定义的 QU 角色以及实施时间表。你公司也没有说明 QU 将如何监督你们的操作，以确保满足所有要求，并在批放行之前识别错误。

An adequate QU overseeing all elements of cGMP is necessary to consistently ensure drug product quality. Your firm's quality systems are inadequate. See FDA's guidance document *Quality Systems Approach to Pharmaceutical cGMP Regulations* at: https://www.fda.gov/regulatory-information/search-fda-guidance-documents/quality- systems-approach-pharmaceutical-current-good-manufacturing-practice-regulations for help in implementing quality systems and risk management approaches to meet the requirements of cGMP regulations 21 CFR parts 210 and 211.

需要有充分的 QU 来监督所有生产操作，以始终如一地确保药品质量。你公司的质量体系不完善。请参阅 FDA 指南，药品 cGMP 法规的质量体系方法，帮助实施质量体系和风险管理方法，以满足 cGMP 法规 21 CFR 第 210 和 211 部分的要求，网址（略，见上）。

In response to this letter, provide a comprehensive assessment and remediation plan to ensure your QU is given the authority and resources to effectively function. The assessment should also include, but not be limited to:

针对本函，请提供全面的评估和整改计划，以确保你公司 QU 获得有效运行的权力和资源。评估还应包括但不限于：

（略）

此处与 FDA 发给 Cosmetic Science Laboratories LLC 的警告信（编号：MARCS-CMS 645558，即 "5 水系统未经充分设计与监控"）中有关 QU 的回应要求部分的内容类似，故略去。

物料检验

2. Your firm failed to withhold from use each lot of components, drug product containers, and closures until the lot had been sampled, tested, or examined, as appropriate,

and released for use by the quality control unit. Your firm failed to conduct at least one test to verify the identity of each component of a drug product. Your firm also failed to validate and establish the reliability of your component supplier's test analyses at appropriate intervals (21 CFR 211.84 (a), 211.84 (d)(1), and 211.84 (d)(2)).

2. 在对批次进行取样、检验或检查（视情况而定）并质量放行以供使用之前，你公司未能停止使用每批物料、药品容器和密封件。你公司未能进行至少一项检验，来确认药品每种原辅料都被鉴别。你公司也未能以适当的时间间隔，来验证和建立物料供应商检验分析的可靠性［21 CFR 211.84 (a)、211.84 (d)(1) 和 211.84 (d)(2)］。

You failed to adequately test incoming components used to manufacture finished drug products. For example,

你公司未能充分检验用于生产成品制剂的进场原辅料，例如，

● You lacked sufficiently specific identity tests for potential diethylene glycol (DEG) and ethylene glycol (EG) contamination of glycerin and propylene glycol ingredients used in the manufacturing of drug products. Some of your firm's products formulated with glycerin or propylene glycol are intended for oral use in pediatric populations.

● 针对药品生产中使用的甘油和丙二醇原辅料存在潜在二甘醇（DEG）和乙二醇（EG）污染，你公司缺乏充分具体的鉴别检验。你公司的一些用甘油或丙二醇配制的产品供儿童口服使用。

In your response, you commit to revise the raw material specifications for glycerin and propylene glycol to include appropriate identity testing prior to release for manufacturing drug products.

在回复中，你公司承诺修订甘油和丙二醇的原料质量标准，以在药品生产放行之前进行适当的鉴别检验。

Your response is inadequate. You do not include appropriate identity testing on glycerin and propylene glycol lots currently in your inventory. Additionally, you fail to provide sufficient evidence demonstrating adequate identity testing on all containers of all lots of glycerin and propylene glycol prior to their use in the manufacture of drug products. You lack appropriate testing of representative samples of each lot of high-risk components. Without appropriate testing of components, you cannot ensure the quality and safety of your drug products.

你公司的回应不够充分。你们没有对库存中当前的甘油和丙二醇批次进行适当的鉴别检验。此外，未能提供充分的证据证明在用于药品生产之前，对所有批次的甘油和丙二醇的所有容器均进行了充分的鉴别检验。你公司对每批高风险原辅料的代表性

样品缺乏适当的检验。如果不对原辅料进行适当的检验，就无法确保药品的质量和安全性。

The use of ingredients contaminated with DEG or EG has resulted in various lethal poisoning incidents in humans worldwide. See FDA's guidance document *Testing of Glycerin, Propylene Glycol, Maltitol Solution, Hydrogenated Starch Hydrolysate, Sorbitol Solution, and Other High-Risk Drug Components for Diethylene Glycol and Ethylene Glycol* to help you meet the cGMP requirements when manufacturing drugs containing ingredients at risk for DEG or EG contamination, at https://www.fda.gov/media/167974/download.

在全球范围内，使用受 DEG 或 EG 污染的原辅料已导致多起人类致命中毒事件。请参阅 FDA 指南，甘油、丙二醇、麦芽糖醇溶液、氢化淀粉水解物、山梨醇溶液和其他高风险药品原辅料中二甘醇和乙二醇的检验，以帮助你公司在生产含有 DEG 或 EG 污染风险原辅料的药品时满足 cGMP 要求，请访问（网址略，见上）。

● Your incoming component tests, including those for your pediatric OTC cough and cold products, did not include identity testing on each component lot prior to their use. Several API lots were released into production without performing adequate acceptance testing, including identity. For example, an API, (b)(4), was used to manufacture (b)(4) without qualifying your supplier and performing identification testing.

● 你公司的进场原辅料检验（包括儿科非处方咳嗽和感冒产品的原辅料检验）未能包括每个原辅料批次在使用前的鉴别项目。一些 API 批次在没有进行充分验收检验（包括鉴别检验）的情况下就投入生产。例如，API（b）（4）用于生产（b）（4），但未对你公司供应商进行确认并进行鉴别检验。

In your response, you commit to outsource the testing of all incoming components to a local laboratory as well as updating procedures for acceptance of incoming components. You also plan to revise your procedures to include all required testing for raw materials and to test retain samples of previously released lots of components.

在回复中，你公司承诺将所有进场物料的检验外包给当地实验室，并更新进场物料的验收程序。你们还计划修订程序，以包括所有必需的原料检验，并检验先前放行的原辅料留样。

Your response is inadequate. You fail to address the full scope and impact of the cGMP deficiencies as well as the associated risks to drug product quality, including addressing the risks posed to batches already in distribution. Without appropriate testing of components and ingredients, you cannot ensure the quality and safety of your drug products.

你公司的回应不够充分。你们未能解决 cGMP 缺陷的全部范围和影响以及药品质量的相关风险，包括解决已流通批次所带来的风险。如果不对原辅料和成分进行适当的检验，你公司就无法确保药品的质量和安全性。

● You did not adequately establish the reliability of your raw material suppliers, including your API suppliers. For example, you acknowledged that you have not qualified your suppliers and you did not follow your written procedure, LAB 06 Version #3.

● 你公司没有充分确定原料供应商（包括原料药供应商）的可靠性。例如，你公司承认没有对供应商进行确认，并且没有遵循书面程序 LAB 06 第 3 版。

In your response, you commit to perform supplier qualification.

在回复中，你公司承诺执行供应商确认。

Your response is inadequate because you do not provide a detailed plan to evaluate supplier reliability. Your procedure does not specify the need to comprehensively assess component attributes and it did not establish appropriate intervals for requalification.

你公司的回复不充分，因为没有提供评估供应商可靠性的详细计划。你公司的程序没有指定全面评估物料属性的必要性，也没有建立适当的再确认间隔时间要求。

We acknowledge that, after the inspection and a discussion with FDA on May 12, 2023, you sent for analysis retains of bulk glycerin, propylene glycol, (b)(4), (b)(4) and (b)(4) that you had used to manufacture drug products that are in distribution and within expiry. Based on the provided results, you concluded there was no DEG/EG contamination in the samples of retains tested.

我们知晓，在 2023 年 5 月 12 日进行检查并与 FDA 讨论后，对于正在流通且在有效期内的药品，就其生产涉及的甘油、丙二醇、（b）（4）、（b）（4）和（b）（4），你公司将留样送去检验。根据提供的结果，你们得出结论，检验的留样中不存在 DEG/EG 污染。

From the discussion with FDA, you also stated you would test appropriate representative samples of incoming high-risk component lots for potential DEG/EG contamination prior to manufacturing drug products.

在与 FDA 的讨论中，你公司还表示，在生产药品之前，将对进场的高风险原辅料批次的适当代表性样品进行潜在的 DEG/EG 污染检验。

In response to this letter, provide：

在回复本函时，请提供：

● A full risk assessment for drug products that are within expiry which may contain any ingredient at risk for DEG or EG contamination（including but not limited to glycerin）. Take

147

prompt and appropriate actions to determine the safety of all lots of the component（s）and any related drug product that could contain DEG or EG, including customer notifications and product recalls for any contaminated lots. Identify additional appropriate corrective actions and preventive actions that secure supply chains in the future, including but not limited to ensuring that all incoming raw material lots are from fully qualified manufacturers and free from unsafe impurities. Detail these actions in your response to this letter.

● 就任何含有 DEG 或 EG 污染风险的原辅料（包括但不限于甘油），且在效期内的药品，提供全面的风险评估。立即采取适当的措施，就任何可能含有 DEG 或 EG 的原辅料或相关药品批次，确定其安全性，包括通知客户和召回任何受污染批次的产品。确定其他适当的 CAPA，以确保未来的供应链安全，包括但不限于：确保所有进场原料批次均来自有充分资质的生产商，且不含不安全的杂质。在你公司对本函的回复中详细说明这些行动。

● A description of how you will test each component lot for conformity with all appropriate specifications for identity, strength, quality, and purity. Include a list of test specifications and test methods for each component. If you intend to accept any results from your supplier's Certificate of Analysis（COA）instead of testing each component lot for strength, quality, and purity, specify how you will robustly establish the reliability of your supplier's results through initial validation as well as periodic revalidation. In addition, include a commitment to conduct at least one specific identity test for each incoming component lot, as required. In the case of glycerin, propylene glycol, and certain additional high-risk components we note that this includes the performance of parts A, B, and C of the United States Pharmacopeia（USP）monograph for identity.

● 说明如何检验每个批次，确定是否符合有关鉴别、规格、质量和纯度质量标准。如果你公司打算接受供应商 COA 的结果，而不是检验每个物料批次的规格、质量和纯度，请说明如何进行初始验证和定期再验证，从而稳健地确定供应商结果的可靠性。此外，还应承诺对于每个进场原辅料批次，至少进行一个专属鉴别检验。就甘油、丙二醇和其他高风险原辅料而言，我们注意到这包括 USP 专论 A、B 和 C 部分的性能表现。

● A risk assessment of components qualified and released for use in manufacturing without appropriate testing for purity, strength, and quality.

● 就用于生产的物料进行风险评估，这些物料被判为合格并放行，但未对纯度、规格和质量进行适当的检验。

● The chemical quality control specifications you use to test and determine suitability of each incoming lot of high-risk drug components to determine acceptability for use in manufacturing.

● 化学质量控制标准，其用于检验和确定每批进场高风险药物原辅料的适用性，以确定其在生产中使用的可接受性。

● A comprehensive, independent review of your material system to determine whether all suppliers of components, containers, and closures are each qualified and the materials are assigned appropriate expiration or retest dates. The review should also determine whether incoming material controls are adequate to prevent use of unsuitable components, containers, and closures.

● 对你公司的物料系统进行全面、独立的审查，以确定所有物料、容器和密封件的供应商是否均合格，并为物料指定了适当的有效期或复验日期。审查还应确定进场物料控制是否足以防止使用不合适的物料、容器和密封件。

● A summary of results obtained from testing all components to evaluate the reliability of the COA from each component manufacturer.

● 结果汇总：对所有物料进行检验，以评估每个物料生产商的 COA 可靠性。

● A summary of your program for qualifying and overseeing contract facilities that test components and the drug products you manufacture.

● 你公司对检验所生产的原辅料和药品的外包设施进行确认和监督的计划的总结。

生产和过程控制的书面程序

3. Your firm failed to establish written procedures for production and process control designed to assure that the drug products you manufacture have the identity, strength, quality, and purity they purport or are represented to possess, and your firm's quality control unit did not review and approve those procedures, including any changes(21 CFR 211.100(a)).

3. 你公司未建立用于生产和过程控制的书面程序，以确保所生产的药品具有其声称或声称拥有的鉴别、规格、质量和纯度，且你公司的质量部门未审查和批准这些程序，包括任何变更〔21 CFR 211.100(a)〕。

Your firm lacked an adequate process validation program and sufficient validation studies for your drug product manufacturing processes. For example, your process validation program was not inclusive for all products you manufacture. During the inspection, you acknowledged your process performance qualification(PPQ)studies were incomplete.

你公司缺乏适当的工艺验证计划和充分的药品生产工艺验证研究。例如，工艺验证计划并不包括你们生产的所有产品。在检查过程中，你公司承认工艺性能确认（PPQ）研究不完整。

In your response you state a lack of a validation plan is the root cause of the problems and you commit to complete process validation activities. You also note that you will provide a procedure and timelines for completion of validation studies.

在回复中，你公司指出缺乏验证计划是问题的根本原因，并且你们承诺完成工艺验证活动。你公司还表示，你们将提供完成验证研究的程序和时间表。

Your response does not commit to ensuring prospective PPQ studies are completed prior to distribution of products, nor do you include a risk assessment for any marketed drug products.

在回复中，你公司并没有承诺确保在产品流通之前完成前瞻性 PPQ 研究，也不包括对任何上市药品的风险评估。

（略）

此处与 FDA 发给 Profounda, Inc. 的警告信（编号：MARCS-CMS 642595, 即"2 未能提供生产工艺的验证数据"）中有关工艺验证的重要性部分的内容类似，故略去。

In your response to this letter, provide：

在你公司对本函的回复中，请提供：

（略）

此处与 FDA 发给 Dunagin Pharmaceuticals Inc. dba Massco Dental 的警告信（编号：MARCS-CMS 644335, 即"3 与非药用产品的共线生产问题"）中工艺验证回应要求类似, 故略去。

设备问题

4. Your firm failed to routinely calibrate, inspect, or check according to a written program designed to assure proper performance of automatic, mechanical, electronic equipment, or other types of equipment, including computers, used in the manufacture, processing, packing, and holding of a drug product. Your firm also failed to exercise appropriate controls over computer or related systems to assure that only authorized personnel institute changes in master production and control records, or other records（21 CFR 211.68（a）and（b））.

4. 你公司未能按照书面程序进行例行校准、核查或检定，该程序针对用于生产、加工、包装和储存的自动、机械、电子设备或其他类型设备（包括计算机），旨在确保其正常性能。你公司也未能对计算机或相关系统实施适当的控制，以确保只有授权人员才能更改主生产和控制记录或其他记录［21 CFR 211.68（a）和（b）］。

● You could not provide documentation that your OTC drug product manufacturing equipment was suitable for its intended use and that it was qualified. You acknowledged that you did not qualify your OTC drug production equipment.

● 你公司无法提供文件证明 OTC 药品生产设备适合其预期用途并且经确认。你公司承认，非处方药生产设备未经确认。

In your response, you commit to providing an equipment qualification plan. You also state you have qualification protocols that have not been completed.

在回复中，你公司承诺提供设备确认计划。还声明你们有尚未完成的确认方案。

Your response is inadequate. Your response does not include your equipment qualification plan, equipment qualification protocols, a timeline for completion, and a risk assessment for the drug products you produced using unqualified equipment.

你公司回应不够充分。你们的回复不包括设备确认计划、设备确认方案、完成时间表以及你们使用未经确认设备生产的药品的风险评估。

● Laboratory equipment used to generate analytical data for finished drug product release lacked restricted access and sufficient controls. For example, some laboratory staff had administrator rights allowing uncontrolled access to delete or modify high performance liquid chromatography（HPLC）files. You had no mechanism to facilitate traceability of individuals who deleted or modified data generated by computerized systems. Furthermore, your firm did not adequately maintain backups of data generated by your laboratory equipment.

● 用于生成成品制剂放行分析数据的实验室设备缺乏限制访问和充分的控制。例如，一些实验室工作人员拥有管理员权限，允许不受控制的访问，来删除或修改高效液相色谱（HPLC）文件。你公司没有任何机制，可以方便地追踪删除或修改计算机系统生成数据的个人。此外，你公司没有充分维护实验室设备生成的数据备份。

In your response, you acknowledge your lack of knowledge regarding the use of the HPLC software.

在回复中，你公司承认你们缺乏有关 HPLC 软件的使用知识。

Your response is inadequate. Your response does not provide adequate details of required improvements and expertise（e.g., management oversight, competencies）to assure data integrity. Your response also does not include provisions for retrospective review and CAPA for the accuracy and integrity of data to support the safety, effectiveness, and quality of the drugs you manufacture. Additionally, your response does not address data retention.

你公司的回应不够充分。就确保数据可靠性所需的改进和专业知识（例如管理监督、胜任力），你们的回复没有提供的足够详细信息。你们的回复也不包括确保数据的准确性和可靠性的回顾性审查和 CAPA 规定，以支持所生产药品的安全性、有效性和质量。此外，你公司的回复并未解决数据保存问题。

- You did not routinely calibrate your production scales used for weighing drug product components, including API, to reflect actual operating ranges. For example, your（b）（4）calibration check only documented one weight.

- 你公司没有定期校准用于称量药物原辅料（包括 API）的生产用秤，以反映实际操作范围。例如，你们的（b）（4）校准检查仅记录了一个重量。

In your response, you acknowledge that you failed to adequately calibrate your production scales.

在回复中，你公司承认未能充分校准生产用秤。

Your response is inadequate. Your response does not include sufficient details on how you will calibrate scales and you do not provide procedures for calibration or a plan to assess previously manufactured drug product batches that may have been impacted by inconsistencies with specified production weights. You also do not provide a plan to assess other equipment that may not have been calibrated appropriately.

你公司的回应不够充分。你们的回复没有包含有关如何校准秤的足够详细信息，也没有提供校准程序，或评估先前生产的药品批次的计划，这些批次可能受到与指定生产重量不一致的影响。就评估可能未适当校准的其他设备，你公司也没有提供相应的计划。

Without complete and accurate records, you cannot ensure your firm makes appropriate batch release, stability, and other decisions that are fundamental to ongoing assurance of drug product quality.

如果没有完整、准确的记录，就无法确保你公司做出适当的批放行、稳定性以及对持续保证药品质量至关重要的其他决策。

See FDA's guidance document *Data Integrity and Compliance With Drug cGMP* for guidance on establishing and following cGMP compliant data integrity practices at https://www.fda.gov/regulatory-information/search-fda-guidance-documents/data- integrity-and-compliance-drug-cGMP-questions-and-answers.

有关建立和遵循 cGMP 合规数据可靠性实践的指南，请参阅 FDA 指南，数据可靠性和药品 cGMP 合规性，网址（略，见上）。

In response to this letter, provide:

在回复本函时，请提供：

● A complete assessment of documentation systems used throughout your manufacturing and laboratory operations to determine where documentation practices are insufficient. Include a detailed CAPA plan that comprehensively remediates your firm's documentation practices to ensure you retain attributable, legible, complete, original, accurate, contemporaneous records throughout your operation.

● 对整个生产操作中使用的文档系统进行全面评估，以确定记录规范的不足之处。包括详细的 CAPA 计划，以全面整改你公司的记录规范，以确保在整个运营过程中保存可追溯的、清晰的、完整的、原始的、准确的和同步的记录。

● A comprehensive, independent assessment and corrective action and preventive action (CAPA) plan for computer system security and integrity. Include a report identifying design and control vulnerabilities and appropriate remediations for each of your laboratory and manufacturing computer systems. This should include, but not be limited to:

● 针对计算机系统安全性和完整性的全面、独立的评估和 CAPA 计划。包括识别设计和控制漏洞的报告，以及针对你公司每个实验室计算机系统的相应整改措施。这应包括但不限于：

○ A list of all hardware and equipment (standalone and network) in your laboratory.

○ 实验室中所有硬件和设备（单机和联网）的清单。

○ Identification of vulnerabilities in hardware and software, encompassing both networked and non-networked systems (e.g., programmable logic controller (PLC)).

○ 识别硬件和软件中的漏洞，包括联网和非联网系统［例如可编程逻辑控制器（PLC）］。

○ A list of all software configurations (both equipment software and laboratory information management system (LIMS)) and versions, details of all user privileges, and oversight responsibilities for each of your laboratory systems. Regarding user privileges, specify user roles and associated user privileges (including the specific permissions allowed for anyone who has administrative rights) for all staff who have access to the laboratory computer systems, their organizational affiliation, and title. Also describe how you will ensure laboratory staff are not given administrative rights, or other permissions that compromise data retention or reliability.

○ 所有软件配置［包括设备软件和实验室信息管理系统（LIMS）］和版本的清单、所有用户权限的详细信息以及每个实验室系统的监督责任。关于用户权限，为有权访问实验室计算机系统的所有工作人员指定用户角色和相关用户权限（包括允许任何具有管理权限的人的特定权限），以及他们的组织隶属关系和职称，并说明你公司将如何确保实验室工作人员不被授予管理权限或其他损害数据保存或可靠性的权限。

○ System security provisions including, but not limited to, whether unique usernames and passwords are always used, and their confidentiality safeguarded.

○ 系统安全规定，包括但不限于是否始终使用唯一的用户名 / 密码，并保护其机密性。

○ Detailed procedures for robust use and review of audit trail data, and current status of audit trail implementation for each of your systems.

○ 健全地使用并审查审计追踪数据的细化程序，以及每个系统审计追踪实施的当前状态。

○ Interim control measures and procedural changes for the control, review, and full retention of laboratory data.

○ 用于控制、审查和完全保存实验室数据的临时控制措施和程序变更。

○ Technological improvements to increase the integration of data generated through electronic systems from standalone equipment（e.g., balances, pH meters, water content testing）into the LIMS network.

○ 技术改进，以增加通过电子系统从单机设备（例如天平、pH 计、水含量检验）生成的数据与 LIMS 网络的集成。

○ A detailed summary of your procedural updates and associated training, including, but not limited to, system security control to prevent unauthorized access, appropriate user role assignments, secondary review of all analyses, and other system controls.

○ 你公司程序更新和相关培训的详细汇总，包括但不限于：防止未经授权访问的系统安全控制、适当的用户角色分配、所有分析的复核以及其他系统控制。

○ Your remediated program for ensuring strict ongoing control over electronic and paper-based data to ensure all additions, deletions, or modifications of information in your records are authorized, and all data is retained. Provide your full CAPA plan and any improvements made to date.

○ 确保对电子和纸质数据进行严格持续控制的整改计划，以确保对记录中信息的所有添加、删除或修改均获得授权，并保存所有数据。提供你公司的完整 CAPA 计划以及迄今为止所做的任何改进。

○ Provisions for oversight from quality assurance (QA) managers, executives, and internal auditors with appropriate IT expertise (e.g., understanding of infrastructure, configuration, network requirements, strict segregation of administrative rights).

○ 提供对质量保证（QA）经理、管理人员和具有适当 IT 专业知识的内部审计员监督的规定（例如，了解基础设施、配置、网络要求、管理权限的严格隔离）。

○ An independent, thorough retrospective assessment into the impact of laboratory system design, control, and staff practices on your data accuracy, completeness, and retention for the last three years.

○ 就过去三年实验室系统设计、控制和员工实践对数据准确性、可靠性和保存的影响，进行独立、彻底的回顾性评估。

● Your CAPA plan and updated SOPs to implement routine, vigilant operations management oversight of facilities and equipment. This plan should ensure, among other things, prompt detection of equipment/facilities performance issues, adherence to appropriate preventive maintenance schedules, and improved systems for ongoing management review.

● 你公司的 CAPA 计划和更新的 SOP，以便对设施和设备实施常规的、警戒性的运营管理监督。该计划应确保及时发现设备 / 设施性能问题，遵守适当的预防性维护计划以及改进持续管理评审系统。

● Your remediated calibration program, including but not limited to scale calibrations (e.g., daily calibration checks with certified weights; ensuring routine checks represent actual operational ranges).

● 你公司的整改校准计划，包括但不限于秤校准（例如，使用经过认证的砝码进行日常校准检查；确保例行检查代表实际操作范围）。

Quality Unit Authority | 质量部门授权

Your inspectional history indicates that your quality unit is not able to fully exercise its authority and/or responsibilities. Your firm must provide the quality unit with the appropriate authority and sufficient resources to carry out its responsibilities and consistently ensure drug quality.

检查历史表明，你公司的质量部门无法充分行使其授权和（或）责任。你公司必须为质量部门提供相应的授权和充分的资源，以履行其职责并始终如一地确保药品质量。

Repeat Violations at Facility | 设施中的重复违规情况

In a previous warning letter（FLA-05-13）and previous inspections, dated June 28 to July 8, 2004; August 15 to August 24, 2005; June 15 to June 23, 2009; January 25 to March 1, 2011; and September 10 to September 16, 2016, FDA cited similar cGMP violations. You proposed specific remediation for these violations in your response. Repeated failures demonstrate that executive management oversight and control over the manufacture of drugs is inadequate.

在之前的警告信（FLA-05-13）和检查中（日期为 2004 年 6 月 28 日至 7 月 8 日；2005 年 8 月 15 日至 8 月 24 日；2009 年 6 月 15 日至 6 月 23 日；2011 年 1 月 25 日至 3 月 1 日；2016 年 9 月 10 日至 9 月 16 日），FDA 列举了类似的 cGMP 违规情况。你公司在回复中提出了针对这些违规情况的具体整改措施。屡次不合格表明高级管理层对药品生产的监督和控制不到位。

14 MAH 未能对委托生产进行充分监督

警告信编号： MARCS-CMS 654879

签发时间： 2023-10-20；**公示时间：** 2023-11-21

签发机构： 药品质量业务四处（Division of Pharmaceutical Quality Operations IV）

公　　司： Elemental Herbs Inc. dba ALL good

所在国家 / 地区： 美国

主　　题： cGMP/ 成品制剂 / 掺假（cGMP/Finished Pharmaceuticals/Adulterated）

简　　介： FDA 于 2023 年 1 月至 2 月对该药品生产设施进行了检查。FDA 指出，该公司的质量部门未能对其药品生产进行充分的监督。举例来说，该公司未对其委托实验室产生的 OOS 结果进行适当的调查，也未及时向为其生产该药品的 CMO 传达这些 OOS 结果，以便进行生产调查。在其回复中，该公司计划聘请一名顾问来建立质量体系，并承诺制定 SOP，其中包括正确处理 OOS 结果的程序。然而，FDA 认为该公司的回应不够充分，因为其未确定或实施任何临时措施，来整改或防止重大的质量保证违规情况，也并未提供采取纠正和预防措施的时间表。

本警告信以下部分与本书此前其他警告信内容类似，故略去：前言、合同商的责任（Contractor's Responsibilities）、cGMP 顾问推荐（cGMP Consultant Recommended）、未经批准的新药和标识错误违规情况（Unapproved New Drug and Misbranding Violations）、结论（Conclusion）。

质量部门未能履责

1. Your firm failed to establish an adequate quality unit and the responsibilities and

procedures applicable to the quality control unit are not in writing and fully followed（21 CFR 211.22（a）and 211.22（d））.

1. 你公司未能建立适当的质量部门，适用于质量部门的责任和程序未以书面形式呈现且未得到完全遵守 ［21 CFR 211.22（a）和 211.22（d）］。

Your quality unit（QU）did not provide adequate oversight for the manufacture of your drug products, for example：

你公司质量部门（QU）没有对药品的生产提供充分的监督，例如：

● Adequate procedures were not in place describing and defining the roles and responsibilities between your QU and your contract manufacturing organizations（CMOs）. For example, there were inadequate or no procedures for：

● 没有适当的程序，来描述和定义 QU 和合同生产组织（CMO）之间的角色和责任。例如，以下方面的程序不充分或没有：

○ Qualification of CMOs to manufacture your drug products

○ CMO 生产药品的资质确认

○ Establishment of drug product specifications

○ 制定药品质量标准

○ Sharing complaints with CMOs

○ 与 CMO 分享投诉

○ Management of changes

○ 变更管理

○ Investigation of product returns

○ 产品退货调查

● Out-of-specification（OOS）results generated by your contract laboratories were not appropriately investigated by your firm. For example, an investigation was not conducted by your firm when OOS results for Zinc Oxide assay were reported at multiple timepoints during real time stability testing of your "ALL good" SPF-20Coconut lip balm. Furthermore, your firm did not communicate these OOS results in a timely manner to the CMO that manufactured this drug product for you.

● 你公司没有对委托实验室生成的不合格（OOS）结果进行适当的调查。例如，在对"ALL Good"SPF-20椰子润唇膏进行实时稳定性检验期间，在多个时间点报告了氧化锌测定的OOS结果，但你公司并未进行调查。此外，你公司没有及时向为你们生产该药品的CMO传达这些OOS结果。

Without adequate quality procedures and oversight, you cannot ensure the consistency of your manufacturing processes and the purported identity, strength, quality, and purity of drug products released to the market.

如果没有充分的质量程序和监督，就无法确保生产工艺的一致性，也无法确保在市药品所声称的鉴别、规格、质量和纯度。

In your response, you plan to hire a consultant to establish Quality Systems and commit to develop standard operating procedures (SOPs) including, but not limited to, the proper handling of OOS results.

在回复中，你公司计划聘请一名顾问来建立质量体系，并承诺制定标准操作程序（SOP），包括但不限于正确处理OOS结果。

Your response is inadequate. You do not identify or implement any interim actions that will be undertaken to correct or prevent the significant QU violations and do not provide a timeframe for when corrective actions and preventive actions (CAPAs) will be instituted.

你公司回应不够充分。你们没有确定或实施任何为整改或防止重大QU违规情况而采取的临时措施，也没有提供采取纠正和预防措施（CAPA）的时间表。

Your firm's quality systems are inadequate. See FDA's guidance document *Quality Systems Approach to Pharmaceutical cGMP Regulations* for help implementing quality systems and risk management approaches to meet the requirements of cGMP regulations 21 CFR, parts 210 and 211, at https://www.fda.gov/media/71023/download.

你公司的质量体系不完善。请参阅FDA指南，药品cGMP法规的质量体系方法，帮助实施质量体系和风险管理方法，以满足cGMP法规21 CFR第210和211部分的要求，网址（略，见上）。

For more information about handling failing OOS, out-of-trend, or other unexpected results and documentation of your investigations, see FDA's Guidance document *Investigating Out-of-Specification (OOS) Test Results for Pharmaceutical Production* at https://www.fda.gov/regulatory-information/search-fda-guidance-documents/investigating-out-specification-oos-test-results-pharmaceutical-production-level-2-revision

有关处理不合格、OOS、超常或其他非预期结果以及你公司调查记录的更多信息，请参阅FDA指南，调查药品生产的不合格（OOS）检验结果，网址（略，见上）。

In response to this letter, provide：

在回复本函时，请提供：

（略）

此处与 FDA 发给 Dunagin Pharmaceuticals Inc. dba Massco Dental 的警告信（编号：MARCS-CMS 644335，即 "3 与非药用产品的共线生产问题"）中 QU 和 OOS 调查要求类似，故略去。

稳定性研究

2. Your firm failed to follow an adequate written testing program designed to assess the stability characteristics of drug products and to use results of stability testing to determine appropriate storage conditions and expiration dates（21 CFR 211.166（a））.

2. 你公司未能遵循适当的书面检验程序，以评估药品的稳定性特征；未能使用稳定性检验结果，来确定适当的储存条件和有效期［21 CFR 211.166（a）］。

Your firm failed to establish an adequate stability program and determine appropriate expiration dates for over-the-counter（OTC）drug products that you own and distribute, specifically：

针对拥有和流通的非处方（OTC）药品，你公司未能为其制定适当的稳定性计划，并确定适当的有效期，特别是：

● Your firm marketed at least seven Sun Protection Factor（SPF）drug products within adequate data to support their labeled expiration date.

● 你公司上市了至少七种防晒系数（SPF）药品，并有充分的数据支持其标签上的有效期。

● Your firm failed to establish an adequate stability program for OTC drug products.

● 你公司未能为非处方药产品建立充分的稳定性计划。

● Your firm failed to put a representative sample of all drugs in unique container closure systems in a stability testing program.

● 就具有独特性容器封闭系统的所有药品，你公司未能将其代表性样品纳入稳定性检验计划中。

In your response, you commit to doing a complete review of the stability program being performed by your CMOs. You state that this review will take at least（b）（4）from initiation.

However, a proposed initiation date is not provided.

在回复中，你公司承诺对 CMO 正在执行的稳定性计划进行全面审查。你们声明此审查从启动起至少需要（b）（4）。但是，没有提供拟议的启动日期。

Your response is inadequate. You fail to provide updated stability protocols to ensure all unique product types are included in your stability program. Additionally, your response does not include a timeline for remediation of your stability program.

你公司的回应不够充分。你们未能提供更新的稳定性方案，来确保所有独特的产品类型都包含在稳定性计划中。此外，你公司回复不包括整改稳定性计划的时间表。

In response to this letter, provide the following:

在回复本函时，请提供以下信息：

（略）

此处与 FDA 发给 Cosmobeauti Laboratories & Manufacturing Inc. 的警告信（编号：MARCS-CMS 657682，即"3 与非药用产品的共线生产问题"）中有关稳定性的回应要求部分的内容类似，故略去。

第四部分

生物制品

1 生物制品上市前未进行审批

警告信编号： MARCS-CMS 631303

签发时间： 2023-6-5；**公示时间：** 2023-7-25

签发机构： 药品质量业务二处（Division of Biological Products Operations Ⅱ）

公　　司： Stratus Biosystems，LLC dba CellGenuity Regenerative Science

所在国家 / 地区： 美国

主　　题： 偏差 /CFR/ 人类细胞、组织和细胞产品（HCT/Ps）的法规 [Deviations/CFR/Regulations for Human Cells，Tissues & Cellular Products（HCT/Ps）]

简　　介： 在 2021 年 10 月至 11 月期间，FDA 对位于得克萨斯州的一家公司进行了检查，检查对象是该公司生产的同种异体用途产品，包括羊水衍生产品，这些产品属于 21 CFR 中定义的人体细胞、组织或基于细胞或组织的产品（HCT/P）。根据 FD&C 法案，用于治疗人类疾病或病症的羊水产品通常被视为药品进行监管。而根据 PHS 法案的规定，这类产品在上市前需要进行审查和批准。因此，该公司的产品被视为药品和生物制品进行监管。FDA 指出，作为生物制品的药物必须具有有效的生物制品许可证（BLA），而许可证只有在产品被证明安全、纯净和有效后才会被颁发。在开发阶段，这类产品只有在申办人持有有效的研究性新药申请（IND）的情况下，才能被流通供人类临床使用。然而令人担忧的是，该公司的产品均未获得批准的 BLA，也没有有效的 IND。基于这些信息，FDA 认定该公司的行为违反了 FD&C 法案和 PHS 法案。

本警告信以下部分与本书此前其他警告信内容类似，故略去：结论（Conclusion）

During an inspection of your firm，Stratus Biosystems，LLC（dba CellGenuity Regenerative Science or CellGenuity），located at 913 S Main St，Ste 215，Grapevine，TX

76051-7575, conducted between October 26, 2021 and November 10, 2021, the United States Food and Drug Administration（FDA）documented your manufacture of products for allogeneic use, including an umbilical cord and amniotic membrane derived product, AmnioAMP-WJ™, and an amniotic fluid derived product, AmnioAllograft（collectively, "your products"）. You distribute your products to healthcare providers and facilities throughout the United States. These products are intended for injection and are purported to be sterile.

2021 年 10 月 26 日至 2021 年 11 月 10 日，FDA 对你公司 Stratus Biosystems, LLC（以下名义经营：dba CellGenuity Rgenesis Science 或 CellGenuity）进行检查，其位于得克萨斯州（略，见上）。检查期间，FDA 记录了你公司生产的同种异体用途产品，包括脐带和羊膜衍生产品 AmnioAMP-WJ™ 以及羊水衍生产品 AmnioAllograft（统称为"你公司产品"）。你公司产品流通向美国各地的医疗健康提供者和机构。这些产品用于注射，标识是无菌的。

Information and records gathered at the time of and after the inspection, including information regarding your products available online at cellgenuity.com, reflect that your products are intended to treat various diseases or conditions. Additionally, information collected indicates your products fit within the definition of a biological product in the Public Health Service Act（PHS Act）[42 U.S.C. 262（i）]. Your products are drugs as defined in section 201（g）of the Federal Food, Drug, and Cosmetic Act（FD&C Act）[21 U.S.C. 321（g）] and biological products as defined in section 351（i）of the Public Health Service Act.

检查时和检查后收集的信息和记录，包括 cellgenuity.com 上提供的有关你公司产品的信息，反映了其旨在治疗各种疾病或病症。此外，收集的信息表明，你公司产品符合《公共卫生服务法案》（PHS 法案）[42 U.S.C. 262（i）] 中生物制品的定义。你公司产品是《联邦食品、药品和化妆品法案》（FD&C 法案）201（g）条 [21 U.S.C. 321（g）] 界定的药品，以及《公共卫生服务法案》351（i）条 [42 U.S.C. 262（i）] 界定的生物制品。

Your product derived from both umbilical cord and amniotic membrane, AmnioAMP-WJ™, is also a human cell, tissue, or cellular or tissue-based product（HCT/P）as defined in 21 CFR 1271.3（d）and is subject to regulation under 21 CFR Part 1271, issued under the authority of section 361 of the PHS Act [42 U.S.C. 264]. HCT/Ps that do not meet all the criteria in 21 CFR 1271.10（a）, and when no exception in 21 CFR 1271.15 applies, are not regulated solely under section 361 of the PHS Act [42 U.S.C. 264] and the regulations in 21 CFR Part 1271. Such products are regulated as drugs, devices, and/or biological products under the FD&C Act and/or the PHS Act, and are subject to additional regulation, including appropriate premarket review.

你公司源自脐带和羊膜的产品 AmnioAMP-WJ™ 也是 21 CFR 1271.3（d）中定义的人体细胞、组织或基于细胞或组织的产品（HCT/P），并受 21 CFR 第 1271 部分的监管，该部分是根据 PHS 法案第 361 节 ［42 U.S.C. 264］的授权发布的。不符合 21 CFR 1271.10（a）中所有标准的 HCT/P，并且当 21 CFR 1271.15 中的例外情况不适用时，仅在 PHS 法案第 361 条 ［42 U.S.C. 264］和 21 CFR 第 1271 部分中的规定下，其不受监管。此类产品根据 FD&C 法案和（或）PHS 法案作为药物、医疗器械和（或）生物制品进行监管，并受到额外监管，包括适当的上市前审查。

Based on a review of materials described above, Stratus Biosystems, LLC does not qualify for any exception in 21 CFR 1271.15, and your HCT/P derived from umbilical cord and amniotic membrane fails to meet all the criteria in 21 CFR 1271.10（a）. Therefore, this HCT/P is not regulated solely under section 361 of the PHS Act ［42 U.S.C. 264］and the regulations in 21 CFR Part 1271.

根据对上述物料的审查，Stratus Biosystems, LLC 不符合 21 CFR 1271.15 中的任何例外条件，并且你公司源自脐带和羊膜的 HCT/P 不符合 21 CFR 1271.10（a）中的所有标准。因此，该 HCT/P 不仅仅受 PHS 法案第 361 条 ［42 U.S.C. 264］和 21 CFR 第 1271 部分的规定管辖。

Specifically, an HCT/P meets the criterion established by 21 CFR 1271.10（a）（2）if it is "intended for homologous use only, as reflected by the labeling, advertising, or other indications of the manufacturer's objective intent." AmnioAMP-WJ™ is not intended to perform the same basic function or functions of umbilical cord and amniotic membrane in the recipient as in the donor, such as serving as a conduit（for umbilical cord）or serving as a selective barrier for the movement of nutrients between the external and in utero environment, protecting the fetus from the surrounding maternal environment, and serving as a covering to enclose the fetus and retain fluid in utero（for amniotic membrane）. Rather, using your product to treat orthopedic diseases or conditions, for example, is not homologous use as defined in 21 CFR 1271.3（c）.

具体而言，如果 HCT/P "仅用于同源用途，如标签、广告或生产商客观意图的其他指示所反映的那样"，则该 HCT/P 符合 21 CFR 1271.10（a）（2）制定的标准。AmnioAMP-WJ™ 尤意在受体中发挥与供体相同的脐带和羊膜的基本功能，例如充当导管（用于脐带）；或作为营养物质在子宫外环境和子宫内环境之间移动的选择性屏障，保护胎儿免受周围母体环境的影响，并作为包裹胎儿和保留子宫内液体（用于羊膜）的覆盖物。相反的例子有，将你公司产品用于治疗骨科疾病或病症，这并不属于 21 CFR 1271.3（c）中定义的同源用途。

Be advised that the definition of HCT/Ps in 21 CFR 1271.3（d）excludes secreted or extracted human products. Accordingly, secreted bodily fluids, such as amniotic fluid, are generally not considered HCT/Ps subject to regulation under 21 CFR Part 1271. Amniotic fluid intended to treat diseases or conditions in humans is generally regulated as a drug under the FD&C Act and a biological product under the PHS Act and requires premarket review and approval. As such, your product derived from amniotic fluid, AmnioAllograft™, is regulated as a drug and biological product under section 351 of the PHS Act and the FD&C Act.

请注意，21 CFR 1271.3（d）中 HCT/P 的定义不包括分泌或提取的人类产品。因此，分泌的体液（例如羊水）通常不被视为受 21 CFR 第 1271 部分监管的 HCT/P。根据 FD&C 法案，用于治疗人类疾病或病症的羊水通常作为药品进行监管。产品符合 PHS 法案，需要上市前审查和批准。因此，根据 PHS 法案第 351 条和 FD&C 法案，你公司羊水衍生产品 AmnioAllograft™ 作为药品和生物制品进行监管。

To lawfully market a drug that is a biological product, a valid biologics license application（BLA）must be in effect [42 U.S.C. 262（a）]. Such licenses are issued only after showing that the product is safe, pure, and potent. While in the development stage, such products may be distributed for clinical use in humans only if the sponsor has an investigational new drug application（IND）in effect as specified by FDA regulations [21 U.S.C. 355（i）; 42 U.S.C. 262（a）（3）; 21 CFR Part 312]. None of your products are the subject of an approved BLA nor is there an IND in effect for any of them. Based on this information, we have determined that your actions have violated the FD&C Act and the PHS Act.

要合法销售属于生物制品的药品，必须具有有效的生物制品许可证 [42 U.S.C. 262（a）]。只有在证明产品安全、纯净和有效之后，才会颁发此类许可证。在开发阶段，只有在申办人按照 FDA 法规规定 [21 U.S.C. 355（i）; 42 U.S.C. 262（a）（3）; 21 CFR 第 312 部分]，在持有有效的研究性新药申请（IND）的情况下，这类产品才可以流通供人类临床使用。你公司产品均未获得批准的 BLA，也没有有效的 IND。根据这些信息，我们确定你公司的行为违反了 FD&C 法案和 PHS 法案。

Additionally, during the inspection, FDA investigators documented evidence of significant deviations from current good manufacturing practice（cGMP）requirements, including deviations from section 501（a）（2）（B）of the FD&C Act and 21 CFR Parts 210 and 211.

此外，在检查过程中，FDA 调查员记录了与现行药品生产质量管理规范（cGMP）要求存在严重不符合项的证据，包括与 FD&C 法案第 501（a）（2）（B）条以及 21 CFR 第 210 和 211 部分的偏差。

At the conclusion of the inspection, FDA investigators issued a Form FDA-483, List of Inspectional Observations, which described significant cGMP deviations applicable to your products. FDA identified additional significant deviations upon further review of the information collected during inspection, as discussed below. These deviations, involving over (b)(4) vials of your products manufactured since March 2019, include, but are not limited to, the following:

检查结束时，FDA 调查员发布了一份 FDA 483 表格（检查观察清单），其中描述了适用于你公司产品的重大 cGMP 偏差。FDA 在进一步审查检查期间收集到信息后，还发现了其他严重不符合项，如下所述。这些偏差涉及自 2019 年 3 月以来生产的超过（b）（4）瓶产品，包括但不限于以下内容。

无菌工艺验证

1. Failure to establish and follow appropriate written procedures designed to prevent microbiological contamination of drug products purporting to be sterile, including procedures for validation of all aseptic and sterilization processes [21 CFR 211.113(b)]. For example:

1. 未能建立并遵循适当的书面程序，包括验证所有无菌和灭菌工艺的程序，以防止声称无菌的药品受到微生物污染 [21 CFR 211.113(b)]。例如：

a. The aseptic processes used to manufacture your products have not been validated(i.e., by performing media fill simulations). By the nature of their routes of administration, your products purport to be sterile and are expected to be sterile.

a. 用于生产你公司产品的无菌工艺尚未经过验证（即通过执行培养基模拟灌装）。根据其给药途径的性质，你公司产品声称是无菌的，并且要求是无菌的。

b. You have not established appropriate written procedures for environmental monitoring in the aseptic processing areas where your products are manufactured. For example, you do not have written procedures that require surface sampling, personnel monitoring, viable air monitoring, and non-viable particulate monitoring to be performed in association with each production run. Such procedures are important to detect problems and demonstrate control of the aseptic processing areas.

b. 你公司尚未在生产产品的无菌工艺区建立适当的环境监测书面程序。例如，没有书面程序要求与每次生产运行相关的表面取样、人员监测、空气微生物监测和悬浮粒子监测。对于监测问题和确保无菌工艺区的控制来说，此类程序非常重要。

c. Your written gowning procedure for personnel who perform aseptic processing is inadequate to protect your products from contamination. For example, in accordance with your written procedure:

c. 你公司为执行无菌工艺操作的人员编写的更衣程序不足以保护产品免受污染。例如，按照你们的书面程序：

i. Personnel wear non-sterile gowning components, such as surgical masks and hairnets, while processing your products without any barrier between open products and personnel. Additionally, during the inspection, FDA investigators observed a technician with exposed skin processing your products.

i. 工作人员在加工产品时穿着非无菌的防护服套装组件，例如外科口罩和发网，开放的产品和人员之间没有任何屏障。此外，在检查过程中，FDA 调查员观察到一名操作员在处理产品的时候暴露了皮肤。

ii. Personnel don gowning in the unclassified shipping and receiving room prior to entering the cleanroom, which may increase the risk of introducing product contaminants.

ii. 进入洁净室之前，人员在无洁净级别的收发室中穿戴防护服，这可能会增加产品中引入污染物的风险。

d. You have not established and followed written procedures for the（b）（4）sterilization of the（b）（4）filter that comes into direct contact with your AmnioAllograft and AmnioAMP-WJ products during processing.

d. 你公司尚未制定并遵循书面程序，来对加工过程中与 AmnioAllograft 和 AmnioAMP-WJ 产品直接接触的（b）（4）过滤器进行（b）（4）灭菌。

环境监测

2. Failure to have an adequate system for cleaning and disinfecting the room and equipment to produce aseptic conditions［21 CFR 211.42（c）（10）（v）］. For example：

2. 没有充分的系统，对房间和设备进行清洁和消毒，以产生无菌条件［21 CFR 211.42（c）（10）（v）］。例如：

a. You have not validated your process for cleaning and disinfecting the cleanrooms, the critical processing areas where your products are manufactured.

a. 你公司尚未验证洁净室（你公司产品生产的关键加工区域）的清洁和消毒工艺。

b. According to your Standard Operating Procedure（SOP）SB-024 titled "Clean Environment Cleaning and Maintenance", your cleanrooms require cleaning with a（b）（4）only（b）（4）.（b）（4）-forming microorganisms are routinely detected in your environmental samples.

b. 根据标题为"清洁环境清洁和维护"的标准操作规程（SOP）SB-024，你公司洁净室需要仅使用（b）（4）进行清洁。（b）（4）产生的微生物通常会在你们的环境样品中检测到。

c. Standard Operating Procedure（SOP）SB-024 titled "Clean Environment Cleaning and Maintenance" lacks adequate instructions for cleaning and disinfection of your cleanrooms, including the disinfectant contact time and cleaning agents used. Additionally, this procedure does not require cleaning（b）（4）manufacture of batches nor is there data or rationale for the cleaning agents used.

c. 标题为"清洁环境清洁和维护"的标准操作规程（SOP）SB-024 缺乏有关洁净室清洁和消毒的充分说明，包括消毒剂接触时间和使用的清洁剂。此外，该规程不需要清洁（b）（4）批次生产，也没有所用清洁剂的数据或理论依据。

d. Your SOP SB-027 titled "Equipment Management and Cleaning" lacks adequate cleaning procedures for the equipment（e.g., incubators）used during aseptic processing operations, including but not limited to, use of a（b）（4）agent, frequency of disinfectants used, and disinfectant contact times. Additionally, this procedure does not address cleaning between batches.

d. 你公司标题为"设备管理和清洁"的 SOP SB-027 缺乏对无菌工艺操作期间使用的设备（例如培养箱）的适当清洁程序，包括但不限于（b）（4）试剂的使用、消毒剂的频率使用情况和消毒剂接触时间。此外，该程序不涉及批次之间的清洁。

质量标准

3. Failure to establish laboratory controls that include scientifically sound and appropriate specifications designed to assure that drug products conform to appropriate standards of identity, strength, quality, and purity [21 CFR 211.160（b）]. For example, you have not established scientifically sound and appropriate specifications and test procedures to assure that your products conform to appropriate standards of identity, strength, quality, and purity. Your finished product testing is limited to sterility testing and endotoxin testing as measurements of product attributes.

3. 未能建立实验室控制措施，其中包括科学合理和相应的质量标准，旨在确保药品符合适当的鉴别、规格、质量和纯度标准 [21 CFR 211.160（b）]。例如，你公司尚未建立科学合理且相应的质量标准和检验程序，以确保你公司产品符合适当的鉴别、规格、质量和纯度标准。你们的成品检验仅限于无菌检验和内毒素检测，将其作为产品属性的检验。

生产工艺验证

4. Failure to establish written procedures for production and process control designed to assure that the drug products have the identity, strength, quality, and purity they purport or are represented to possess［21 CFR 211.100（a）］. For example：

4. 未能建立书面的生产和过程控制程序，旨在确保药品具有其声称或陈述的鉴别、强度、质量和纯度［21 CFR 211.100（a）］。例如：

a. The manufacturing processes for your products have not been validated with respect to identity, strength, quality, and purity.

a. 你公司产品的生产工艺尚未在鉴别、强度、质量和纯度方面得到验证。

b. Prior to June 2021, you had not established written procedures for manufacturing AmnioAllograft™ or AmnioAMP-WJ™.

b. 2021 年 6 月之前，你公司尚未制定生产 AmnioAllograft™ 或 AmnioAMP-WJ™ 的书面程序。

调查不充分

5. Failure to thoroughly investigate any unexplained discrepancy, or the failure of a batch or any of its components to meet any of its specifications whether or not the batch has been already distributed，［21 CFR 211.192］. For example, you failed to thoroughly investigate the following sterility and environmental monitoring failures：

5. 无论批次是否已经流通，对于该批次或其原辅料无法解释的偏差、未能满足其质量标准，你公司未能进行彻底调查［21 CFR 211.192］。例如，你公司未能彻底调查以下无菌和环境监测不合格：

a. From January 2021 and November 2021, your firm has had approximately（b）（4）sterility failures and（b）（4）endotoxin failures；however, you did not conduct any investigations to determine root cause or determine if any other product lots/batches were affected by the failures. Examples of organisms identified in the sterility failures include *Cutibacterium acnes*, *Staphylococcus pasteuri*, and *Corynebacterium acnes*.

a. 从 2021 年 1 月到 2021 年 11 月，你公司大约发生了（b）（4）次无菌不合格和（b）（4）次内毒素不合格；但是没有进行任何调查，来确定根本原因，或确定是否有任何其他批次受其影响。在无菌检验中鉴别出的不合格微生物包括痤疮皮肤杆菌、巴氏葡萄球菌和痤疮棒杆菌等。

b. From July 2021 and August 2021, your firm has had approximately (b)(4) environmental monitoring failures in your critical processing areas where your products are manufactured. While you identified the contaminating organisms, you failed to provide evidence that you investigated these failures to determine the root cause, product impact, or corrective and preventative actions. Examples of organisms identified in your critical processing areas include Bacillus species non-anthracis, Paenbacillus species, and fungi.

b. 从 2021 年 7 月到 2021 年 8 月,在生产产品的关键加工区域中,你公司发生了大约 (b)(4) 次环境监测不合格。虽然你公司确定了污染微生物,但未能提供证据证明你们调查了这些不合格,以确定根本原因、产品影响或纠正和预防措施。在关键加工区域中发现的微生物包括非炭疽芽孢杆菌、类芽孢杆菌和真菌。

稳定性研究

6. Failure to establish and follow a written testing program designed to assess the stability characteristics of drug products and to use the results of such stability testing to determine appropriate storage conditions and expiration dates [21 CFR 211.166(a)]. Specifically, you assigned a (b)(4) – to (b)(4) –year expiration date to your products without stability testing.

6. 未能遵循适当的书面检验程序,以评估药品的稳定性特征;未能使用稳定性检验结果,来确定适当的储存条件和有效期 [21 CFR 211.166(a)]。具体来说,在未进行稳定性研究的情况下,你公司为产品指定了 (b)(4) 至 (b)(4) 年的效期。

We have reviewed your written response, dated December 2, 2021, to FDA's inspectional observations on the FDA-483 and have determined your response is inadequate to address the above-noted deficiencies. We acknowledge that you represent that "Stratus has stopped manufacture of products until such time as the FDA inspector observations can be addressed." We also acknowledge your statement that Stratus "has responded to the facts cited in the observation and formulated its plans for action upon the most similar applicable rules under 21 CFR 1271 et seq."

你公司于 2021 年 12 月 2 日针对 FDA 483 表格的检查观察项进行了书面回复,对此我们已审查,并确定你公司的回复不足以解决上述缺陷。我们知晓,你们声明 "Stratus 已停止生产产品,直到 FDA 检查员的观察项得到解决"。我们还知晓你们的如下声明,即 Stratus "已对观察中引用的事实做出回应,并根据 21 CFR 1271 及以下最相似的适用规则制定了行动计划。"

While you assert that your products should only be regulated under section 361 of the PHS Act, the available evidence shows that your products do not meet the relevant criteria. Your response also does not adequately address your failure to have an IND in effect to study your products and your lack of an approved BLA to lawfully market your products. As noted above, to lawfully market a drug that is also a biological product, a valid biologics license must be in effect [42 U.S.C. 262(a)]. Such licenses are issued only after a demonstration that the product is safe, pure, and potent. While in the development stage, such products may be distributed for clinical use in humans only if the sponsor has an investigational new drug application (IND) in effect for that product, as specified by FDA regulations, that covers such clinical use [21 U.S.C. 355(i); 42 U.S.C. 262(a)(3); 21 CFR Part 312].

虽然你公司声称产品应仅受 PHS 法案第 361 条的监管，但现有证据表明你公司产品不符合相关标准。你们的回复也没有充分解决未能拥有有效的 IND 来研究你公司产品，或者缺乏经批准的 BLA 来合法上市你公司产品的问题。如上所述，要合法上市同时也是生物制品的药品，必须持有有效的生物制品许可证 [42 U.S.C. 262(a)]。只有在证明产品安全、纯净和有效后，才会颁发此类许可证。在开发阶段，只有申办人对该产品具有有效的研究性新药申请（IND）（按照 FDA 法规的规定，涵盖此类临床用途），此类产品才可以流通用于人类临床用途 [21 U.S.C. 355(i)、42 U.S.C. 262(a)(3)、21 CFR 第 312 部分]。

Your response also does not address the quantity of product inventory you may still have at your facility and your plans for its disposition. Furthermore, your response does not describe actions you have taken or plan to take to address the impact of the above-noted cGMP deficiencies on your distributed products that carry a (b)(4) - to (b)(4) -year shelf life and were manufactured under the above-described conditions.

你公司回复也没有说明：你们设施中可能仍有的产品库存数量以及处置计划。此外，你公司回复未描述你们已经采取或计划采取的措施，以解决上述 cGMP 不足对已流通的产品所产生的影响。这些产品具有（b）（4）到（b）（4）年的效期，且是在上述描述的条件下生产的。

2 细胞产品的无菌保证问题

警告信编号： MARCS-CMS 638823

签发时间： 2023-6-21；**公示时间：** 2023-7-11

签发机构： 生物制品业务一处（Division of Biological Products Operations I）

公　　司： Row1 Inc. dba Regenative Labs

所在国家 / 地区： 美国

主　　题： 偏差 /CFR/ 人类细胞、组织和细胞产品（HCT/Ps）的法规 [Deviations/CFR/Regulations for Human Cells，Tissues & Cellular Products（HCT/Ps ）]

简　　介： 2022 年 3 月，FDA 对该公司进行了检查。FDA 注意到，该公司生产的源自人类脐带的细胞产品已经流通至美国各地的医生和医疗诊所。这些产品适用于多种给药途径，包括注射，并声称是无菌的。然而，FDA 指出该公司未能建立并遵循适当的书面程序，包括验证所有无菌和灭菌工艺的程序，以防止声称无菌的药品受到微生物污染的风险。在检查过程中，FDA 调查员观察到员工的行为未能充分预防产品受到微生物污染的情况。例如，在无菌操作期间，操作员未更换或消毒在 ISO 8 级别的走廊中佩戴的外层无菌手套。

本警告信以下部分与本书此前其他警告信内容类似，故略去：前言、结论（Conclusion）。

无菌工艺

1. Failure to establish and follow appropriate written procedures designed to prevent microbiological contamination of drug products purporting to be sterile，including procedures for validation of all aseptic and sterilization processes [21 CFR 211.113（ b ）]．For example：

1. 未能建立并遵循适当的书面程序，包括验证所有无菌和灭菌工艺的程序，以防止声称无菌的药品受到微生物污染［21 CFR 211.113（b）］。例如：

a. The aseptic processes used to manufacture your products have not been validated（e.g., by performing（b）（4））since your firm's manufacturing operations began in February 2020. Your products purport to be sterile and are expected to be sterile.

a. 自你公司于 2020 年 2 月开始生产操作以来，用于生产的无菌工艺尚未经过验证［例如，通过执行（b）（4）］。你公司产品声称是无菌的，并且要求是无菌的。

b. You have not established appropriate written procedures for environmental monitoring in your firm's aseptic processing area where your products are manufactured. For example：

b. 针对生产你公司产品的无菌工艺区，你们尚未建立适当的环境监测书面程序。例如：

i. Your action limits for microbiological monitoring（i.e., active viable air, surface samples, and personnel gloved fingertips）within the critical area（i.e., inside the biological safety cabinet（BSC））were observed to be（b）（4）colony forming units（CFUs）per m3, greater than（b）（4）CFUs per "plate and floor", and（b）（4）CFUs per plate, respectively. Such high numbers of microorganisms could contribute to product contamination and pose a potentially significant safety concern.

i. 观察到关键区域［即生物安全柜（BSC）内部］内微生物监测（即主动空气微生物取样、表面样品和人员戴手套的指尖）的行动限为每一立方米（b）（4）个菌落形成单位（CFU），分别大于（b）（4）每个"培养皿和地面"的 CFU 和（b）（4）每个培养皿的 CFU。存在如此大量的微生物，可能会导致产品污染，并造成潜在的重大安全问题。

ii. Your action limit for active viable air samples within the cleanroom was observed to be greater than or equal to（b）（4）CFUs per m3. Such high numbers of microorganisms could contribute to product contamination and also pose a potentially significant safety concern.

ii. 据观察，洁净室内空气微生物样品的行动限大于或等于（b）（4）CFU/m3。存在如此大量的微生物，可能会导致产品污染，并造成潜在的重大安全问题。

iii. You do not perform non-viable particulate monitoring, active or passive viable air sampling, or sampling of critical surfaces in the BSC for microorganisms in association with each production batch.

iii. 你公司没有对每个生产批次进行空气悬浮粒子监测、主动或被动空气微生物取样，或生物安全柜中关键表面的微生物取样。

c. During the inspection, FDA investigators observed personnel practices that do not adequately protect against microbiological contamination of your products. For example:

c. 在检查过程中，FDA 调查员观察到人员行为未能充分防止产品受到微生物污染。例如：

i. Operators were observed processing ProTextTM (ID：(b)(6), (b)(7)(C)) without changing or disinfecting the outer pair of sterile gloves donned in the ISO 8 hallway. Processing steps include (b)(4) of birth tissue, including removing debris and aseptic transfer of in-process material.

i. 据观察，在处理 ProTextTM［ID：(b)(6), (b)(7)(C)］时，操作员没有更换或消毒 ISO 8 走廊中佩戴的外层无菌手套。处理步骤包括 (b)(4) 分娩组织，包括清除碎片和在制品的无菌转移。

ii. Operators performing aseptic processing of ProTextTM (ID：(b)(6), (b)(7) (C)) were also observed repeatedly passing gloved hands and sleeves over containers of open, in-process umbilical cord tissue within the BSC as well as using gloved hands as a seal to cover open containers of in-process umbilical cord tissue during processing.

ii. 对于执行 ProTextTM［ID：(b)(6), (b)(7)(C)］的无菌处理的操作人员，观察到他们在生物安全柜内将戴手套的手和袖子反复经过敞开的、工艺中的脐带组织容器，以及在处理过程中使用戴手套的手封住敞开的脐带组织容器。

生产工艺验证

2. Failure to establish written procedures for production and process control designed to assure that the drug products have the identity, strength, quality, and purity they purport or are represented to possess［21 CFR 211.100 (a)］. Specifically, you have not validated the manufacturing processes for your products with respect to identity, strength, quality, and purity. For example, your validation for umbilical cord processing only included bioburden testing as a measurement of product attributes.

2. 未能建立书面的生产和过程控制程序，旨在确保药品具有其声称或陈述的鉴别、强度、质量和纯度［21 CFR 211.100 (a)］。具体来说，你公司尚未验证生产工艺，以针对产品的鉴别、强度、质量和纯度。例如，你们对脐带加工的验证仅包括微生物负荷检验，将其作为产品属性的衡量标准。

稳定性研究

3. Failure to establish and follow a written testing program designed to assess the stability characteristics of drug products and to use the results of such stability testing to determine appropriate storage conditions and expiration dates [21 CFR 211.166（a）]. Specifically, you assign a five-year expiration date to your products without supporting data regarding the stability characteristics of the products.

3. 未能遵循适当的书面检验程序，以评估药品的稳定性特征；未能使用稳定性检验结果，来确定适当的储存条件和有效期 [21 CFR 211.166（a）]。具体来说，你公司为产品指定了五年有效期，但没有相关稳定性特征的支持数据。

We have received and reviewed your written responses, dated April 20, 2022 and August 22, 2022, to FDA's inspectional observations on the Form FDA-483. We acknowledge that you represent that you have corrected the cGMP deficiencies documented on the FDA-483. However, the corrective actions described in your responses are not adequate to address the above-noted violations. For example, your response does not address your failure to validate your aseptic manufacturing process. Additionally, you contend that your manufacturing process does not require process validation, and your proposed stability study does not include all stability-indicating characteristics of your products. As another example, your revised gowning procedure indicates exam gloves should be removed in the ISO-7 cleanroom prior to performing a（b）（4）hand scrub and donning sterile gloves. We have concerns that this may result in exposure of skin in the aseptic processing area, which may increase the risk of contamination during the manufacturing process.

你公司于 2022 年 4 月 20 日和 2022 年 8 月 22 日对 FDA 483 表格的检查意见进行了书面回复，我们已收到并已审核。我们知晓，你公司声明已整改 FDA 483 表格中记录的 cGMP 缺陷。但是，你公司的回复中描述的整改措施不足以解决上述违规情况。例如，并未解决你们未能验证无菌生产工艺的问题。此外，你公司认为你们的生产工艺不需要工艺验证，并且提出的稳定性研究不包括产品的所有稳定性指示特性。再举一个例子，你公司修订后的更衣程序表明，在执行（b）（4）手部擦洗和戴上无菌手套之前，应在 ISO 7 洁净室中脱掉检查手套。我们担心这可能会导致无菌工艺区的皮肤暴露，从而可能增加生产工艺中的污染风险。

Additionally, your responses do not address your firm's continued manufacture and distribution of your products or your plans for disposition of your current inventory manufactured under the violative conditions outlined above.

此外，你公司的回复并未涉及你公司继续生产和流通产品，也未涉及你们对在上述违规条件下生产的当前库存的处置计划。

While you assert that your products should be regulated solely under section 361 of the PHS Act, as explained above, the available evidence shows that your products do not meet all the criteria in 21 CFR 1271.10(a) for regulation solely under section 361 of the PHS Act and the regulations in 21 CFR Part 1271. Your response also does not adequately address your failure to have an IND in effect to study your products addressed in this letter or your lack of an approved BLA to lawfully market your products. As noted above, to lawfully market a drug that is a biological product, a valid biologics license must be in effect [42 U.S.C. 262 (a)]. Such licenses are issued only after showing that the product is safe, pure, and potent. While in the development stage, such a product may be distributed for clinical use in humans only if the sponsor has an IND in effect for that product, as specified by FDA regulations, that covers such clinical use [21 U.S.C. 355(i); 42 U.S.C. 262(a)(3); 21 CFR Part 312].

虽然你公司声称产品应仅根据 PHS 法案第 361 条进行监管（如上所述），但现有证据表明，你公司产品不符合 21 CFR 1271.10(a)，即仅根据 PHS 法案第 361 条和 21 CFR 第 1271 部分进行监管的所有标准。你们的回复也没有充分解决你公司未能拥有有效的 IND 来研究你们的产品，或者缺乏经批准的 BLA 来合法上市你们的产品。如上所述，要合法上市属于生物制品的药品，必须持有有效的生物制剂品许可证 [42 U.S.C. 262(a)]。只有在证明产品安全、纯净和有效后，才会颁发此类许可证。在开发阶段，只有申办人对该产品具有有效的研究性新药申请（IND）（按照 FDA 法规的规定，涵盖此类临床用途），此类产品才可以流通用于人类临床用途 [21 U.S.C. 355(i)、42 U.S.C. 262(a)(3)、21 CFR 第 312 部分]。

3 未通过无菌检验，产品依然放行

警告信编号： MARCS-CMS 646353

签发时间： 2023-6-1；**公示时间：** 2023-8-1

签发机构： 生物制品业务一处（Division of Biological Products Operations I）

公　　司： RenatiLabs Inc.

所在国家 / 地区： 美国

主　　题： 偏差 /CFR/ 人类细胞、组织和细胞产品（HCT/Ps）的法规 [Deviations/CFR/Regulations for Human Cells，Tissues & Cellular Products（HCT/Ps）]

简　　介： 2022 年 8 月，FDA 对该公司进行了检查。该公司生产一种源自人类脐带的同种异体用途产品。该公司已将产品直接流通向美国各地的医生。这些产品旨在通过关节内注射或局部开放伤口进行给药，并声称是无菌的。然而，FDA 指出，该公司在产品放行方面存在严重问题。该公司未拒绝放行那些未符合既定标准、质量标准或任何其他相关质量控制标准的药品。FDA 注意到，根据其委托实验室的最终报告，某个批次的产品未通过无菌检验。尽管如此，该公司的质量代表和高级管理层却批准了这批产品的放行，并开始进行流通。在 FDA 对该公司进行检查时，已经有大量该批次产品售出。

本警告信以下部分与本书此前其他警告信内容类似，故略去：前言、结论（Conclusion）。

不符合质量标准

1. Drug products failing to meet established standards or specifications and any other relevant quality control criteria are not rejected［21 CFR 211.165（f）］. For example：

1. 对于不符合既定标准或质量标准以及任何其他相关质量控制标准的药品，并未被拒绝放行［21 CFR 211.165（f）］。例如：

You failed to reject WJMAX™ lot REN20210205 after this lot failed sterility testing, due to contamination with Staphylococcus epidermidis, according to the final report from your contract laboratory dated March 22, 2021. Your Quality Representative and Management with Executive Responsibility approved this lot for release for distribution on June 14, 2021, and June 22, 2021, respectively. You have sold numerous vials of this lot, as recently as（b）（4）.

根据你公司委托实验室2021年3月22日的最终报告，WJMAX™批次REN20210205未通过无菌检验，原因是表皮葡萄球菌污染，但你们未能拒绝放行。分别于2021年6月14日和2021年6月22日，你公司质量代表和高级管理层批准了该批次的放行，并用于流通。你们已销售大量该批次产品，最近已售出（b）（4）。

无菌和灭菌工艺验证

2. Failure to establish and follow appropriate written procedures designed to prevent microbiological contamination of drug products purporting to be sterile, including procedures for validation of all aseptic and sterilization processes［21 CFR 211.113（b）］. For example：

2. 未能建立并遵循适当的书面程序，包括验证所有无菌和灭菌工艺的程序，以防止声称无菌的药品受到微生物污染［21 CFR 211.113（b）］。例如：

a. Your firm failed to validate the aseptic process used to manufacture WJMAX™（i.e., by performing media fill simulations）. By the nature of its route of administration, and per your product labeling, your product purports to be sterile and is expected to be sterile.

a. 你公司未能验证用于生产WJMAX™的无菌工艺（即通过执行培养基模拟灌装）。根据其给药途径的性质以及你公司产品标签，其声称是无菌的并且要求是无菌的。

b. You failed to conduct environmental monitoring for any of the（b）（4）processing runs of WJMAX™ in the aseptic processing areas.

b. 就无菌工艺区中WJMAX™的所有（b）（4）加工活动，你公司未能进行环境监测。

生产工艺验证

3. Failure to establish written procedures for production and process control designed to assure drug products have the identity, strength, quality, and purity they purport or are represented to possess［21 CFR 211.100（a）］. For example：

3. 未能建立书面的生产和过程控制程序，旨在确保药品具有其声称或陈述的鉴别、强度、质量和纯度［21 CFR 211.100（a）］。例如：

The manufacturing process for WJMAX™ has not been validated with respect to identity, strength, quality, and purity.

WJMAX™ 的生产工艺尚未在鉴别、规格、质量和纯度方面得到验证。

实验室控制

4. Failure to establish laboratory controls that include scientifically sound and appropriate specifications, standards, sampling plans, and test procedures designed to assure that components, drug product containers, closures, in-process materials, labeling, and drug products conform to appropriate standards of identity, strength, quality, and purity［21 CFR 211.160（b）］. For example：

4. 未能建立实验室控制措施，其中包括科学合理且相应的规范、标准、取样计划和检验程序，旨在确保原辅料、药品容器、密封件、在制品、标签和药品符合适当标准下的鉴别、规格、质量和纯度［21 CFR 211.160（b）］。例如：

a. Sterility samples of WJMAX™ are stored at（b）（4）prior to sterility testing. Freezing in this manner has the potential to destroy any microbial content in the samples before testing; therefore, contamination, if present, may not be detected.

a. 在无菌检验之前，WJMAX™ 的无菌样品储存在（b）（4）中。以这种方式冷冻有可能在检验前破坏样品中的微生物水平；因此，如果存在污染，可能无法检测到。

b. You have not collected and tested sterility samples that are representative of the lot size. You have tested（b）（4）vials for sterility regardless of lot size, which may consist of as many as（b）（4）vials.

b. 你公司尚未收集和检验代表批次的无菌样品。无论批次如何，你们都检验（b）（4）个西林瓶的无菌性，即使批次可能包含多达（b）（4）个西林瓶。

批记录

5. Failure to prepare batch production and control records for each batch of drug product produced that include documentation that each significant step in the manufacture, processing, packing, or holding of the batch was accomplished [21 CFR 211.188(b)]. For example：

5. 你公司未能为每批药品准备批生产和控制记录，其中包括该批次生产、加工、包装或放置中每个重要步骤的完成情况[21 CFR 211.188(b)]。例如：

a. Your batch records do not include documentation of all investigations made according to 21 CFR 211.192. For example：

a. 你公司的批记录不包括根据 21 CFR 211.192 进行的所有调查的记录。例如：

i. Your batch record for WJMAX™ lot REN20210205 does not include documentation of any investigation into the sterility failure for this lot reported to you on March 22, 2021.

i. 你公司的 WJMAX™ 批次 REN20210205 的批记录：其未包含 2021 年 3 月 22 日向你们报告的该批次无菌不合格的任何调查记录。

ii. The batch record for WJMAX™ lot REN20210205 does not include documentation of any investigation into the umbilical cord described as "Slightly yellow in areas" under the "Abnormal/Additional Findings" section of the batch record. Your Quality Representative and Management with Executive Responsibility approved this lot for release for distribution on June 14, 2021, and June 22, 2021, respectively.

ii. WJMAX™ 批次 REN20210205 的批记录：针对批记录的"异常 / 其他发现项"段落下脐带"区域略黄"描述，未能包括任何调查记录。分别于 2021 年 6 月14 日和 2021 年 6 月 22 日，你公司质量代表和高级管理层批准了该批次的放行流通。

b. Your batch record for WJMAX™ does not include documentation of each significant step described in QP220.101a, "Wharton Jelly/Umbilical Cord Suspension Procedure"(dated 09/01/2020), such as the addition of (b)(4) for homogenization, the (b)(4)program used for tissue dissociation, and the (b)(4) as required for cryopreservation.

b. 你公司的 WJMAX™ 批记录：其未包括 QP220.101a 中描述的每个重要步骤的文件记录，QP220.101a 为"沃顿胶 / 脐带混悬程序"（日期为 2020 年 9 月 1 日），重要步骤例如有：添加（ b ）（ 4 ）进行匀浆、组织解离所使用的（ b ）（ 4 ）程序，以及冷冻保存所需的（b）(4)。

稳定性研究

6. Failure to establish and follow a written testing program designed to assess the stability characteristics of drug products and to use results of such stability testing to determine appropriate storage conditions and expiration dates [21 CFR 211.166 (a)]. For example：

6. 未能遵循适当的书面检验程序，以评估药品的稳定性特征；未能使用稳定性检验结果，来确定适当的储存条件和有效期 [21 CFR 211.166 (a)]。例如：

You assigned a four-year expiration date to batches of WJMAX™ without supporting stability testing data.

你公司为 WJMAX™ 批次指定了四年有效期，但没有支持性的稳定性检验数据。

FDA has reviewed your written response, dated September 1, 2022, to the inspectional observations on the Form FDA-483 issued at the conclusion of the inspection. The corrective actions described in your response are not adequate to address the above-noted violations. We note that some planned corrective actions did not include a timeline for completion and cannot be evaluated because of a lack of supporting documentation. Our concerns regarding your response to specific FDA-483 observations include but are not limited to, the following：

你公司于 2022 年 9 月 1 日对检查结束时发布的 FDA 483 表格中的检查意见做出了书面回复，对此 FDA 已进行审查。你公司回复中描述的整改措施不足以解决上述违规情况。我们注意到，一些计划的整改措施没有包括完成时间表，并且由于缺乏支持文件而无法评估。就你公司对 FDA 483 表格观察项的回复，我们对此存有疑问，包括但不限于以下内容：

a. In response to FDA-483 Observation 2, your proposal to "perform the tissue dispersion or reduction purely (b)(4)" or "quantify total protein" "if deemed necessary" would not alter the regulatory status of your product as a drug and biological product. Moreover, the method suitability test referenced in your response is insufficient to assure that your product has the identity, strength, quality, and purity it purports or is represented to possess as required by 21 CFR 211.100 (a).

a. 针对 FDA 483 表格观察项 2，你公司提出，"如果认为有必要时"，"以仅仅（b）(4）方式，进行组织弥散或还原""量化总蛋白"，这不会改变你公司产品的监管状态，即作为药品和生物制品监管。此外，你公司回复中引用了方法适用性检验，这不足以确保你们的产品具有其声称或表示具有 21 CFR 211.100 (a) 要求的鉴别、规格、质量和纯度。

b. In response to FDA-483 Observation 3, you state that storage of sterility samples at (b)(4)not affect detection of microbial contamination. FDA disagrees. There is no assurance that microorganisms, which may be weakened by the manufacturing process, would survive freezing and be reliably detected by sterility testing.

b. 针对 FDA 483 表格观察项 3，你公司声明，在（b）（4）处储存无菌性样品不会影响微生物污染的检测。对此，FDA 不同意。微生物可能因生产工艺而被弱化，无法保证其能够在冷冻中存活，并通过无菌检验可靠地检测到。

c. In response to FDA-483 Observation 5, you stated that you have a "robust system for environmental monitoring which is documented in[your]SOPs" and it was developed with(b) (4), a third-party microbiology lab. You also stated that your firm "intends to adhere to[your] robust environmental monitoring for future tissue processing" and that testing would be conducted(b)(4). Your environmental monitoring procedure provided during the inspection, QP 195.102 Air, Surface, & Personnel Environmental Monitoring, Revision 00(Effective Date 09/01/2020), is inadequate to detect problems and demonstrate control of the aseptic processing area. For example, this procedure does not specify the frequency of non-viable particulate monitoring, surface sampling, or use of settle plates to ensure this monitoring is performed in association with each production batch. Additionally, this procedure does not sufficiently address alert and action levels and the appropriate response to deviations from alert and action levels.

c. 针对 FDA 483 表格观察项 5，你公司表示你们拥有 "稳健的环境监测系统，并在 ［你公司的］SOP 中有规定"，且系统是与第三方微生物实验室（b）（4）开发的。你公司还表示 "此后，打算为组织工艺继续贯彻［你们这一］稳健的环境监测"，并且将进行检验（b）（4）。你公司在检查期间提供了环境监测程序，QP 195.102 空气、表面和人员环境监测，修订版 00（生效日期 2020 年 9 月 1 日），其不足以检测出问题并证明对无菌工艺区的控制。例如，该程序没有指定悬浮粒子监测、表面取样或使用沉降皿的频率，以确保与每个生产批次相关联地执行该监测。此外，该程序没有充分解决警戒限和行动限，以及对偏离警戒和行动限的适当回应。

Notably, your response does not address your firm's plans regarding product that has been distributed or that remains in inventory that was manufactured under the violative conditions noted above. We note, according to your firm's materials, your products carry a four-year shelf life.

值得注意的是，就已流通的产品或在上述违规条件下生产的库存中的产品，你公司的回复并未涉及相关计划。我们注意到，根据你公司的资料，产品有四年的有效期。

Regarding your plans to continue manufacturing and distributing your product, your response states, "RenatiLabs is committed to adhere to the compliance regime to process and deliver tissue products under section 361 of the FDA compliance regulations." As noted above, WJMAX™ is not regulated solely under section 361 of the PHS Act［42 U.S.C. 264］.

关于你公司继续生产和流通产品的计划，回复指出，"RenatiLabs 致力于遵守 FDA 合规法规第 361 条规定的合规制度，来加工和交付组织产品。"如上所述，WJMAX™ 不仅受 PHS 法案第 361 条（42 U.S.C. 264）的监管。

Your response states that you intend "to eventually engage in IRB and IND directed studies." As noted above, to lawfully market a drug that is a biological product, a valid biologics license must be in effect［42 U.S.C. 262（a）］. Such licenses are issued only after showing that the product is safe, pure, and potent. While in the development stage, such a product may be distributed for clinical use in humans only if the sponsor has an IND in effect as specified by FDA regulations［21 U.S.C. 355（i）; 42 U.S.C. 262（a）（3）; 21 CFR Part 312］.

你公司的回复表明，你们打算"最终参与 IRB 和 IND 定向研究"。如上所述，要合法上市属于生物制品的药品，必须持有有效的生物制品许可证［42 U.S.C. 262（a）］。只有在证明产品安全、纯净和有效后，才会颁发此类许可证。在开发阶段，只有申办人对该产品具有有效的研究性新药申请（IND）（按照 FDA 法规的规定），此类产品才可以流通用于人类临床用途［21 U.S.C. 355（i）; 42 U.S.C. 262（a）（3）; 21 CFR 第 312 部分］。

4 偏差调查不完善

警告信编号： MARCS-CMS 657085

签发时间： 2023-9-14；**公示时间：** 2023-9-29

签发机构： 生物制品业务一处（Division of Biological Products Operations I）

公　　司： Fresenius Kabi AG

所在国家/地区： 德国

主　　题： cGMP 偏差（cGMP Deviations）

简　　介： 该集团是一家成立于 1912 年的德国医疗技术公司，总部位于黑森州巴特洪堡。作为《财富》杂志评选的全球 500 强企业之一，该集团也是德国最大的制药公司和私立医院运营商。FDA 对其在波多黎各的子公司进行了检查。在检查期间，FDA 调查员发现了该公司生产血包单位和血液相关产品过程中严重偏离了 cGMP 要求。FDA 指出，该公司未能按照已建立并获得批准的书面程序操作，对于那些存在未解释差异的批次或其原辅料，以及未能达到其质量标准的情况，该公司没有进行适当的全面调查。具体来说，在 2021 年至 2022 年产品年度回顾期间，在约 28 个批次的最终灭菌产品，其料液或称为"未灭菌成品"中采集的样品超出了微生物负荷行动限。大约有 21 个批次的结果被认为是多不可计（TNTC）。此外，约有 31 批次的未灭菌成品超出了孢子计数行动限。截止 FDA 检查时，该公司对这些偏差的调查并不完善，因调查没有包括对根本原因的全面评估，尽管这些批次已经被放行。

本警告以下部分与本书此前其他警告信内容类似，故略去：结论（Conclusion）

The United States Food and Drug Administration（FDA）conducted an inspection of your firm, Fenwal International, Inc.（a Fresenius Kabi company）, located at Road 357, Km 0.8, Maricao, PR 00606, between September 12, 2022 and September 24, 2022. During the inspection, the FDA investigators documented significant deviations from current good manufacturing practice（cGMP）requirements in the manufacture of your blood-pack units （BPUs）with and without in-line leukoreduction filters, as well as Alyx component solutions, Amicus component solutions, and InterSol, a platelet additive solution（collectively, "your products" or "your terminally sterilized products"）*1*. These deviations from cGMP requirements include failure to conform to applicable requirements of Section 501（a）（2）（B） of the Federal Food, Drug, and Cosmetic Act（FD&C Act）［21 U.S.C. § 351（a）（2）（B）］ and Title 21, Code of Federal Regulations（21 CFR）, Parts 210 and 211.

2022 年 9 月 12 日至 9 月 24 日期间，FDA 对你公司 Fenwal International, Inc. 进行了检查，该公司位于波多黎各（详细地址略，见上）。在检查期间，FDA 调查员记录了你公司在制造含和不含离线白细胞减少过滤器的血包单位（BPU），以及 Alyx 组分溶液，Amicus 组分溶液和 InterSol（一种血小板添加剂溶液）（以下统称为"你公司产品"或"你公司最终灭菌产品"）的过程中，与 cGMP 要求存在显著偏差。这些与 cGMP 要求的偏差包括：未能遵守《联邦食品、药品和化妆品法案》（FD&C 法案）［21 U.S.C. 351（a）（2）（B）］，以及《联邦法规》第 21 篇（21 CFR），第 210 和 211 部分。

At the close of the inspection, FDA issued and discussed with your firm a Form FDA-483, List of Inspectional Observations, which described significant deviations from cGMP requirements noted during the inspection. FDA identified additional significant deviations upon further review of the information collected during the September 2022 inspection, as discussed below. The cGMP deviations include, but are not limited to, the following:

检查结束时，FDA 发布并与你公司讨论了 FDA 483 表格（检查观察清单），其中描述了检查期间发现的与 cGMP 要求的重大偏差。在进一步审查 2022 年 9 月检查期间收集的信息后，FDA 发现了其他重大偏差，如下所述。cGMP 偏差包括但不限于以下内容。

调查不充分

1. Failure to follow established, approved written procedures and thoroughly investigate any unexplained discrepancy or the failure of a batch or any of its components to meet any of its specifications, whether or not the batch has already been distributed［21 CFR 211.192］. Specifically:

1. 未按照已建立并批准的书面程序进行操作，无论批次是否已经流通，对于该批次或其原辅料无法解释的偏差，未能满足其质量标准，你公司未能进行彻底调查［21 CFR 211.192］。具体来说：

a. During the annual product review periods ranging from January 01, 2021 to February 28, 2022, approximately 28 batches/lots of your terminally sterilized products exceeded your firm's action limit for bioburden samples taken from bulk solutions(i.e., "mixing tanks")or "finished unsterilized units." Results for approximately 21 lots were considered too numerous to count(TNTC). Additionally, approximately 31 lots of finished unsterilized units exceeded the spore count action limit. At the time of the inspection, your investigations into these excursions were not thorough because the investigations did not include an evaluation to determine the root cause, although batches had been released.

a. 在 2021 年 1 月 1 日至 2022 年 2 月 28 日的产品年度回顾期间，在约 28 个批次的最终灭菌产品，其料液（即"混合罐"）或"未灭菌成品"中采集的样品超出了的微生物负荷行动限。 约 21 个批次的结果被认为多不可计（TNTC）。此外，约 31 批次未灭菌成品超出了孢子计数行动限。截至检查时，你公司对这些偏差的调查并不彻底，因为调查没有包括确定根本原因的评估，尽管批次已经放行。

b. Your firm does not investigate "swarming organisms" as a TNTC result, as required by your established, written *Procedure for Plate Counting of Microbiological Samples* applicable to bioburden testing, water testing, and environmental monitoring among other tests.

b. 你公司未按照已建立的、书面的《微生物样品的平板计数程序》的要求，对"游走菌"TNTC 结果进行调查，该程序适用于生物负荷测试、水质测试、环境监测等其他检验。

Your firm's failure to conduct adequate failure investigations is a repeat deficiency noted during our 2010, 2012, 2013 and 2021 inspections.

你公司未能进行充分的调查，这是我们在 2010 年、2012 年、2013 年和 2021 年检查期间所注意到的重复缺陷。

产品放行

2. Failure to test in-process materials for identity, strength, quality, and purity, as appropriate, and approve or reject by the quality control unit, during the production process [21 CFR 211.110(c)]. For example, your firm failed to reject lots of your bulk solutions (i.e., "mixing tanks")and finished unsterilized units with in-process bioburden results of TNTC.

2. 在生产过程中，质量控制部门未能对中间物料酌情检验鉴别、规格、质量和纯度，以及批准或拒收[21 CFR 211.110(c)]。例如，对于微生物负荷结果为 TNTC 的料液（即"混合罐"）或"未灭菌成品"批次，你公司未能拒放。

灭菌前微生物污染水平

3. Failure to establish and follow appropriate written procedures designed to prevent microbiological contamination of drug products purporting to be sterile, including procedures for validation of all aseptic and sterilization processes [21 CFR 211.113（b）]. For example：

3. 未能建立并遵循适当的书面程序，包括验证所有无菌和灭菌工艺的程序，以防止声称无菌的药品受到微生物污染 [21 CFR 211.113（b）]。例如：

a. Your firm has failed to establish that your sterilization process can achieve your established minimum sterility assurance level（SAL）of（b）（4）when TNTC bioburden levels are present in your finished unsterilized units.

a. 就未灭菌成品中存在 TNTC 微生物负荷水平的情况，你公司未能确定你们的灭菌工艺可以达到（b）（4）的既定最低无菌保证水平（SAL）。

b. Your firm has failed to establish and follow appropriate written procedures to prevent microbiological contamination of finished units of your products prior to terminal sterilization. Bioburden control is critical for preventing a challenge to your validated sterilization process and to minimize bioburden-associated byproducts.

b. 你公司未能建立并遵循适当的书面程序，来防止最终灭菌之前成品受到微生物污染。微生物负荷控制对于防止已验证灭菌工艺受到挑战，并最大限度地减少与微生物负荷相关的副产品来说至关重要。

消毒灭菌

4. Failure to clean, maintain, and, as appropriate for the nature of the drug, sanitize and/or sterilize equipment and utensils at appropriate intervals to prevent contamination that would alter the safety, identity, strength, quality, or purity of the drug product beyond the official or other established requirements [21 CFR 211.67（a）]. For example：

4. 未能根据药品的性质，按照适当的时间间隔，对设备和器具进行消毒和（或）灭菌，以防止污染，从而改变药品的安全性、鉴别、规格、质量、纯度，使其超过药典或其他既定要求 [21 CFR 211.67（a）]。例如：

a. Inspection of filling module（b）（4）on September 13, 2022, revealed an approximate two-inch hole on top of the HEPA box, broken edges and residue on the diffusion grate above the filling nozzles, tubing ports with missing tubing connections, and brown residue on filling equipment surfaces near the filling nozzle. This filling area is used to manufacture Amicus component solutions, Alyx component solutions, and Intersol.

a. 2022 年 9 月 13 日对灌装模具（b）(4)进行的检查发现，HEPA 盒顶部有一个大约两英寸的孔，灌装喷嘴上方的扩散格栅上有破损的边缘和残留物，管道端口缺少管道连接，灌装喷嘴附近的灌装设备表面上有棕色残留物。该灌装区用于生产 Amicus 组分溶液、Alyx 组分溶液和 Intersol。

b. Inspection of mixing room (b)(4) on September 22, 2022, revealed apparent black growth on room-supply HEPA filters and black residue inside mixing tank(b)(4).

b. 2022 年 9 月 22 日对混合室（b）(4)进行检查，发现供应房间的 HEPA 过滤器上有明显的黑色生长物，混合罐（b）(4)内有黑色残留物。

厂房状态

5. Failure to maintain buildings used in the manufacture, processing, packing, or holding of drug products in a good state of repair [21 CFR 211.58]. For example, FDA's inspection of mixing room(b)(4)revealed gaps in the ceiling that connect to the unclassified utility space, cracked and peeling surfaces on the floors and walls, flaking paint on the ceiling near air return vents, and a tarp collecting pooling water in the ceiling space approximately fifty feet from filling room(b)(4). It is essential that your facility is in a good state of repair to protect drug products from potential routes of contamination.

5. 未能使用于生产、加工、包装或储存药品的厂房保持良好的维修状态 [21 CFR 211.58]。例如，FDA 对混合室（b）(4)的检查发现：天花板上有与无洁净级别公用设施场所有相连的缝隙、地板和墙壁上出现了裂纹和脱落的表面、回风口附近的天花板上出现了剥落的油漆，以及一个防水布在离灌装室（b）(4)约五十英尺的天花板空间汇集积水。你公司的设施必须处于良好的维修状态，以保护药品免受潜在污染途径的影响。

质量标准

6. Failure to establish laboratory controls that include scientifically sound and appropriate specifications, standards, and test procedures designed to assure that components, in-process material, and drug products conform to appropriate standards of identity, strength, quality, and purity [21 CFR 211.160(b)]. For example：

6. 未能建立实验室控制措施，其中包括科学合理和相应的质量标准，旨在确保药品符合适当的鉴别、规格、质量和纯度标准 [21 CFR 211.160(b)]。

a. Your approach to calculating the SAL for lots of finished unsterilized units of your products with TNTC pre-sterilization bioburden results is not scientifically sound. Your firm calculated the SAL using a value of (b)(4) when the results obtained were TNTC. As noted by your firm during the inspection, TNTC is not a number and cannot be used to calculate the SAL. Your firm has used this erroneous calculation to determine the impact of TNTC results on the sterility assurance of the involved lots.

a. 你公司使用 TNTC 预灭菌微生物负荷结果，来计算大量未灭菌成品单位的 SAL，这一方法在科学上并不合理。当获得的结果为 TNTC 时，你公司使用（b）(4) 值计算 SAL。正如你公司在检查期间指出的，TNTC 不是数字，不能用于计算 SAL。但你公司使用此错误计算，来确定 TNTC 结果对相关批次无菌保证的影响。

b. You did not conduct a study to demonstrate the suitability of your bioburden test method for Anticoagulant Citrate Dextrose Solution, USP, Formula A (ACD-A) that demonstrates your ability to detect a variety of organisms in the presence of ACD-A. Your bacteriostatic study, performed in 1988, only included Bacillus subtilis and Candida Albicans as test organisms. ACD-A is one of your Alyx and Amicus component solutions.

b. 你公司没有对抗凝枸橼酸葡萄糖溶液 USP 处方 A（ACD-A）的微生物负荷检验方法进行研究，来证明其适用性，从而说明你们在 ACD-A 存在的情况下检测多种微生物的能力。你公司于 1988 年进行的抑菌研究仅包括枯草芽孢杆菌和白色念珠菌作为检验微生物。ACD-A 是 Alyx 和 Amicus 组分溶液之一。

c. During the inspection, our investigator observed microbial growth over the majority of the test plate and around the perimeter with no defined edges for bioburden tank sample 71643 for Citrate Phosphate Dextrose (CPD) bulk solution. Your Quality Manager stated that the observed plate growth would only be documented as 1 CFU. CPD is part of your BPU product.

c. 在检查过程中，我们的调查员观察到，就枸橼酸磷酸酯葡萄糖（CPD）料液的微生物负荷罐样品 71643，大部分检验皿都有微生物生长，出现在周边且没有明确的边缘。你公司质量经理表示，对于观察到的培养皿生长，只会记录为 1 CFU。CPD 是 BPU 产品的一部分。

We acknowledge receipt of your letters dated October 17, 2022, November 14, 2022, December 16, 2022, January 19, 2023, February 14, 2023, March 17, 2023, April 17, 2023, May 12, 2023, and July 25, 2023, which respond to the Form FDA-483 and set forth your corrective actions. We have reviewed your represented corrective actions. For some of your corrective actions, you have not provided sufficient detail to assess their adequacy. For example, your firm has not provided sufficient evidence that corrective actions to reduce bioburden in mixing tanks and filled units are effective. More notably, your commitments do not adequately resolve your recurring violations, including your firm's failure to conduct adequate failure investigations.

我们知晓并收到你公司于 2022 年 10 月 17 日、2022 年 11 月 14 日、2022 年 12 月 16 日、2023 年 1 月 19 日、2023 年 2 月 14 日、2023 年 3 月 17 日、2023 年 4 月 17 日、2023 年 5 月 12 日和 2023 年 7 月 25 日的来信，对 FDA 483 表格做出回应，并阐述你公司的整改措施。我们已审查了你们所提出的整改措施。你公司没有提供充分的细节来评估一些整改措施的充分性。例如，没有提供充分的证据，来证明减少混合罐和已灌装单元中微生物负荷的整改措施是有效的。更值得注意的是，你公司的承诺并不能充分解决你们反复出现的违规情况，包括你公司未能进行充分的不合格调查。

Your firm, including your quality unit, continuously has failed to adequately correct your violations and—for those violations that FDA has observed during previous inspections—prevent their recurrence. Indeed, the nature of your violations demonstrates that your quality control unit has failed to ensure that your firm manufactures drug products that meet established specifications for identity, strength, quality, and purity.

你公司，包括你们的质量部门，一直未能充分整改违规情况，并且对于 FDA 在之前的检查中发现的违规情况，也未能防止其再次发生。事实上，你公司的违规情况表明质量控制部门未能确保所生产的药品符合既定的鉴别、规格、质量和纯度质量标准。

Additionally, the cGMP deviations cited in this letter pose a significant risk that the products may be contaminated with microorganisms. We note that organisms previously recovered in your facility and bioburden samples of your products were genetically matched to isolates from clinical cases of septic reactions involving Acinetobacter species and Staphylococcus saprophyticus. In addition, an instance of TNTC in bioburden testing occurred in Amicus lot（b）（4）, which was used to collect platelets implicated in a septic transfusion reaction. More recently, according to your April 2023 response, *Acinetobacter baumanni* was recovered from a tank used for Amicus lot（b）（4）on March 24, 2023, and an environmental monitoring sample on November 01, 2022.

此外，本函中引用的 cGMP 偏差构成了产品可能被微生物污染的重大风险。我们注意到，之前在你公司的设施中回收到微生物和你公司产品样品中存在微生物负荷，这与来自涉及不动杆菌属和腐生葡萄球菌的败血症反应临床病例的分离株在基因上相匹配。此外，微生物负荷检验中的 TNTC 实例发生在 AMICUS 批次（b）（4）中，该批次用于收集与败血性输血反应有关的血小板。最近，根据你公司 2023 年 4 月的回复，鲍曼不动杆菌是在 2023 年 3 月 24 日和 2022 年 11 月 1 日分别从 Amicus 批次（b）（4）使用的储罐中和环境监测样品中回收到的。

5 培养基模拟灌装的灌装数量不足

警告信编号： MARCS-CMS 631039

签发时间： 2023-9-18；**公示时间：** 2023-9-29

签发机构： 药品质量业务二处（Division of Biological Products Operations Ⅱ）

公　　司： Signature Biologics，LLC

所在国家／地区： 美国

主　　题： 偏差/CFR/人类细胞、组织和细胞产品（HCT/Ps）的法规［Deviations/CFR/Regulations for Human Cells，Tissues & Cellular Products（HCT/Ps）］

简　　介： 在 2021 年 12 月，FDA 对该公司进行了检查。该公司生产一种源自人类脐带的同种异体用途产品。在警告信中，FDA 首先指出公司未能建立并遵循适当的书面程序，以防止声称无菌的药品受到微生物污染。公司未能充分验证用于生产他们产品的无菌工艺，因为用于验证研究的培养基灌装批次不能代表最大商业批量。此外，该公司在环境监测、质量标准、热原检验、工艺与清洁验证和稳定性研究等方面存在严重的 cGMP 缺陷。

本警告信以下部分与本书此前其他警告信内容类似，故略去：前言、结论（Conclusion）。

无菌和灭菌工艺验证

　　1. Failure to establish and follow appropriate written procedures designed to prevent microbiological contamination of drug products purporting to be sterile［21 CFR 211.113（b）］. Your firm failed to adequately validate the aseptic processes used to manufacture your Signature Cord™ product in that the media fill batches used for your validation studies did not

represent the maximum commercial batch size. For example, your validation studies entitled "Aseptic Processing Validation Report—Signature Cord" utilized a maximum of (b)(4) vials per batch. However, from November 2018 through February 2020, your firm manufactured (b)(4) commercial batches of Signature Cord™ with (b)(4) vials.

1. 未能建立并遵循适当的书面程序，以防止声称无菌的药品受到微生物污染［21 CFR 211.113（b）］。你公司未能充分验证用于生产你公司产品（ Signature Cord™ ）的无菌工艺，因为用于验证研究的培养基灌装批次并不代表最大商业批量。例如，你公司验证研究标题为"无菌工艺验证报告 – Signature Cord"，其中每批次最多使用（b）（4）瓶。然而，从 2018 年 11 月到 2020 年 2 月，你公司生产了（b）（4）商业批次的 Signature Cord™，其批量（b）（4）瓶。

环境监测

2. Failure to have an adequate system for monitoring environmental conditions in an aseptic processing area［21 CFR 211.42（c）（10）（iv）］. Your firm has not established an adequate system for environmental monitoring in the aseptic processing areas where your products are manufactured. For example:

2. 没有充分的系统，来监测无菌工艺区的环境条件［21 CFR 211.42（c）（10）（iv）］。针对生产产品的无菌工艺区，你公司尚未建立适当的环境监测系统。例如：

a. You have not performed microbiological monitoring of viable air in the ISO 7 supporting cleanrooms in association with each production run.

a. 对于 ISO 7 支持的洁净室中与每次生产周期相关的空气，你公司尚未进行微生物监测。

b. Your environmental monitoring procedure describes the following as acceptable results for microbiological monitoring: (b)(4) colony forming units (CFUs) for surfaces within the ISO 7 supporting cleanrooms, (b)(4) CFUs for settling plate samples within the ISO 7 supporting cleanrooms, (b)(4) CFUs for personnel glove samples within the ISO 7 supporting cleanrooms, and (b)(4) CFUs for personnel garment samples within the ISO 7 supporting cleanrooms. Your allowance for such high numbers of microorganisms could contribute to product contamination and pose a potentially significant safety concern.

b. 在你公司的环境监测程序中，将以下内容描述为可接受的微生物监测结果：ISO 7 支持性洁净室表面 ——（b）（4）菌落形成单位（CFU），ISO 7 支持性洁净室内的沉降皿样品——（b）（4）CFU，ISO 7 支持性洁净室中人员手套样品——（b）（4）CFU，以及 ISO 7 支持性洁净室中人员服装样品——（b）（4）CFU。允许如此大量的微生物数量可能会导致产品污染，并造成潜在的重大安全问题。

质量标准

3. Laboratory controls do not include the establishment of scientifically sound and appropriate specifications designed to assure that the drug products conform to appropriate standards of identity, strength, quality, and purity [21 CFR 211.160 (b)]. For example, at the time of the inspection, your finished product testing was limited to sterility testing as a measurement of product attributes.

3. 实验室控制未能包括建立科学合理且相应的质量标准，旨在确保药品符合适当的鉴别、规格、质量和纯度标准 [21 CFR 211.160 (b)]。例如，在检查时，你公司的成品检验仅限于无菌检验，将其作为产品属性的衡量标准。

热原检验

4. Each of batch of drug product purporting to be pyrogen-free is not laboratory tested to determine conformance to such requirements [21 CFR 211.167 (a)]. For example, your firm failed to perform endotoxin testing as a release criterion on (b) (4) units of Signature Cord™ product manufactured and distributed by your firm since November 2018. By the nature of the route of administration, your product is purported to be pyrogen-free and is expected to be pyrogen-free.

4. 对于声称无热原的每批药品，其均未经过实验室检验，以确定是否符合此类要求 [21 CFR 211.167 (a)]。例如，自 2018 年 11 月以来，对于生产和流通的 (b) (4) 件 Signature Cord™ 产品，你公司未进行内毒素检测，以将其作为放行标准。根据给药途径的性质，你公司产品声称无热原，并且要求无热原。

工艺验证

5. Failure to establish written procedures for production and process controls designed to assure that the drug products have the identity, strength, quality, and purity they purport or are represented to possess [21 CFR 211.100 (a)]. For example, the manufacturing process for your product has not been validated.

5. 未能建立书面的生产和过程控制程序，旨在确保药品具有其声称或陈述的鉴别、强度、质量和纯度 [21 CFR 211.100 (a)]。例如，你公司产品的生产工艺尚未经过验证。

清洁验证

6. Failure to have an adequate system for cleaning and disinfecting the room and equipment to produce aseptic conditions [21 CFR 211.42 (c)(10)(v)]. For example, at the time of the inspection, you had not validated your process for cleaning and disinfecting the Biological Safety Cabinets (BSCs) and supporting cleanrooms where your product was manufactured.

6. 没有充分的系统，对房间和设备进行清洁和消毒，以产生无菌条件[21 CFR 211.42 (c)(10)(v)]。例如，在检查时，你公司没有验证生产你公司产品的生物安全柜（BSC）和辅助洁净室的清洁和消毒的工艺。

稳定性研究

7. Failure to establish a written testing program designed to assess the stability characteristics of drug products and to use results of such stability testing to determine appropriate storage conditions and expiration dates [21 CFR 211.166 (a)]. Specifically, you assigned a two-year expiration date to your product without supporting data.

7. 未能遵循适当的书面检验程序，以评估药品的稳定性特征；未能使用稳定性检验结果，来确定适当的储存条件和有效期[21 CFR 211.166 (a)]。具体来说，你公司在没有支持数据的情况下为产品指定了两年的有效期。

FDA received your written responses dated January 10, 2022, March 1, 2022, April 1, 2022, May 24, 2022, June 30, 2022, August 31, 2022, and November 2, 2022, to the inspectional observations on the Form FDA-483. The corrective actions described in your responses are not adequate to address the above-referenced deficiencies. We note that certain corrective actions cannot be evaluated because they lack supporting documentation. In addition, your responses do not address your specific plans for disposition of the inventory of Signature Cord™ at your facility. Additionally, for your previously distributed product, you do not describe actions you have taken or plan to take that adequately address the impact of the above-noted deficiencies on your distributed product that carries a two-year shelf life and was manufactured under the above-described conditions.

于 2022 年 1 月 10 日、2022 年 3 月 1 日、2022 年 4 月 1 日、2022 年 5 月 24 日、2022 年 6 月 30 日、2022 年 8 月 31 日和 2022 年 11 月 2 日，你公司对 FDA 483 表格上的检查意见进行了书面回复，对此 FDA 已收到。你公司回复中描述的整改措施不足以解决上述缺陷。我们注意到，因其缺乏支持性记录，某些整改措施无法评估。此外，你公司的回复并未涉及如何处置 Signature Cord™ 库存的具体计划。此外，对于之前流通的产品，你公司没有描述已经采取或计划采取的措施，以充分解决上述缺陷对你公司流通产品的影响，该产品的有效期为两年，并且是在上述描述的条件下生产的。

We acknowledge your commitment to voluntarily suspend the manufacture and distribution of Signature Cord™. However, your responses do not adequately address your failure to have an IND in effect to study your product addressed in this letter or your lack of an approved BLA to lawfully market your product. As noted above, to lawfully market a drug that is a biological product, a valid biologics license must be in effect [42 U.S.C. 262(a)]. Such licenses are issued only after showing that the product is safe, pure, and potent. While in the development stage, such a product may be distributed for clinical use in humans only if the sponsor has an IND in effect for that product, as specified by FDA regulations, that covers such clinical use [21 U.S.C. 355(i); 42 U.S.C. 262(a)(3); 21 CFR Part 312].

我们知晓，你公司承诺自愿暂停生产和流通 Signature Cord™。然而，你公司的回复并没有充分解决你们未能拥有有效的 IND 来研究你公司产品，或者你们缺乏经批准的 BLA 来合法上市你公司产品。如上所述，要合法上市属于生物制品的药品，必须持有有效的生物制品许可证 [42 USC 262(a)]。只有在证明产品安全、纯净和有效后，才会颁发此类许可证。在开发阶段，只有申办人对该产品具有有效的研究性新药申请（IND）（按照 FDA 法规的规定，涵盖此类临床用途），此类产品才可以流通用于人类临床用途 [21 U.S.C. 355(i)、42 U.S.C. 262(a)(3)、21 CFR 第 312 部分]。

第五部分

无菌制剂

1 眼科药品未满足无菌要求

警告信编号： MARCS-CMS 648269

签发时间： 2023-4-28；**公示时间：** 2023-5-16

签发机构： 药品质量业务四处（Division of Pharmaceutical Quality Operations IV）

公　　司： Pharmedica USA, LLC

所在国家 / 地区：美国

主　　题： cGMP/ 成品制剂 / 掺假（cGMP/Finished Pharmaceuticals/ Adulterated）

摘　　要： 2022 年 11 月，FDA 对该药品生产设施进行了检查。调查员指出，该公司生产的药品被设计或预期为无菌，但在不卫生的条件下制备、包装或放置，这可能导致药品被污染或对健康有害。因此，根据 FD&C 法案，这些药品被视为掺假。举例来说，调查员观察到设施缺乏用于无菌药品生产的 ISO 洁净区域，同时也发现设施年久失修。在检查期间，该公司告知 FDA，他们并不了解眼科药品需要无菌条件，同时也承认他们的设施没有相应的设计和设备，用于处理或生产无菌药品，尽管他们的药品被标识为"眼药水"。随后，在 2023 年 2 月，FDA 与该公司举行了电话会议。FDA 建议该公司考虑下架目前在美国市场上市的相关产品。随后，在 2023 年 3 月，该公司自愿在全球范围内召回了这些产品，因为这些药品未能达到无菌标准。公司也承诺停止在该设施生产所有药品。

本警告信以下部分与本书此前其他警告信内容类似，故略去：结论（Conclusion）。

Insanitary Conditions ｜ 不卫生条件

The FDA investigator noted that drug products intended or expected to be sterile were prepared, packed, or held under insanitary conditions, whereby they may have become contaminated with filth or rendered injurious to health, causing your drug products to be adulterated under section 501 (a)(2)(A) of the FD&C Act. For example, the investigator observed that your facility lacked ISO classified areas, including ISO 5, for sterile drug product manufacturing, and your manufacturing facility was in a state of disrepair.

FDA 调查员指出，药品旨在或预期为无菌，但其是在不卫生的条件下制备、包装或储存的，其可能被污物污染或对健康有害，因此根据 FD&C 法案第 501 (a)(2)(A) 条，你公司的药品被视为掺假。例如，调查员观察到，你公司的设施缺乏用于无菌药品生产的 ISO 洁净区域，包括 ISO 5，并且你公司的生产设施年久失修。

cGMP Violations │ cGMP 违规

During our inspection, our investigators observed specific violations including, but not limited to, the following.

在检查过程中，我们的调查员发现了具体的违规情况，包括但不限于以下内容。

无菌控制

1. Your firm failed to establish and follow appropriate written procedures that are designed to prevent microbiological contamination of drug products purporting to be sterile, and that include validation of all aseptic and sterilization processes. Your firm also failed to perform operations within specifically defined areas of adequate size and to have separate or defined areas or such other control systems necessary to prevent contamination or mix-ups in aseptic processing areas (21 CFR 211.113 (b) & 211.42 (c)(10)).

1. 你公司未能建立并遵循适当的书面程序，来防止声称无菌的药品受到微生物污染，其中包括对所有无菌和灭菌工艺的验证。你公司也未能在足够面积的特定区域内进行操作，也未能拥有单独或界定的区域或其他必要的控制系统，来防止无菌工艺区的污染或混淆［21 CFR 211.113 (b) 和 211.42 (c)(10)］。

You manufactured a multi-dose, preservative-free, over-the-counter (OTC) ophthalmic drug product for the product owner, Purely Soothing, without adequate facility design, controls, and procedures to ensure sterility of containers/closures and finished ophthalmic drug product. If ophthalmic drugs are not sterile, they pose an unacceptable risk to patients including infection and potential for vision loss.

你们为产品所有者 Purely Soothing 生产了多剂量、不含防腐剂的非处方（OTC）眼科药品，但没有充分的设施设计、控制和程序，来确保容器 / 密封件和眼科成品制剂的无菌性。如眼科药品不是无菌的，它们会给患者带来不可接受的风险，包括感染和潜在的视力丧失。

Furthermore, it is essential that multi-dose ophthalmic drug products contain one or more suitable substances that will preserve a product and minimize the hazard of injury resulting from incidental contamination during use.

此外，多剂量眼科药品制剂必须含有一种或多种合适的物料，以确定产品的防腐性，并且最大限度地减少使用过程中偶然污染造成的伤害隐患。

During the inspection, you informed us that you were unaware that ophthalmic drug products are required to be sterile, and acknowledged that your facility is not designed and equipped to handle or manufacture sterile drug products, even though your drug products are intended for use as "eye drops".

在检查期间，你公司告诉我们，不知道眼科药品需要无菌，并承认你公司的设施没有相应的设计和设备，来处理或生产无菌药品，即使你公司的药品旨在用作"眼药水"。

To help you meet the cGMP requirements when manufacturing sterile drugs using aseptic processing, see FDA's guidance document *Sterile Drug Products Produced by Aseptic Processing—Current Good Manufacturing Practice* at https://www.fda.gov/media/71026/download.

请参阅 FDA 指南，通过无菌工艺生产的无菌药品 – 现行药品生产质量管理规范，以帮助你公司在使用无菌工艺生产无菌药品时满足 cGMP 要求，网址（略，见上）。

确认与验证

2. Your firm failed to establish adequate written procedures for production and process control designed to assure that the drug products you manufacture have the identity, strength, quality, and purity they purport or are represented to possess(21 CFR 211.100(a)).

2. 你公司未能建立充分的书面生产和过程控制程序，旨在确保你公司生产的药品具有其声称或陈述的鉴别、规格、质量和纯度［21 CFR 211.100(a)］。

You failed to adequately qualify the equipment and validate the processes used to manufacture your drug products. You have not performed process performance qualification (PPQ) studies, nor do you have an ongoing program for monitoring process control, to ensure stable manufacturing operations and consistent drug quality for products in U.S. distribution.

你公司未能充分确认设备并验证用于生产药品的工艺。尚未进行工艺性能确认

（PPQ）研究，也没有持续的工艺控制监测计划，以确保在美国流通的产品具有稳定的生产操作和始终一致的药品质量。

（略）

此处与 FDA 发给 Profounda, Inc. 的警告信（编号：MARCS–CMS 642595，即"2 未能提供生产工艺的验证数据"）中有关工艺验证的重要性部分的内容类似，故略去。

产品检验

3. Your firm failed to have, for each batch of drug product, appropriate laboratory determination of satisfactory conformance to final specifications for the drug product, including the identity and strength of each active ingredient, prior to release, and conduct for each batch of drug product, appropriate laboratory testing, as necessary, required to be free of objectionable microorganisms(21 CFR 211.165(a)and 21 CFR 211.165(b)).

3. 你公司没有对每批药品进行适当的实验室确认，以在放行之前确定其是否符合最终产品的质量标准要求，包括每种原料药的鉴别和规格。也未能根据需要，对每批药品进行适当的实验室检验，以确保不含有害微生物［21 CFR 211.165(a) 和 21 CFR 211.165(b)］。

Your firm failed to conduct adequate release testing of all your drug products. For example：

你公司未能对所有药品进行充分的放行检验。例如：

● You did not conduct appropriate laboratory testing, including sterility testing, for each batch of drug product(e.g., ophthalmic)that are required to be sterile.

● 对于对每批要求无菌的药品（例如眼科药品），你公司没有进行适当的实验室检验，包括无菌检验。

● You did not conduct appropriate laboratory testing of each batch of drug product(e.g., nasal spray)required to be free of objectionable microorganisms.

● 对于要求不含有害微生物的每批药品（例如鼻喷雾剂），你公司没有进行适当的实验室检验。

Full release testing, including for identity, strength, and purity, must be performed prior to batch release and distribution. Without adequate testing, you do not have adequate scientific evidence to assure that your drug products conform to appropriate specifications before release.

在批放行和流通之前，必须进行全面的放行检验，包括鉴别、规格和纯度。如果没有充分的检验，你公司就没有充分的科学证据，来确保药品在放行前符合相应的质量标准。

物料检验

4. Your firm failed to test samples of each component for identity and conformity with all appropriate written specifications for purity, strength, and quality. Your firm also failed to validate and establish the reliability of your component supplier's test analyses at appropriate intervals（21 CFR 211.84（d）（1）and 211.84（d）（2））.

4. 你公司未进行至少一项检验来确认药品中每种原辅料都被鉴别，并使其符合所有适当纯度、规格和质量的书面标准。你公司也未能在适当的时间间隔内，验证和确定你公司物料供应商的检验分析的可靠性［21 CFR 211.84（d）（1）和（2）］。

Your firm failed to conduct adequate testing on the components used to manufacture your finished drug products（e.g., ophthalmic product, nasal spray）. Additionally, your firm accepts components from your suppliers without establishing the reliability of your suppliers' test analyses, and you did not obtain or review the suppliers' certificate of analysis（COA）for all components（e.g., methylsulfonylmethane（MSM）,（b）（4）water）.

对于用于生产成品（例如眼科产品、鼻喷雾剂）的原辅料，你公司未能进行充分的检验。此外，在没有确定供应商检验分析可靠性的情况下，你公司接受了供应商的物料，并且你公司没有获取或审查所有物料的供应商分析证书（COA）［例如，甲基磺酰甲烷（MSM），（b）（4）水］。

Without adequate testing, you do not have scientific evidence that the components conform to appropriate specifications prior to use in the manufacture of your drug products.

如果没有充分的检验，你公司就没有科学证据证明这些原辅料在用于药品生产之前符合相应的质量标准。

质量部门

5. Your firm's quality control unit failed to exercise its responsibility to ensure drug products manufactured are in compliance with cGMP, and meet established specifications for identity, strength, quality, and purity（21 CFR 211.22）.

5. 你公司的质量控制部门未能履行职责，以确保所生产的药品符合 cGMP 要求，并符合有关鉴别、规格、质量和纯度的既定质量标准（21 CFR 211.22）。

Your firm failed to establish an adequate quality unit（QU）with the responsibilities and authority to oversee the manufacture of your drug products. For example，you failed to ensure：

你公司未能建立一个胜任的质量部门（QU），来负责监督药品的生产。例如，你公司未能确保：

● Adequate procedures describing roles and responsibilities of the QU，including but not limited to supplier qualification，batch release，complaints，process validation，equipment cleaning，and cGMP training（21 CFR 211.22（a）and（d）).

● 描述 QU 角色和职责的适当程序，包括但不限于供应商资质确认、批放行、投诉、工艺验证、设备清洁和 cGMP 培训［21 CFR 211.22（a）和（d）］。

● Adherence to a stability program（21 CFR 211.166（a）).

● 遵守稳定性计划［21 CFR 211.166（a）］。

● Consistent and complete batch records（21 CFR 211.188）.

● 一致且完整的批记录（21 CFR 211.188）。

● Adequate investigations and deviations（21 CFR 211.192）.

● 充分的调查和偏差（21 CFR 211.192）。

Even when a QU consists of one or only a few，those persons are still accountable for overseeing ongoing effectiveness of all systems and procedures，and review of the results of manufacture to ensure that product quality standards have been met.

即使 QU 由一个或几个人组成，这些人员仍然负责监督所有系统和程序的持续有效性，并审查生产结果，以确保满足产品质量标准。

Drug Recall & Production Ceased ｜药品召回和生产停止

On February 2，2023，FDA held a teleconference with you. We recommended you consider removing any batches of Purely Soothing 15% MSM Drops and Purely Soothing MSM Nasal Spray drug products currently in distribution from the U.S. market.

2023 年 2 月 2 日，FDA 与你公司召开了电话会议。建议你公司考虑移除目前在美国市场上市的所有批次的纯舒 15% MSM 滴剂和纯舒 MSM 鼻喷雾剂药品。

On February 14, 2023, you communicated your commitment to cease the manufacturing and distribution of all drug products with no intention of producing drug products in the future and agreed to voluntary recall all drug products manufactured with active ingredient MSM.

2023 年 2 月 14 日，你公司表达了停止生产和流通所有药品的承诺，未来也无意再生产药品，并同意自愿召回所有使用原料药 MSM 生产的药品。

On March 3, 2023, you issued a voluntary worldwide recall of Purely Soothing, 15% MSM Drops（i.e., ophthalmic）due to non-sterility. The company announcement was posted to the FDA website: https://www.fda.gov/safety/recalls-market-withdrawals-safety-alerts/pharmedica-usa-llc-issues-voluntary-worldwide-recall-purely-soothing-15-msm-drops-due-non-sterility.

2023 年 3 月 3 日，你公司因未无菌而在全球范围内自愿召回纯舒 15% MSM 滴剂（眼用）。公司公告已发布在 FDA 网站上：网址（略，见上）。

We acknowledge your commitment to cease production of all drugs at this facility.

我们知晓，你公司承诺停止在该设施生产所有药品。

If you plan to resume any operations regulated under the FD&C Act, notify this office prior to resuming your drug manufacturing operations. If you resume cGMP activities, you are responsible for resolving all deficiencies and systemic flaws to ensure your firm is capable of ongoing cGMP compliance. In your notification to the agency, provide a summary of your remediations to demonstrate that you have appropriately completed all corrective action and preventive action（CAPA）.

如果你公司计划恢复 FD&C 法案规定的任何运营，请在恢复药品生产运营之前通知本办公室。如果你公司恢复 cGMP 活动，则有责任解决所有缺陷和系统性问题，以确保你公司能够持续遵守 cGMP。在向 FDA 发出的通知中，请提供你公司的整改措施汇总，以证明已正确完成所有纠正和预防措施（CAPA）。

If you resume cGMP activities, you should engage a consultant qualified as set forth in 21 CFR 211.34 to assist your firm in meeting cGMP requirements. The qualified consultant should also perform a comprehensive six-system audit of your entire operation for cGMP compliance and evaluate the completion and efficacy of all CAPA before you pursue resolution of your firm's compliance status with FDA.

如果你公司恢复 cGMP 活动，应该聘请符合 21 CFR 211.34 规定的有资质的顾问，来协助你公司满足 cGMP 要求。有资质的顾问还应对你公司的整个运营进行全面的六大系统审核，以确保 cGMP 合规性，并在与 FDA 寻求解决你公司的合规状态之前评估所有 CAPA 的完成情况和有效性。

2 无菌洁净室的压差问题

警告信编号： MARCS-CMS 655666

签发时间： 2023-7-20；**公示时间：** 2023-8-1

签发机构： 药品质量业务二处（Division of Pharmaceutical Quality Operations II）

公　　司： Iso-Tex Diagnostics，Inc.

所在国家／地区： 美国

主　　题： cGMP／成品制剂／掺假（cGMP/Finished Pharmaceuticals/Adulterated）

摘　　要： 2023 年 1 月，FDA 对该药品生产设施进行了检查。首先，FDA 指出，该公司设施设计、设备适用性和环境条件的缺陷显著增加了无菌药品的污染风险。在设施条件的设计和控制方面，该公司未能确保洁净室材料在设计和建造上合理，易于清洁和消毒。在环境条件监测和控制方面，也未能确保设施的设计、控制和维护能够防止低质量空气进入并污染无菌工艺操作洁净室，导致整个洁净室偏离其既定的限度。在检查前至少两个月的记录显示，无菌工艺操作洁净室与相邻更衣室之间经常出现负压差，导致进入无菌工艺操作洁净室的空气质量较低。此外，该公司也未能对这些反复出现的偏移进行调查。

本警告信以下部分与本书此前其他警告信内容类似，故略去：前言、cGMP 顾 问 推 荐（cGMP Consultant Recommended）、结 论（Conclusion）。

无菌药品的污染风险

1. Your firm failed to have buildings used in the manufacture，processing，packing，or holding of drug products of a suitable size，construction，and location to facilitate cleaning，

maintenance, and proper operations (21 CFR 211.42 (a)). Your firm also failed to establish an adequate system for monitoring environmental conditions in aseptic processing areas, and an adequate system for cleaning and disinfecting the room and equipment to produce aseptic conditions (21 CFR 211.42 (c)(10)(iv)&(v)).

1. 你公司未能拥有适当大小、结构和位置的厂房，用于生产、加工、包装或放置药品，以方便清洁、维护和正确操作 [21 CFR 211.42 (a)]。你公司也未能建立适当的系统，来监测无菌工艺区的环境条件，以及适当的系统来清洁和消毒房间和设备，以产生无菌条件 [21 CFR 211.42 (c)(10)(iv)&(v)]。

Your deficient facility design, equipment suitability, and environmental conditions significantly increased contamination risk to drugs intended to be sterile.

设施设计、设备适用性和环境条件的缺陷显著增加了无菌药品的污染风险。

■ Inadequate Design and Control of Facility Conditions
设施条件的设计和控制不充分

You failed to ensure that cleanrooms are properly designed and constructed of materials that allow for the ease of cleaning and disinfection. For example, our investigators observed:

你公司未能确保洁净室材料在设计和建造上合理，易于清洁和消毒。例如，我们的调查员观察到：

● The door of your (b)(4) connection to your aseptic processing cleanroom and gowning room was in disrepair and unable to fully close.

● 你公司的（b)(4）与无菌工艺操作洁净室和更衣室连接的门年久失修，无法完全关闭。

● Foreign particulates hanging from two ceiling HEPA Filters within your aseptic processing cleanroom.

● 无菌工艺操作洁净室内的两个天花板 HEPA 过滤器悬挂着异物颗粒。

● Inadequately sealed fluorescent light fixtures in aseptic processing cleanrooms.

● 无菌工艺操作洁净室中的荧光灯装置密封不充分。

● Exposed electrical lightbulb sockets and an emergency light within aseptic processing cleanroom without a cover.

● 无菌工艺操作洁净室内没有盖子的外露电灯泡插座和应急灯。

Inadequate Monitoring and Control of Environmental Conditions
环境条件监测和控制不充分

You failed to ensure that your facility is designed, controlled, and maintained to prevent lower quality air from entering and contaminating your aseptic processing cleanrooms, resulting in departures from your established limits throughout your clean rooms. For example:

你公司未能确保：设施的设计、控制和维护能够防止低质量空气进入并污染无菌工艺操作洁净室，从而导致整个洁净室偏离既定的限度。例如：

- Since at least December 1, 2022, negative differential pressure was frequently documented between your sterile drug processing cleanroom containing aseptic processing hoods and the adjacent gowning room, that allows for lower quality of air to move into your aseptic processing cleanroom. You lacked investigations into these recurring excursions.

- 至少自 2022 年 12 月 1 日起，包含无菌工艺操作罩的无菌工艺操作洁净室与相邻更衣室之间经常记录到负压差，导致进入无菌工艺操作洁净室的空气质量较低。你公司缺乏对这些反复出现的偏移的调查。

- From at least August 10, 2022, you failed to maintain the relative humidity below (b)(4) as established in your "Environmental Quality and Control Program" procedure. Your relative humidity data reveals repetitive and extended excursions. For example, in aseptic processing cleanroom (b)(4), from January 15, 2023, starting at 7: 40pm, and ending January 18, 2023, at 7: 10pm, the relative humidity ranged from 60.1 to 94.8%, and averaged 73.5%. Upon request for additional information on April 26, 2023, you did not provide any investigations into the excursions. You were also unable to provide procedures, use logs, or qualification documentation for a (b)(4) dehumidifier operating in gowning cleanroom, suite (b)(4), used to control relative humidity. Your use of a (b)(4) dehumidifier in a cleanroom indicates a poorly designed HVAC system.

- 至少从 2022 年 8 月 10 日起，你公司未能将相对湿度保持在"环境质量和控制计划"程序中规定的（b）（4）以下。你公司的相对湿度数据揭示了重复和长时间的偏移。例如，在无菌工艺操作洁净室（b）（4）中，从 2023 年 1 月 15 日晚上 7：40 开始，到 2023 年 1 月 18 日晚上 7：10 结束，相对湿度范围为 60.1%~94.8%，平均相对湿度 73.5%。在 2023 年 4 月 26 日要求提供更多信息时，你们没有提供任何有关偏移的调查。对于在更衣洁净室、套间（b）（4）中运行、用于控制相对湿度的（b）（4）除湿机，你公司也无法提供其程序、使用台账或确认文件。你公司在洁净室中使用（b）（4）除湿机表明 HVAC 系统设计不当。

Aseptic processes should be designed to minimize exposure of sterile articles to potential contamination hazards, including, but not limited to, variation in environmental conditions. It is vital for rooms of higher air cleanliness to have a substantial positive pressure differential relative to adjacent rooms of lower air cleanliness. A suitable facility monitoring system is critical to maintain appropriate environmental conditions throughout all of your cleanrooms. All deviations from established limits should be appropriately investigated to rapidly detect atypical changes that can compromise the facility's environment. Prompt detection of an emerging problem is essential to preventing contamination of your aseptic production operations.

无菌工艺的设计应尽量减少无菌物品暴露于潜在污染危害的情况，包括但不限于环境条件的变化。对于空气洁净度较高的房间来说，相对于空气洁净度较低的相邻房间需要具有显著的正压差，这是至关重要的。对于在所有洁净室中保持适当的环境条件来说，合适的设施监控系统至关重要。应适当调查所有与既定限度有关的偏差，以快速检测可能损害设施环境的异常变化。对于防止无菌生产操作受到污染来说，及时发现新出现的问题是至关重要的。

Your response is inadequate because you fail to address systemic issues to ensure your facility is suitable for the aseptic processing for sterile drugs. You also do not provide meaningful evidence that your manufacturing environment is under an ongoing state of control.

你公司的回应是不充分的，因为你们未能解决系统性问题，以确保设施适合无菌药品的无菌工艺操作。你公司也没有提供有意义的证据，来证明生产环境处于持续的受控制状态。

In response to this letter, provide:

在回复本函时，请提供：

● A comprehensive risk assessment of all contamination hazards with respect to your aseptic processes, equipment, and facilities, including an independent assessment that includes, but is not limited to:

● 就你公司的无菌工艺、设备和设施的所有污染危害，进行全面的风险评估，包含独立评估，这包括但不限于：

○ All human interactions within the ISO 5 area

○ ISO 5 区域内的所有人员交互

○ Equipment placement and ergonomics

○ 设备放置和人体工程学

○ Air quality in the ISO 5 area and surrounding room

○ ISO 5 区域和周围房间内的空气质量

○ Facility layout

○ 设施布局

○ Personnel Flows and Material Flows（throughout all rooms used to conduct and support sterile operations）

○ 人流和物流（用于执行和支持无菌操作的所有房间）

● A detailed remediation plan with timelines to address the findings of the contamination hazards risk assessment. Describe specific tangible improvements to be made to aseptic processing operation design and control.

● 详细的整改计划和时间表，以解决污染危害风险评估所发现的问题。描述要对无菌工艺操作设计和控制进行的具体切实改进。

● A thorough, independent assessment, and corrective action and preventive action（CAPA）for your pressure differential system and environmental temperature and humidity conditions. Include a comprehensive evaluation of monitoring, recording, alarm documentation, deviation investigation, data retention and overall system control in your assessment. Provide a CAPA that includes, but is not limited to：

● 针对你公司的压差系统以及环境温湿度条件进行彻底、独立的评估，以及纠正和预防措施（CAPA）。在评估中应包括对监控、记录、警报记录、偏差调查、数据保存和整体系统控制的全面评估。提供 CAPA，包括但不限于：

○ The state of control of air balance between clean areas and adequacy of integration of each of the HVAC systems

○ 洁净区之间风量平衡的控制状态以及每个 HVAC 系统集成的充分性

○ Documentation for all alarms, irrespective of the length or location of the event, and retention of this data

○ 所有警报的记录，无论事件的持续时间或位置，以及该数据的保存情况

○ Remediated procedures for investigating deviations from established limits, including but not limited to specific provisions for handling instances in which a pressure reversal occurs

○ 调查与既定限度偏差的整改程序，包括但不限于处理发生反向压差情况的具体规定

○ Remediated facility monitoring systems that will rapidly detect atypical changes of pressure, temperature, and humidity, in your cleanrooms simultaneously

○ 整改设施监控系统，可同时快速检测洁净室中压力、温湿度的异常变化

● A comprehensive, independent assessment of the design and control of your firm's manufacturing operations, with a detailed and thorough review of all microbiological hazards.

● 对你公司生产操作的设计和控制进行全面、独立的评估，并对所有微生物危害进行详细、彻底的审查。

● A detailed risk assessment addressing the hazards posed by distributing drug products with potential contamination. Specify actions you will take in response to the risk assessment, such as customer notifications and product recalls.

● 针对流通具有潜在污染的药品所造成的危害，进行详细的风险评估。指定你公司将针对风险评估采取的行动，例如客户通知和产品召回。

● Complete investigations into all batches with potential microbial contamination. The investigations should detail your findings regarding the root causes of the contamination.

● 对所有可能存在微生物污染的批次进行全面调查。调查应详细说明有关污染根本原因的调查结果。

● All microbial test methods and specifications used to analyze each of your drug products.

● 用于分析你公司的每种药品的所有微生物检验方法和质量标准。

● Your CAPA plan to implement routine, vigilant operations management oversight of facilities and equipment. This plan should ensure, among other things, prompt detection of equipment/facilities performance issues, effective execution of repairs, adherence to appropriate preventive maintenance schedules, timely technological upgrades to the equipment/facility infrastructure, and improved systems for ongoing management review.

● 你公司的 CAPA 计划，包括对设施和设备实施日常、警戒性的运营管理监督。至少，该计划应确保及时发现设备 / 设施性能问题，有效执行维修，遵循相应的预防性维护计划，及时对设备 / 设施进行技术升级，并对持续管理评审的系统进行改进。

● Your complete investigation into failed cleanroom certification study data relating to air changes. Include all original and corrected calculations regarding air changes, the location of all air inlets and exhaust outlets in the room, and a detailed description of the BSC design (e.g., intake of air) and its position in the room. You should also provide an independent assessment of the investigation, and the adequacy of air changes in all of your cleanrooms, by a qualified consult.

● 你公司对与换气相关的洁净室认证研究不合格数据的完整调查。包括有关空气变化的所有原始和修正计算、房间内所有进气口和排气口的位置，以及 BSC 设计（例如，进气）及其在房间内位置的详细描述。你公司还应该由有资质的顾问对调查结果以及所有洁净室换气的充分性进行独立评估。

● Smoke studies that evaluate the suitability of your biological safety cabinets（BSC）used for the aseptic manufacturing of your drug products.

● 烟雾研究，其评估用于药品无菌生产的生物安全柜（BSC）的适用性。

无菌工艺验证

2. Your firm failed to establish and follow appropriate written procedures that are designed to prevent microbiological contamination of drug products purporting to be sterile, and that include validation of all aseptic and sterilization processes（21 CFR 211.113（b））.

2. 你公司未能建立并遵循适当的书面程序，包括验证所有无菌和灭菌工艺的程序，以防止声称无菌的药品受到微生物污染［21 CFR 211.113（b）］。

Your firm manufactures sterile radiopharmaceutical drug products that are aseptically filled. You failed to have appropriate gowning for aseptic production of sterile injectable drug products. For example, investigators observed your production personnel：

你公司生产无菌灌装的无菌放射性药品制剂。没有为无菌注射药品的无菌生产提供合适的防护服。例如，调查员观察到你公司的生产人员：

● With exposed facial skin and hair entering your ISO 5 production environment while performing aseptic manual filling of Volumex I-131, Lot # V230102-1107.

● 在暴露面部皮肤和头发的状态下进入 ISO 5 生产环境，并对 Volumex I-131（批号 V230102-1107）进行无菌人工灌装。

● On multiple instances, failing to disinfect their sterile gloves before returning to the ISO 5 area.

● 多次情况下，在返回 ISO 5 区域之前未能对无菌手套进行消毒。

● Use poor sterile gowning behavior and practices（e.g., sterile gown touched the floor while donning the gowning）.

● 使用不良的无菌更衣行为和实践（例如，穿无菌服时无菌服接触地板）。

- Gowning without using suitable sterile gloves.

- 未使用合适的无菌手套进行更衣。

Your firm's failure to ensure that personnel gown appropriately and strictly adhere to acceptable aseptic procedures significantly increases the risk of drug product contamination.

你公司未能确保人员穿着适当并严格遵守可接受的无菌程序，这会显著增加药品污染的风险。

In addition, your production staff and equipment (e.g., active air monitor, analytical balance printer) blocked the path of unidirectional airflow in your ISO 5 production environment during filling operations of Volumex I–131, Lot # V230102–1107. Unidirectional airflow design is used to protect sterile equipment surfaces, container– closures, and drug product, and should not be obstructed by personnel or equipment. Disruption of unidirectional air in the critical area poses a significant risk to product sterility.

此外，在 Volumex I–131（批号 V230102–1107）的灌装操作过程中，你公司的生产人员和设备（例如空气监测器、分析天平打印机）阻挡了 ISO 5 生产环境中的单向气流路径。单向气流设计用于保护无菌设备表面、容器密闭件和药品，并且不应被人员或设备阻碍。关键区域单向空气的破坏会对产品无菌造成重大风险。

Your response is inadequate because you do not commit to conducting a retrospective review of drug product manufactured under these conditions for potential quality and safety impact. Additionally, your response does not include supporting documentation of CAPA activities.

你公司的回复是不充分的，因为你公司没有承诺对在这些条件下生产的药品进行潜在的质量和安全影响回顾性审查。此外，你公司的回复不包括 CAPA 活动的支持文档。

In response to this letter, provide：

在回复本函时，请提供：

- Your plan to ensure appropriate aseptic practices and cleanroom behavior during production. Include steps to ensure routine and effective supervisory oversight for all production batches. Also, describe the frequency of quality unit oversight (e.g., audit) during aseptic processing and supporting operations.

- 确保生产工艺中采取适当的无菌操作和洁净室行为的计划。包括确保对所有生产批次进行常规和有效监督的步骤。另外，描述无菌工艺操作和支持操作期间质量部门监督（例如审计）的频率。

● A thorough retrospective review and risk assessment that evaluates how poor aseptic technique and cleanroom behavior may have affected the quality and sterility of your drugs.

● 彻底的回顾性审查和风险评估，评估不良的无菌技术和洁净室行为可能如何影响药品的质量和无菌性。

● A gowning qualification program that establishes, both initially and on a periodic basis, the capability of an individual to adequately don the complete sterile gown in an aseptic manner.

● 更衣确认计划，用于初始和定期确认人员以无菌方式充分穿戴完整无菌更衣的能力。

● Details regarding how you will establish adequate gowning, training, gowning qualification, and supervision on an ongoing basis.

● 有关如何建立适当的更衣、培训、更衣资质确认和持续监督的详细信息。

实验室控制措施

3. Your firm failed to establish laboratory controls that include scientifically sound and appropriate specifications, standards, sampling plans, and test procedures designed to assure that components, drug product containers, closures, in-process materials, labeling, and drug products conform to appropriate standards of identity, strength, quality, and purity (21 CFR 211.160 (b)).

3. 你公司未能建立实验室控制措施，包括科学合理且相应的规范、标准、取样计划和检验程序，以确保物料、药品容器、密封件、中间体、标签和药品符合相关规定，即鉴别、规格、质量和纯度的标准 [21 CFR 211.160(b)]。

Our investigators observed inadequately controlled laboratory reagents (i.e., inadequate labeling), as well as expired testing materials. The use of uncontrolled and expired testing materials may impact the validity of your testing results used to support the release of your drug products.

我们的调查员观察到实验室试剂控制不充分（即贴标不充分）以及过期的检测用物料。使用不受控制和过期的检验物料，这可能会影响用于支持药品放行的检验结果的有效性。

Your response is inadequate because you do not conduct or commit to conducting an investigation to determine product impact nor do you commit to determining whether your corrective actions require extension to other related procedures.

你公司的回复不充分，没有进行或承诺进行调查，以确定产品影响，也没有承诺确定你公司的整改措施是否需要扩展到其他相关程序。

In response to this letter, provide a comprehensive, independent assessment of your laboratory practices, procedures, methods, equipment, documentation, and analyst competencies. Based on this review, provide a detailed plan to remediate and evaluate the effectiveness of your laboratory system.

在回复本函时，请对你们的实验室实践、程序、方法、设备、文件和分析人员能力进行全面、独立的评估。根据此审查，提供详细的计划来整改和评估实验室系统的有效性。

Additional Guidance on Aseptic Processing
无菌工艺的更多指南

See FDA's guidance document *Sterile Drug Products Produced by Aseptic Processing—Current Good Manufacturing Practice* to help you meet the cGMP requirements when manufacturing sterile drugs using aseptic processing at https://www.fda.gov/media/71026/download.

请参阅 FDA 指南，通过无菌工艺生产的无菌药品 – 现行药品生产质量管理规范，以帮助你公司在使用无菌工艺生产无菌药品时满足 cGMP 要求，网址（略，见上）。

Repeat Violations and Observations at Facility
设施中的重复违规情况和观察项

In a previous warning letter, 2011-DAL-WL-03, issued on December 3, 2010, and previous inspections ending on January 31, 2018, July 10, 2015, and September 12, 2011, FDA cited similar cGMP violations and observations. You proposed specific remediation for these violations and observations in your responses. Repeated failures demonstrate that executive management oversight and control over the manufacture of drugs is inadequate.

在之前于 2010 年 12 月 3 日发出的警告信 2011-DAL-WL-03 以及于 2018 年 1 月 31 日、2015 年 7 月 10 日和 2011 年 9 月 12 日结束的检查中，FDA 引用了类似的 cGMP 违规情况和观察项。你公司在回复中提出了针对这些违规情况和观察项的具体整改措施。屡次不合格表明高级管理层对药品生产的监督和控制不够。

3 注射剂药品的颗粒物检查存在缺陷

警告信编号： MARCS-CMS 654136

签发时间： 2023-7-25；**公示时间：** 2023-8-1

签发机构： 药物审评与研究中心 | CDER（Center for Drug Evaluation and Research | CDER）

公　　司： Baxter Healthcare Corporation

所在国家 / 地区： 美国

主　　题： cGMP/ 成品制剂 / 掺假（cGMP/Finished Pharmaceuticals/ Adulterated）

摘　　要： 百特医疗是一家总部位于美国的全球医疗健康公司，成立于 1931 年。该公司于 1971 年首次跻身财富美国 500 强，总部位于美国伊利诺伊州，并在全球范围内设有多个办事处和制造设施。2023 年 1 月，FDA 对其位于印度的药品生产设施展开了检查。在这次检查中，FDA 发现了一些重要问题，尤其是在关于注射剂药品中的颗粒物检查中，发现自动检查机存在故障情况。然而，该公司并未充分调查这一问题，反而继续使用自动检查机来检查商业流通的产品。FDA 指出，长期以来，该公司一直完全依赖这种自动目检系统，用于检测各种缺陷，包括颗粒污染，但并未对所有缺陷进行 100% 的人工目检，因此失效问题屡次出现，属于重复缺陷。在 2018 年 7 月向该公司发出警告信后，该公司曾承诺评估并实施改进程序，以改善调查活动。然而，FDA 发现该公司未采取有力的措施，来及时调查这些反复出现和持续存在的缺陷，也未能充分解决其不合格问题。

本警告信以下部分与本书此前其他警告信内容类似，故略去：前言、质量体系失效（Ineffective Quality System）、工艺控制（Process Controls）、cGMP 顾问推荐（cGMP Consultant Recommended）、结论（Conclusion）。

偏差调查

1. Your firm failed to thoroughly investigate any unexplained discrepancy or failure of a batch or any of its components to meet any of its specifications, whether or not the batch has already been distributed（21 CFR 211.192）.

1. 无论批次是否已经流通，对于该批次或其原辅料不满足质量标准、存在无法解释的偏差或不合格，你公司未能进行彻底调查（21 CFR 211.192）。

You failed to conduct adequate investigations into endotoxin testing and your 100% automated visual inspection system. You conducted investigations that were not thorough, expanded to an appropriate scope, or based on scientifically supported root cause（s）. You did not identify and implement appropriate corrective actions and preventive actions（CAPA）. Specifically,

你公司未能对内毒素检测和 100% 自动目检系统进行充分的调查。你公司进行的调查不彻底，未扩展到适当的范围，或基于科学支持的根本原因。没有确定并实施适当的纠正和预防措施（CAPA）。具体来说，

● Your firm invalidated multiple endotoxin tests for finished products upon discovery of particulate matter in one or more wells used to perform the kinetic-turbidimetric assay（KTA）method. You failed to characterize the particulate matter and attributed the particulates to environmental and laboratory conditions, such as air ducts and activities being performed by personnel in the immediate vicinity of the analysis. You did not definitively identify the source or sources of the particulate matter, define the scope of potentially impacted operations（including potential manufacturing causes）, and implement scientifically justified CAPA in a timely manner.

● 在用于执行动态浊度法（KTA）的一个或多个孔中发现颗粒物质后，你公司判定成品的多项内毒素检验无效。你公司未能描述颗粒物的特征，并将颗粒物归因于环境和实验室条件，例如空气管道和检验时附近人员进行的活动。没有明确确定颗粒物的一个或多个来源，定义可能受影响的操作范围（包括潜在的生产原因），并及时实施科学合理的 CAPA。

In a previous inspection（May 2022）, FDA cited your firm for inadequate investigations into these and other similar out-of-specification（OOS）endotoxin testing that you invalidated due to uncharacterized particulate contamination in one or more wells during KTA analyses. Prior to and during an October 5, 2022 regulatory meeting with your firm, we requested you perform a retrospective assessment of investigations associated with OOS endotoxin results or endotoxin testing deviations. During the current inspection, your personnel explained that these investigations were not reopened or otherwise reassessed. Although you retained a third-party consultant to perform a retrospective assessment of endotoxin investigations associated with OOS endotoxin result investigations, you did not provide the third-party consultant with an investigation cited during the May 2022 inspection. You also did not ensure the assessment included approximately 20 invalidated laboratory tests generated in 2021 and 2022 (including multiple investigations since the May 2022 inspection).

在之前的一次检查（2022 年 5 月）中，FDA 指出你公司对这些和其他类似的不合格（OOS）内毒素检测调查不充分：在 KTA 分析期间一个或多个孔中存在未表征的颗粒污染，你公司将内毒素检测判为无效。在 2022 年 10 月 5 日与你公司召开监管会议之前和期间，我们要求你公司对与内毒素 OOS 结果或内毒素检测偏差相关的调查进行回顾性评估。在本次检查期间，你公司的人员解释说，这些调查并未重新启动或以其他方式重新评估。尽管你公司聘请了第三方顾问，对与 OOS 内毒素结果调查相关的内毒素调查进行回顾性评估，但你们没有向第三方顾问提供 2022 年 5 月检查期间引用的调查结果。也没有确保评估包括 2021 年和 2022 年生成的约 20 项无效实验室检验（包括自 2022 年 5 月检查以来的多项调查）。

● Your firm did not adequately investigate failures of the (b)(4) automatic inspection machine to detect known defects, including particulate matter in injectable drug products. Despite the data indicating significant deficiencies in the machine's ability to detect known defects during its use, you continued to employ the (b)(4) automatic inspection machine to inspect commercially distributed products (e.g., several batches of (b)(4) injection (b)(4) mg/mL USP). Notably, you fully relied on this automated visual inspection system to detect various defects including particulate contamination for an extended period and did not perform a 100% manual visual inspection for all defects.

● 对于自动检查机检测已知缺陷（包括注射药品中的颗粒物质）的故障问题，你公司没有进行充分调查（b）（4）。尽管数据表明机器在使用过程中检测已知缺陷的能力存在重大不足，但你公司仍继续使用（b）（4）自动检查机，来检查商业流通的产品［例如，多批（b）（4）注射剂，规格为（b）（4）mg/ml USP］。值得注意的是，长期以来，你公司完全依赖这种自动目检系统，来检测包括颗粒污染在内的各种缺陷，并没有对所有缺陷进行 100% 人工目检。

Challenges with defect kits indicated failing rejection rates or other deficiencies. For example, an October 2022 challenge excluded the use of (b)(4) particles despite their lower detectability than other "dark" particles in (b)(4) mL amber glass vials. The challenge also used a highly detectable particle range of (b)(4) μm, but still indicated detection and capability issues. Similar challenges to the (b)(4) automatic inspection machine utilized commercial inspection parameters. You did not initiate adequate investigations into these detection issues. You lacked adequate assurance that sterile injectable drug batches visually inspected with the（b）（4）automatic inspection machine were free from visible particulates.

缺陷样品的挑战试验表明，在拒绝率或其他缺陷上存在不合格。例如，2022 年 10 月的一项挑战排除了（b）（4）颗粒的使用，尽管它们的可检测性低于（b）（4）ml 琥珀色玻璃瓶中的其他"深色"颗粒。该挑战还使用了（b）（4）μm 这一高度可检测颗粒范围，但仍然表明存在检测和能力问题。（b）（4）自动检查机的类似挑战使用了商业检查参数。你公司没有对这些检测问题展开充分的调查。缺乏充分的保证，无法保证用（b）（4）自动检查机目检的无菌注射药品批次不含可见异物。

Your response is inadequate. Your firm previously committed to evaluate and implement improvements to your procedures and practices associated with the conduct of investigations following the conclusion of the July 27 to August 4, 2017, inspection of this facility and in response to the warning letter sent to your firm on July 5, 2018. You also reported significant CAPA activities to address the frequency of endotoxin testing OOS results and deviations following the October 5, 2022, regulatory meeting.

你公司的回应不够充分。在 2017 年 7 月 27 日至 8 月 4 日对该设施进行检查，并在 2018 年 7 月 5 日向你公司发出警告信后，你们曾承诺，评估并实施改进程序和实践，以改善调查活动。在 2022 年 10 月 5 日的监管会议后，你公司还报告了重要的 CAPA 活动，以应对内毒素检测 OOS 结果和偏差的频率。

In your February 17, 2023, response to the Form FDA 483 issued at the conclusion of the most recent inspection, you commit to further revisions of your investigation procedures.

在 2023 年 2 月 17 日，对最近一次检查结束时发布的 FDA 483 表格的回复中，你公司承诺进一步修订调查程序。

However, you do not adequately address your failure to conduct timely investigations into recurring and persistent issues. Your response did not adequately address the use of insufficiently qualified（b）（4）equipment for 100% visual inspection of injectable drug products for approximately five years（until October 2022）and the excessive number of samples contaminated with endotoxins or particles in your laboratory.

但是，就未能及时调查反复出现和持续存在的缺陷，你公司没有充分解决其不合格问题。就大约五年（直到 2022 年 10 月）使用不合格的（b）（4）设备对注射药品进行 100% 目检的问题，以及实验室中被内毒素或颗粒污染的样品数量过多的问题，你公司的回复并没有充分解决。

We encourage the use of automated visual inspection for particulates to augment the 100% manual visual inspection program. Automated methods should be rigorously studied for their capability and robustness under various conditions, machine settings, container-closure sizes, defect types, and other variables. In addition, any use of automated particulate inspection does not supplant the need for 100% manual visual inspection for various other attributes (e.g., cracks).

我们鼓励对颗粒物使用自动目检，以增强 100% 人工目检程序。应严格研究自动化方法在各种条件、机器设置、容器封闭尺寸、缺陷类型和其他变量下的能力和稳健性。此外，任何自动颗粒检查的使用都不能取代对各种其他属性（例如裂纹）进行 100% 人工目检的需要。

In response to this letter, provide：

在回复本函时，请提供：

● A written commitment to have all lots of finished products manufactured at your facility analyzed for endotoxins by a qualified laboratory until you have thoroughly investigated each endotoxin test invalidation event since January 1, 2018, and implemented all necessary CAPA to prevent recurrence of endotoxin result invalidations. This should include but not be limited to assuring CAPA effectiveness for your particulate and pipetting issues.

● 书面承诺：由有资质的实验室对你公司设施生产的所有批次成品进行内毒素分析，直到彻底调查自 2018 年 1 月 1 日以来的每起内毒素检测无效事件，并实施所有必要的 CAPA，以防止内毒素结果无效再次发生。这应包括但不限于：确保 CAPA 有效解决你公司的颗粒和移液问题。

● A comprehensive, independent assessment and remediation plan of your systems for the visual inspection of sterile injectable drugs for defects, including the presence of particulate matter, used for products distributed in the United States that remain within expiry. The assessment should include acceptance and rejection criteria, personnel training, supervision, equipment and personnel qualification, equipment maintenance, and process validation and the procedures governing them. Provide your detailed remediation action plan that includes dates by which each remediation activity will be completed and a periodic independent reassessment of the plan's effectiveness.

● 对你公司的系统进行全面、独立的评估和整改计划，用于目检无菌注射药品的缺陷，包括颗粒物的存在，针对在美国上市的仍在有效期内的产品。评估应包括接受和拒放标准、人员培训、监督、设备和人员资质确认、设备维护、工艺验证及其管理程序。提供详细的整改行动计划，其中包括完成每项整改活动的日期，以及对该计划有效性的定期独立重新评估。

● An independent third-party assessment and remediation plan for your CAPA program. Provide a report that evaluates whether the program includes effective root cause analysis, ensures CAPA effectiveness, analyzes investigation trends, improves the CAPA program when needed, implements final quality unit decisions, and is fully supported by executive management.

● 针对你公司的 CAPA 计划的独立评估和整改计划。提供一份报告，评估是否有效地进行了根本原因分析，确保了 CAPA 的有效性，分析调查趋势，在需要时对 CAPA 计划进行改进，实施质量部门最终决策，并得到高级管理层的充分支持。

● A third-party protocol and the executed protocol final report for the retrospective review of particulate matter investigations associated with distributed in the United States that remain within expiry, irrespective of whether the original investigation resulted in the invalidation of the original result. The protocol should include an evaluation of the investigation's thoroughness; assignment and scientific justification for root cause (s); documentation of CAPA implementation, and documented effectiveness of CAPA.

● 就在美国流通的仍在效期内产品相关颗粒物调查的回顾性审查，无论原调查是否导致原始结果无效，均提供第三方方案和已执行方案的最终报告。方案应包括对调查彻底性的评估；根本原因的确定和科学论证；CAPA 实施的记录，以及 CAPA 有效性的记录。

设备清洁

2. Your firm failed to establish and follow adequate written procedures for cleaning and maintenance of equipment(21 CFR 211.67(b)).

2. 你公司未建立并遵循适当的书面程序，来清洁和维护设备［21 CFR 211.67（ b ）］。

An FDA investigator observed white spots at the bottom of a (b)(4) L bulk solution holding tank used to supply a non-dedicated filling machine despite the vessel being documented as clean. You subsequently analyzed and identified the white spots as (b)(4)(the product previously processed on this equipment) at levels of up to (b)(4) parts per million (ppm). Your limit for post-cleaning residues is not more than (b)(4) ppm.

在用于供应非专用灌装机的（ b ）（ 4 ）L 料液储罐底部，FDA 调查员观察到白点，尽管该容器被记录为清洁的。你公司随后分析并确定了白点为（ b ）（ 4 ）（ 之前在此设备上处理的产品 ），其含量高达百万分之（ b ）（ 4 ）（ ppm ）。清洁后残留物的限度不超过（ b ）（ 4 ） ppm。

Your response is inadequate. Although you revised your cleaning procedure to require vessels to be dry before conducting the visual inspection for cleanliness and implemented visual verification of the vessel interior via a sight glass following the cleaning and (b)(4) activities, you did not provide scientific justification for your use of visual inspection to verify the removal of residues to levels as low as (b)(4) ppm. Your response noted (b)(4) injection, not (b)(4) injection, is the "worst-case product" processed in this vessel, but you did not provide a comprehensive investigation to assess the impact of this cleaning deviation on products previously manufactured on this and other non-dedicated equipment. You also did not propose a systemic assessment of your equipment cleaning program.

你公司的回应不够充分。尽管你们修订了清洁程序，要求容器在进行清洁度目检之前保持干燥，并在清洁和（b）（4）活动之后通过视镜对容器内部进行目视确认，但你公司没有提供科学论证，使用目视来确认残留物的去除，是否低至（b）（4）ppm。你公司的回复指出，（b）（4）注射剂，而不是（b）（4）注射剂，是该容器中处理的"最差情况产品"，但并没有提供全面的调查，来评估这种清洁偏差对以前在此设备和其他非专用设备上生产的产品。也没有提议对你公司的设备清洁计划进行系统评估。

In response to this letter, provide:

在回复本函时，请提供：

● A comprehensive, independent retrospective assessment of your cleaning effectiveness to evaluate the scope of cross-contamination hazards. Include the identity of residues, other manufacturing equipment that may have been improperly cleaned, and an assessment whether cross-contaminated products may have been released for distribution. The assessment should identify any inadequacies of cleaning procedures and practices, and encompass each piece of manufacturing equipment used to manufacture more than one product.

● 对你公司的清洁效果进行全面、独立的回顾性评估，以评估交叉污染危害的范围。包括残留物的鉴别、其他可能未正确清洁的生产设备，以及对交叉污染的药品是否可能已被放行以供流通的评估。评估应确定清洁程序和实践的任何不足之处，并涵盖用于生产一种以上药品的每一台生产设备。

● A CAPA plan, based on the retrospective assessment of your cleaning program, that includes appropriate remediations to your cleaning processes and practices, and timelines for completion. Provide a detailed summary of vulnerabilities in your process for lifecycle management of equipment cleaning. Describe improvements to your cleaning program, including enhancements to cleaning effectiveness; improved ongoing verification of proper cleaning execution for all products and equipment; and all other needed remediations.

● 一项 CAPA 计划，基于对你公司的清洁和预防性维护计划的回顾性评估，其中包括对工艺和实践的相应整改、频率评估和完成时间表。提供设备清洁和预防性维护生命周期管理流程中漏洞的详细汇总。描述对清洁计划的改进，包括提高清洁效果；

改进对所有药品和设备的清洁正确执行的持续确认；以及所有其他需要的整改措施。

工艺验证不充分

3. Your firm failed to establish adequate written procedures for production and process control designed to assure that drug products you manufacture have the identity, strength, quality, and purity they purport or are represented to possess, and to follow all of your written production and process control procedures（21 CFR 211.100（a）and（b））.

3. 你公司未能为生产和过程控制建立适当的书面程序，以确保生产的药品具有其声称或被表示拥有的鉴别、规格、质量和纯度，并没有遵守你公司的所有书面生产和过程控制程序［21 CFR 211.100（a）和（b）］。

Your program for the visual inspection of sterile injectable drug products does not provide adequate assurance that finished products manufactured at your facility possess their purported quality attributes, including that they are free from particulate matter. For example,

你公司的无菌注射药品目检计划无法充分保证设施生产的成品具有其声称的质量属性，包括不含颗粒物。例如，

● Personnel performed 100% manual visual inspection of sterile injectable units for less than the minimum amount of time required by your written procedures.

● 工作人员对无菌注射产品进行 100% 人工目检，其时间少于书面程序所规定的最短时间。

● You lacked scientific justification for removing vials containing（b）（4）particles from the defect kits used to qualify visual inspection processes. For example, although（b）（4）particles were more difficult to reproducibly detect than（b）（4）stopper particles in the（b）（4）mL amber vials, you elected to only use the（b）（4）stopper particles in the defect kits.

● 在用于确认目检工艺的缺陷库中，你公司去除了含有（b）（4）颗粒的西林瓶样品，对此你公司缺乏科学论证。例如，尽管（b）（4）ml 琥珀色西林瓶中的（b）（4）颗粒比（b）（4）胶塞颗粒物更难被重复地检出，但你公司选择仅使用缺陷库中的（b）（4）胶塞颗粒物。

Your response is inadequate. You commit to using a "pacing device" during the 100% manual visual inspections and requiring a supervisor to periodically verify the inspection times. You did not provide a description of the pacing device or commit to requalify operators following implementation of the pacing device. Additionally, you did not commit to evaluate operator performance throughout a（b）（4）.

你公司的回应不够充分。你们承诺在 100% 人工目检期间使用 "配速装置"，并要求主管定期核实检查时间。你公司没有提供配速装置的描述，也没有承诺在实施配速装置后重新对操作人员进行资格确认。此外，你公司没有承诺在整个（b）（4）过程中评估操作员的表现。

You also state a successful qualification program does not evaluate " ··· an inspector's ability to differentiate and identify various types and morphologies of particles." However, it is critical to be able to reproducibly detect particulate defects of different types, morphologies, and sizes.

你公司还指出，成功的确认计划不会评估 "……检查人员区分和识别颗粒的各种类型和形态的能力"。然而，能够重复检测不同类型、形态和尺寸的颗粒缺陷，这是至关重要的。

In response to this letter, provide a comprehensive, independent assessment of each lot of sterile injectable drugs distributed from your facility to the United States that remains within expiry to meet the requirement of being essentially free of visible particles. The assessment should also include consideration of gaps and other deficiencies identified in the independent assessment of your systems for visual inspection of sterile injectable drugs.

作为对本函的回应，就你公司的设施流通到美国的仍在效期内的每批无菌注射药品，请提供一份全面、独立的评估，以满足不含可见异物的要求。对于对无菌注射药品目检系统进行独立评估时发现的差距和其他缺陷，评估也应将其纳入考虑之中。

设备问题

4. Your firm failed to use equipment in the manufacture, processing, packing, or holding of drug products that is of appropriate design, adequate size, and suitably located to facilitate operations for its intended use and for its cleaning and maintenance(21 CFR 211.63).

4. 在药品的生产、加工、包装或储存中，你公司未能使用设计合理、尺寸足够且位置适当的设备，以实现预期用途及清洁和维护操作（21 CFR 211.63 ）。

Equipment used in the manufacture of terminally sterilized drugs at your facility is not designed or maintained appropriately. Our inspection revealed instances of damaged metal and plastic parts, open vials exposed to worn bolt threading, and process flow that required employees to duck underneath the sterile processing line conveyer in order to perform interventions near open vials(e.g., stopper addition on the(b)(4)filling line).

你公司设施中用于生产最终灭菌药品的设备设计或维护不当。我们的检查发现了一些损坏的金属和塑料部件，暴露于磨损的螺栓螺纹的敞开的瓶子，以及工艺流程需要员工蹲下到无菌处理线传送装置下方，以便在敞开的西林瓶附近进行干预（例如，在灌装线上加塞）。

Your response is inadequate. Although you commit to replacing the threaded bolt（b）（4）on the（b）（4）filling line with a different part that will not expose a threading over open vials, you did not commit to evaluate production rooms and production equipment for wear, damage, or poor design that may lead to the generation of particulate matter in the vicinity of open vials. You also plan to install a（b）（4）conveyor at the capping machine outfeed, and merge filling and capping areas, for two filling lines（（b）（4）and（b）（4）），but you did not commit to perform a comprehensive assessment of your facility's production lines to ensure they are appropriately designed and controlled.

你公司的回应不够充分。尽管你公司承诺将用其他部件替换（b）（4）灌装线上的（b）（4）螺纹螺栓，使螺纹不再暴露于打开的瓶子周围，但你公司并未承诺对生产间和生产设备进行评估，以查看是否存在磨损、损坏或不良设计，这些可能会导致在敞开的西林瓶附近产生颗粒物。你公司还计划在加盖机出口处安装（b）（4）输送机，并合并两条灌装线的灌装和封盖区域，但没有承诺对你公司设施的生产线进行全面评估，以确保它们得到适当的设计和控制。

In response to this letter, provide：

在回复本函时，请提供：

● A comprehensive, independent assessment of the design of each sterile drug production line, including facility layout, equipment placement and ergonomics, and personnel and material flow. Provide your detailed remediation plan with timelines to address the findings of the assessment. Describe specific tangible improvements to be made to the sterile processing operation design and control. Include a plan to assess the effectiveness of the improvements.

● 对每条无菌药品生产线的设计进行全面、独立的评估，包括设施布局、设备放置和人体工程学，以及人流和物料。提供详细的整改计划和时间表，以应对评估结果。描述对无菌工艺操作设计和控制要进行的具体切实改进。包括一份评估改进有效性的计划。

● A comprehensive, independent assessment of the condition of equipment including change parts, and the procedures and practices associated with equipment maintenance. Provide your detailed remediation action plan that includes dates by which each remediation activity will be completed and periodic assessment of the plan's effectiveness.

● 对设备状况（包括更换零件）以及与设备维护相关的程序和实践进行全面、独立的评估。提供详细的整改行动计划，其中包括完成每项整改活动的日期和对计划有效性的定期评估。

烟雾研究未充分模拟实际生产条件

警告信编号: MARCS-CMS 654986

签发时间: 2023-8-3; **公示时间:** 2023-8-29

签发机构: 药品质量业务四处(Division of Pharmaceutical Quality Operations IV)

公 司: K.C. Pharmaceuticals Inc.

所在国家/地区: 美国

主 题: cGMP/成品制剂/掺假(cGMP/Finished Pharmaceuticals/ Adulterated)

摘 要: 该公司宣称是自有品牌眼部护理产品的领先制造商。FDA 在 2023 年 1 月至 2 月期间对其药品生产设施进行了检查。在检查中,FDA 首先指出,该公司对无菌生产线的烟雾研究并未在充分模拟实际生产条件下进行。举例来说,2018 年进行的烟雾研究并不能代表无菌灌装线上常规的动态生产条件。此外,自 2020 年以来,两条灌装线都多次出现了培养基灌装不合格的情况。针对 2020 年线上发生的两次不合格情况,该公司未能完成调查,也未能充分解决 2021 年线上不合格情况的根本原因,而是在没有充分科学论证的情况下判定培养基灌装无效。因此,FDA 要求对整个系统进行全面、独立的评估,以调查偏差、差异、OOS(超出规范)结果和不合格事件。同时,该公司需要提供详细的行动计划,以整改这一系统存在的问题。

本警告信以下部分与本书此前其他警告信内容类似,故略去:前言、质量部门失效(Ineffective Quality Unit)、cGMP 顾问推荐(cGMP Consultant Recommended)、结论(Conclusion)。

无菌工艺验证

1. Your firm failed to establish and follow appropriate written procedures that are designed to prevent microbiological contamination of drug products purporting to be sterile, and that includes validation of all aseptic and sterilization processes（21 CFR 211.113（b））.

1. 你公司未能建立并遵循适当的书面程序，包括验证所有无菌和灭菌工艺的程序，以防止声称无菌的药品受到微生物污染［21 CFR 211.113（b）］。

■ Smoke Studies ｜ 烟雾研究

Your smoke studies for your aseptic processing lines were not performed under conditions that adequately simulate actual manufacturing. For example, the smoke study performed in 2018 did not represent routine dynamic manufacturing conditions on the（b）（4）aseptic filling line. During the current inspection, you stated that the 2018 smoke study was the only smoke study performed on the（b）（4）filling line. Your firm began commercial manufacturing using the（b）（4）line in 2020 without adequate smoke studies.

你公司对无菌生产线的烟雾研究并未在充分模拟实际生产的条件下进行。例如，2018 年进行的烟雾研究并不代表（b）（4）无菌灌装线上的常规动态生产条件。在本次检查中，你公司表示 2018 年烟雾研究是在（b）（4）灌装线上进行的唯一烟雾研究。你公司于 2020 年开始使用（b）（4）生产线进行商业生产，但没有进行充分的烟雾研究。

Additionally, during the inspection, and in your response, you acknowledge that your smoke study for line（b）（4）, performed in September 2022, was inadequate. A repeat smoke study was performed in December 2022, however your quality unit had not completed their review at the time of the inspection and this study was not made available for the investigators to review.

此外，在检查期间以及你公司的回复中，你们承认于 2022 年 9 月进行的（b）（4）烟雾研究是不充分的。2022 年 12 月进行了重复烟雾研究，但是你公司的质量部门在检查时尚未完成审核，并且该研究无法供调查员审查。

In your response, you acknowledge that this is a repeat observation. You state that a corrective action and preventive action（CAPA）has been raised to address deficiencies in smoke studies from a holistic perspective with assistance of a third-party consultant. You have decided to repeat smoke studies on both aseptic filling lines to ensure aseptic filling interventions are properly evaluated and documented.

在回复中，你公司承认这种情况是重复出现的。你公司声称已提出纠正和预防措施（CAPA），以便在第三方顾问的协助下，从整体角度解决烟雾研究中的缺陷。你公司决定对两条无菌灌装线重复烟雾研究，以确保无菌灌装干预措施得到正确评估和记录。

Your response is inadequate because it includes plans to perform a product impact assessment without providing detailed information as to how you are determining the impact to products manufactured on lines without adequate smoke studies. Without adequate smoke studies, you cannot substantively assess whether unidirectional ISO 5 airflow is protecting the drug product from contamination.

你公司的回复是不充分的，因为它包括执行产品影响评估的计划，但就如何在没有充分烟雾研究的情况下确定对生产线生产的产品的影响，没有提供有关详细信息。如果没有充分的烟雾研究，你公司无法实质性评估单向 ISO 5 气流是否可以保护药品免受污染。

■ Media Fill Failure Investigations ｜培养基灌装不合格调查

Since 2020, there have been multiple media fill failures representing both filling lines, （b）（4）and（b）（4）. Your firm failed to complete the investigations of two failures in 2020 on line（b）（4）and did not adequately address the root cause of a failure that occurred in 2021 on line（b）（4）, instead invalidating the media fill without adequate scientific justification.

自 2020 年以来，（b）（4）和（b）（4）两条灌装线均出现多次培养基灌装不合格。对于 2020 年（b）（4）线上发生的两次不合格，你公司未能完成调查，也没有充分解决 2021 年（b）（4）线上发生不合格的根本原因，而是在没有充分科学论证的情况下，判定培养基灌装无效。

In your May 23, 2023 response to our request for additional information you provided investigation NCR-20-081, opened on May 15, 2023, which describes the incomplete media fill failure investigations that occurred in October and November 2020 relating to line（b）（4）. Your firm stated that the investigations into these failures had not been closed. The media fill failure in October 2020 occurred after approximately（b）（4）batches of finished drug products were manufactured since May 2020.

在你公司于 2023 年 5 月 23 日对我们提供更多信息的要求的回复中，你公司提供了于 2023 年 5 月 15 日启动的调查 NCR-20-081，该调查描述了与（b）（4）线相关的未完成的培养基灌装不合格调查，这些事件于 2020 年 10 月和 2020 年 11 月发生。你公司表示，对这些不合格的调查尚未关闭。2020 年 10 月的培养基灌装不合格发生时，自 2020 年 5 月后已生产了大约（b）（4）批成品。

In response to this letter, provide:

在回复本函时，请提供:

● A comprehensive, independent assessment of your overall system for investigating deviations, discrepancies, complaints, out-of-specification (OOS) results, and failures. Provide a detailed action plan to remediate this system. Your action plan should include, but not be limited to, significant improvements in investigation competencies, scope determination, root cause evaluation, CAPA effectiveness, quality unit oversight, and written procedures. Address how your firm will ensure all phases of investigations are appropriately conducted.

● 对整个系统进行全面、独立的评估，以调查偏差、差异、投诉、OOS 结果和不合格。提供详细的行动计划，以整改此系统。你公司的行动计划应包括但不限于：调查能力、范围确定、根本原因评估、CAPA 有效性、质量部门监督和书面程序方面的显著提高。说明你公司将如何确保调查的所有阶段都得到适当实施。

● A comprehensive, independent assessment of the design and control of your firm's manufacturing operations, with a detailed and thorough review of all microbiological hazards.

● 对你公司生产操作的设计和控制进行全面、独立的评估，并对所有微生物危害进行详细、彻底的审查。

● Your plan to ensure appropriate aseptic practices and cleanroom behavior during production. Include steps to ensure routine and effective supervisory oversight for all production batches. Also describe the frequency of quality unit oversight (e.g., audit) during aseptic processing and its support operations.

● 你公司确保生产工艺中采取适当的无菌操作和洁净室行为的计划。包括确保对所有生产批次进行常规和有效监督的步骤。另外，描述无菌工艺操作和支持操作期间质量部门监督（例如审计）的频率。

● A thorough retrospective review and risk assessment that evaluates how poor aseptic technique and cleanroom behavior may have affected the quality and sterility of your drugs.

● 彻底的回顾性审查和风险评估，评估不良的无菌技术和洁净室行为可能如何影响药品的质量和无菌性。

● A complete independent assessment of documentation systems used throughout your manufacturing and laboratory operations to determine where documentation practices are insufficient. Include a detailed CAPA plan that comprehensively remediates your firm's documentation practices to ensure you retain attributable, legible, complete, original, accurate, contemporaneous records throughout your operation. This item is especially critical due to the missing documentation described in your May 2023 correspondence.

● 对整个生产和实验室运营中使用的文档系统进行完整的独立评估，以确定记录规范的不足之处。包括一份详细的 CAPA 计划，全面整改你公司的文件记录实践，以确保在整个运营过程中保存可追溯的、清晰的、完整的、原始的、准确的和同步的记录。鉴于你公司 2023 年 5 月的函中描述的文档缺失，此项尤其重要。

无菌工艺操作设计

2. Your firm failed to perform operations within specifically defined areas of adequate size and to have separate or defined areas or such other control systems necessary to prevent contamination or mix-ups in aseptic processing areas(21 CFR 211.42(c)(10)).

2. 你公司未能在足够大小的明确定义区域内进行操作，也未能拥有单独或界定的区域，或其他必要的控制系统，来防止无菌工艺区的污染或混淆［21 CFR 211.42（ c ）（ 10 ）］。

Your aseptic processing operation is inadequately designed to prevent contamination of your ophthalmic drug products.

你公司的无菌工艺操作设计不充分，无法防止眼科药品受到污染。

For example, your firm lacked adequate building management systems (BMS) to monitor and record differential pressures in your aseptic processing facility. You recorded differential pressures by observing photohelic gauges with upper and lower limits that can be (b)(4)accessed and adjusted. Additionally, your operators recorded differential pressures at the (b)(4)of every fill batch, approximately every(b)(4), and at the(b)(4)of filling operations. This frequency is not adequate to detect pressure deviations (e.g., reversals)that could ultimately impact aseptic conditions on the filling line.

例如，你公司缺乏充分的建筑管理系统（BMS），来监控和记录无菌工艺操作设施中的压差。通过观察光电压力计记录了压差，其上下限可以通过（ b ）（ 4 ）访问和调整。此外，你公司的操作员记录了每个灌装批次的（ b ）（ 4 ）处、以（ b ）（ 4 ）频率以及灌装操作的（ b ）（ 4 ）处的压差。该频率不足以检测可能最终影响灌装线上的无菌条件的压力偏差（例如，反向压差）。

In addition, the ISO 5 aseptic processing line, (b)(4), is described as an (b)(4). During the inspection, we observed several (b)(4)in the walls of the enclosure. These(b)(4)were open to the surrounding room during aseptic processing and did not contain any(b)(4). Similarly, the smoke study video that you provided in your May 2023 correspondence showed the (b)(4)line with (b)(4)opened to the surrounding room while the smoke study was being conducted. During this smoke study video, operators are seen conducting interventions on this aseptic filling line with their（b）（4）arms and（b）（4）hands, by reaching through the open ports instead of using installed（b）（4）. While your firm refers to this aseptic processing line as an（b）（4）, both its design and operation does not meet the minimum standards of a（b）（4）.

另外，ISO 5 无菌生产线（b）（4）被描述为（b）（4）。在检查过程中，我们在墙壁上观察到了几个（b）（4）。这些（b）（4）在无菌处理过程中向周围的房间开放，而并未包含任何（b）（4）控制。同样，你公司在 2023 年 5 月的信件中提供的烟雾研究视频显示，在进行烟雾研究时，（b）（4）线与（b）（4）向周围的房间开放。在这段烟雾研究视频中，可以看到操作员用（b）（4）手臂和（b）（4）手对这条无菌灌装线进行干预，方法是穿过开放端口，而不是使用已安装的（b）（4）。虽然你公司将此无菌生产线称为（b）（4），但其设计和操作均不符合（b）（4）的最低标准。

Aseptic processes should be designed to minimize exposure of sterile articles to potential contamination hazards, including, but not limited to, variation in environmental conditions. It is vital for rooms of higher air cleanliness to have a substantial positive pressure differential relative to adjacent rooms of lower air cleanliness. A suitable facility monitoring system is critical to maintain appropriate environmental conditions throughout all of your cleanrooms. All deviations from established limits should be appropriately investigated to rapidly detect atypical changes that can compromise the facility's environment. Prompt detection of an emerging problem is essential to preventing contamination of your aseptic production operations.

无菌工艺的设计应尽量减少无菌物品暴露于潜在污染危害的情况，包括但不限于环境条件的变化。对于空气洁净度较高的房间来说，相对于空气洁净度较低的相邻房间需要有显著的正压差，这是至关重要的。对于在所有洁净室中保持适当的环境条件，合适的设施监控系统意义重大。应对所有偏离既定限度的情况进行适当调查，以快速检测可能损害设施环境的异常变化。对于防止无菌生产操作受到污染，及时发现新出现的问题很有必要。

In your response, you commit to installing a（b）（4）over the photohelic gauges to prevent access. However, in your June 23, 2023 response to our request for additional information, you acknowledge that you have not implemented a continuous monitoring system that ensures differential pressures will be continuously monitored, adequately recorded, and any differential pressure deviations will be detected, documented, and investigated.

在你公司的回复中，你们承诺在光电测量仪上安装（b）（4）以防止进入。然而，在 2023 年 6 月 23 日对我们要求提供更多信息的回复中，你公司承认尚未实施连续监测系统，以确保持续监测、充分记录压差，并且检测、记录和调查任何压差偏差。

In response to this letter, provide the following:

在回复本函时，请提供以下信息：

● Your CAPA plan to implement routine, vigilant operations management oversight of facilities and equipment. This plan should ensure, among other things, prompt detection of equipment/facilities performance issues, effective execution of repairs, adherence to appropriate preventive maintenance schedules, timely technological upgrades to the equipment/facility infrastructure, and improved systems for ongoing management review.

● 你公司的 CAPA 计划对设施和设备实施常规的、警戒性的运营管理监督。至少，该计划应确保及时发现设备 / 设施性能问题，有效执行维修，遵守适当的预防性维护计划，及时对设备 / 设施基础设施进行技术升级，并对持续管理评审的系统进行改进。

● Comprehensive risk assessment of all contamination hazards with respect to your aseptic processes, equipment, and facilities, including an independent assessment that includes, but is not limited to:

● 就你公司的无菌工艺、设备和设施的所有污染危害，进行全面的风险评估，包含独立评估，这包括但不限于：

○ All human interactions within the ISO 5 area

○ ISO 5 区域内的所有人员交互

○ Equipment placement and ergonomics

○ 设备放置和人体工程学

○ Air quality in the ISO 5 area and surrounding room

○ ISO 5 区域和周围区域的空气质量

○ Facility layout

○ 设施布局

○ Personnel Flows and Material Flows (throughout all rooms used to conduct and support sterile operations)

○ 人流和物流（用于执行和支持无菌操作的所有房间）

● A detailed remediation plan with timelines to address the findings of the contamination hazards risk assessment. Describe specific tangible improvements to be made to aseptic processing operation design and control.

● 详细的整改计划和时间表，以解决污染危害风险评估所发现的问题。描述要对无菌工艺操作设计和控制进行的具体切实改进。

清洁验证

3. Your firm failed to establish and follow adequate written procedures for cleaning and maintenance of equipment（21 CFR 211.67（b））.

3. 你公司未建立并遵循适当的书面程序，来清洁和维护设备［21 CFR 211.67（b）］。

Cleaning validation studies for aseptic processing line（b）（4）, used to manufacture multiple formulations of ophthalmic drug products, has not been completed. For example, the（b）（4）compounding tank and product transfer line（b）（4）, used to formulate bulk ophthalmic drugs for filling on line（b）（4）, did not have recovery studies or limits of detection. Additionally, when identifying the（b）（4）conditions under which to conduct the cleaning validation, you relied only on the viscosity of your multiple ophthalmic drug products to make the determination, omitting other factors that can make certain formulations harder to clean. While you chose the product Eye Drops Systane–Ultra Like（EDSU）as （b）（4）, you lacked documented scientific evidence to support use of（b）（4）viscosity as adequate basis for validating the hardest to clean product surface.

针对用于生产眼科药品多种处方的无菌生产线（b）（4），其清洁验证研究尚未完成。例如，对于用于配制用于在线（b）（4）灌装的半成品眼科药品的（b）（4）配制罐和产品传输线（b）（4），其没有回收率研究或检测限。此外，在确定进行清洁验证的（b）（4）条件时，你公司仅依靠多种眼科药品的黏度来做出决定，忽略了可能使某些制剂更难清洁的其他因素。当你公司选择滴眼液产品 Systane–Ultra Like（EDSU）作为（b）（4）时，缺乏书面科学证据，来支持使用（b）（4）黏度作为验证最难清洁产品表面的充分依据。

In your response, you commit to performing a risk assessment and product impact assessment, but lack details regarding what you will evaluate and how you will do so. You did not commit to performing additional verification of cleaning to ensure cross–contamination is not occurring when using the（b）（4）compounding tank, product transfer line（b）（4）, or other equipment. Your response also commits to performing a new study to determine（b）（4） product（s）, without providing details as to what properties would be evaluated and how.

在你公司的回复中，你们承诺进行风险评估和产品影响评估，但就评估什么以及如何评估，你公司缺乏详细的信息。你公司未承诺执行额外的清洁验证，以确保在使用（b）（4）混合罐、产品传输线（b）（4）或其他设备时不会发生交叉污染。你公司的回复还承诺进行一项新的研究，以确定（b）（4）产品，但未提供将评估哪些属性以及如何评估的详细信息。

In response to this letter，provide：

在回复本函时，请提供：

（略）

此处与 FDA 发给 Cosmetic Science Laboratories LLC 的警告信（编号：MARCS-CMS 645558，即"5 水系统未经充分设计与监控"）中有关清洁验证的回应要求部分的内容类似，故略去。

5 培养基灌装中模拟的干预次数不足

警告信编号： MARCS-CMS 658878

签发时间： 2023-9-11；**公示时间：** 2023-9-12

签发机构： 药物审评与研究中心 | CDER（Center for Drug Evaluation and Research | CDER）

公　　司： Similasan AG

所在国家 / 地区： 瑞士

主　　题： cGMP/ 成品制剂 / 掺假 / 标识错误 / 未批准的新药（cGMP/ Finished Pharmaceuticals/Adulterated/Unapproved New Drug）

简　　介： 在查看了公司网站后，FDA 发现很多产品属于未经批准的新药，这引发了 FDA 的担忧。于 2023 年 3 月，FDA 对该生产设施进行了检查。在检查中，FDA 发现其培养基灌装的书面程序存在缺陷，因为这些程序无法准确模拟商业生产。举例来说，商业批次中人工操作频繁且密集，但在培养基灌装过程中模拟的干预次数明显不足。例如，在加盖区域的商业生产中有 38 次干预，而在支持性培养基灌装过程中只模拟了 14 次干预。FDA 强调，这种培养基灌装研究的不足会影响其准确评估验证和过程控制状态的能力。为了确保有效的评估，培养基灌装研究需要准确模拟商业生产过程中发生的干预的数量和类型，这一点非常重要。然而，在该公司的回复中并未包括风险评估或调查，以确定在无菌操作期间过多的人工干预是否影响了其药品的安全性。FDA 强调，公司需要对这些问题进行全面的调查，并提供详细的行动计划来解决这些问题。

本警告信以下部分与本书此前其他警告信内容类似，故略去：前言、未批准的新药（Unapproved New Drugs）、cGMP 顾问推荐（cGMP Consultant Recommended）、结论（Conclusion）。

无菌和灭菌工艺验证

1. Your firm failed to establish and follow appropriate written procedures that are designed to prevent microbiological contamination of drug products purporting to be sterile, and that include validation of all aseptic and sterilization processes.(21 CFR 211.113 (b))

1. 你公司未能建立并遵循适当的书面程序，包括验证所有无菌和灭菌工艺的程序，以防止声称无菌的药品受到微生物污染〔21 CFR 211.113 (b)〕。

The written procedures for your media fills were not appropriate because they failed to accurately simulate commercial manufacturing. Our inspection found that aseptic interventions simulated during your media fills were not sufficiently representative of commercial aseptic manufacturing. For example, the number of interventions conducted during your manually intensive commercial operations exceeded the number performed during your media fills as follows,

你公司培养基灌装的书面程序存在缺陷，因为它们无法准确模拟商业生产。检查发现，在培养基灌装过程中模拟的无菌干预措施不足以代表商业无菌生产。例如，商业批人工操作密集，期间进行的干预次数超过了培养基灌装期间进行的干预次数，如下所示，

- (b)(4), batch(b)(4), documented 38 interventions in the cap(b)(4)area during manufacture and 14 interventions were simulated during your supportive media fill

- (b)(4)，批次（b）(4)，其生产过程中在加盖（b）(4)区域有 38 次干预，而在支持性培养基灌装过程中只模拟了 14 次干预

- (b)(4), batch(b)(4), documented 40 interventions in the cap(b)(4)area during manufacture and 23 interventions were simulated during your supportive media fill

- (b)(4)，批次（b）(4)，其生产过程中在加盖（b）(4)区域有 40 次干预，而在支持性培养基模拟灌装过程中只进行了 23 次干预

Your inadequate media fill studies compromise your ability to accurately assess the state of validation and process control. To ensure a valid assessment, it is critical that media fill studies accurately simulate the number and type of interventions that occur during commercial manufacturing.

你公司对培养基模拟灌装研究不充分，这会影响你们准确评估验证和过程控制状态的能力。为了确保有效的评估，培养基模拟灌装研究需要准确模拟商业生产过程中发生的干预的数量和类型，这一点非常重要。

Furthermore, interventions may increase contamination risks during aseptic manufacturing.

此外，干预措施可能会增加无菌生产过程中的污染风险。

Your response states that you plan to include these and other interventions in the next media fill simulation, scheduled for June 2023. Your response failed to include a risk assessment or investigation to determine whether the safety of your drug products are impacted by the excessive manual interventions during aseptic operations.

你公司的回复指出，在于 2023 年 6 月进行的下一次培养基模拟灌装中，你公司计划纳入这些和其他干预。回复中未能包括风险评估或调查，以确定在无菌操作期间过多的人工干预是否会影响你公司药品的安全性。

You may refer to FDA's guidance document *Sterile Drug Products Produced by Aseptic Processing—Current Good Manufacturing Practice* to help you meet the cGMP requirements when manufacturing sterile drugs using aseptic processing at https://www.fda. gov/media/71026/download.

请参阅 FDA 指南，通过无菌工艺生产的无菌药品 – 现行药品生产质量管理规范，以帮助你们在使用无菌工艺生产无菌药品时满足 cGMP 要求，网址（略，见上）。

In response to this letter, provide:

在回复本函时，请提供：

（略）

此处与 FDA 发给 K.C. Pharmaceuticals Inc. 的警告信（编号：MARCS–CMS 654986，即"4 烟雾研究未充分模拟实际生产条件"）中有关无菌工艺操作设计的回应要求部分的内容类似，故略去。

实验室控制措施

2. Your firm failed to establish laboratory controls that include scientifically sound and appropriate specifications, standards, sampling plans, and test procedures designed to assure that components, drug product containers, closures, in-process materials, labeling, and drug products conform to appropriate standards of identity, strength, quality, and purity.（21 CFR 211.160（b））

2. 你公司未能建立实验室控制措施，其中包括科学合理且相应的规范、标准、取样计划和检验程序，以确保物料、药品容器、密封件、中间体、标签和药品符合相关规定，即鉴别、规格、质量和纯度的标准［21 CFR 211.160（b）］。

You failed to establish and conduct 100% visual inspections of your ophthalmic drug products to ensure that each container is essentially free of visible particulates. Since at least June 23, 2022, your established in-process inspection procedure for in-process inspection for visible particulates was limited to acceptable-quality-limits（AQLs）. The use of AQL sampling is intended as an additional analysis routinely conducted as part of the quality release processes only after performing 100% visual inspection. Your failure to conduct 100% visual inspection increases the risk for the release of ophthalmic drug product with visible particulate contamination.

你公司未能对眼科药品建立并进行100%目检，以确保每个包装不含可见异物。至少自2022年6月23日起，你公司为可见异物进行过程检验而制定了过程检验程序，其仅限于可接受质量水平（AQL）。AQL抽样的使用是作为质量放行程序的一部分而进行的额外分析，只有在进行了100%的目视检查之后才会进行。你公司未进行100%的目视检查，这会增加放行含有可见异物污染的眼药产品的风险。

Your response states that your（b）（4）particle inspection system's imaging processing, that you qualified in 2022 and utilized for 100% visual inspection, "was too slow" and the rejection rate was too high with "false positive［s］" so you suspended its use and implemented manual visual inspections using AQLs, with no 100% visual inspection. As a corrective action, you planned to re-introduce the（b）（4）system on May 1, 2023.

你公司的回复指出，在2022年获得确认并用于100%目检的（b）（4）颗粒检测系统的成像处理"太慢"，拒绝率过高，出现了"误报"，因此你公司暂停了其使用，并基于AQL实施了人工目检，但没有进行100%的目检。作为纠正措施，你公司计划于2023年5月1日重新引入（b）（4）系统。

Your response is inadequate. There is no commitment to conduct a retrospective review for your released drug products that only relied on the AQL sampling to try and assure product quality and limit patient risk. Additionally, your response did not include supportive documentation for routine osmolarity testing of your ophthalmic drug products.

你公司的回应不够充分。没有承诺对你公司已放行的药品进行回顾性审查，这些药品仅依靠AQL抽样来试图确保产品质量并限制患者风险。此外，你公司的回复也没有包括支持文件，证明对眼科药品进行了常规渗透压检验。

In response to this letter, provide:

在回复本函时，请提供:

- Improved in-process testing and monitoring to enhance detection of variation during production of each batch. Include remediated in-process quality standards, including but not limited to enhanced sampling, that will more robustly monitor (b)(4) process control. Describe how the improvements will ensure early detection of process variation and manufacturing defects, and prevent consumer exposure to substandard quality drug products.

● 改进过程检验和监控，以加强对每批生产工艺中变异的检测。包括修正的过程质量标准，这包含但不限于加强取样，以更好地监测（b）（4）过程控制。描述这些改进将如何确保及早发现工艺变异和生产缺陷，并防止消费者接触到质量不合格的药品。

● Given that your container closure system uses an (b)(4) vial, provide data supporting that your (b)(4) particle inspection system can adequately detect particles within your container closure.

● 鉴于你公司的容器密闭系统使用（b）（4）西林瓶，请提供数据支持你公司的（b）（4）颗粒检测系统能够充分检测容器密闭内的颗粒。

● For all batches that you have not conducted 100% visual inspection, conduct 100% visible inspection of your retain samples. If you obtain out-of-specification (OOS) results, conduct investigations and provide your completed investigations, including conclusions and take appropriate market action for all batches of drug products confirmed not meeting specifications.

● 对于未进行 100% 目检的所有批次，对留样进行 100% 目检。如果你公司获得不合格（OOS）结果，请进行调查并提供已完成的调查，包括结论，并对所有确认不符合质量标准的药品批次采取适当的市场行动。

● Supportive documentation clarifying whether you are conducting routine osmolarity testing for your topical ophthalmic drug products for release and stability testing.

● 支持性记录，阐明你公司是否正在对外用眼科药品制剂进行常规渗透压检验，以便放行和稳定性检验。

数据可靠性

3. Your firm failed to ensure that laboratory records included complete data derived from all tests necessary to ensure compliance with established specifications and standards (21 CFR 211.194(a)).

3. 你公司未能确保实验室记录包含所有检验的完整数据，以确保符合既定规范和标准［21 CFR 211.194（a）］。

Your laboratory records do not include complete testing data to support the analysis performed. For example, negative controls for sterility testing are not documented at the time of performance. The absence of concurrently performed negative controls during sterility testing does not allow full assessment of the suitability of the testing performed.

你公司的实验室记录不包括支持所执行分析的完整检验数据。例如，在执行时没有记录无菌检验的阴性对照。在无菌检验期间缺乏同时进行的阴性对照，这导致无法对所进行的检验的适用性进行全面评估。

All cGMP-related data must be retained to enable appropriate assessments and decisions by the QU and to demonstrate ongoing control. The lack of complete testing records compromises the integrity of the testing results.

必须保存所有 cGMP 相关数据，以便 QU 能够进行适当的评估和决策，并证明持续的控制。缺乏完整的检验记录会对检验结果的可靠性产生负面影响。

In your response, you state that you will implement new test method records for standard preparations. You also state that you will follow your test procedures in accordance with the compendial method, and finished product test results reported by the quality control unit for sterile drug products will be accurately recorded. Your response is inadequate because there is no commitment to conduct retrospective reviews for tested products and training of employees to correct deficient practices.

在你公司的回复中，你们声称将为标准试剂实施新的检验方法记录。此外，你公司还将按照药典方法执行检测程序，由质量控制部门报告无菌药品制剂检测结果，并将准确记录。你公司的回应是不充分的，因为没有承诺对已检验产品进行回顾性审查，也没有对员工进行培训，以纠正有缺陷的实践。

In response to this letter, provide：

在回复本函时，请提供：

● A complete assessment of documentation systems used throughout your manufacturing and laboratory operations to determine where documentation practices are insufficient. Include a detailed CAPA plan that comprehensively remediates your firm's documentation practices to ensure you retain attributable, legible, complete, original, accurate, contemporaneous records throughout your operation.

● 对整个生产操作中使用的文件记录系统进行全面评估，以确定记录实践的不足之处。包括详细的 CAPA 计划，以全面整改公司的记录实践，确保你公司在整个运营过程中保存可追溯的、清晰的、完整的、原始的、准确的和同步的记录。

● Your action plan to address any product quality or patient safety risks for your drug products in U.S. distribution, including potential customer notifications and recalls.

● 你公司的行动计划，以解决你们的药品在美国流通时的任何产品质量或患者安全风险，包括潜在的客户通知和召回。

质量部门未能履责

4. Your firm failed to establish an adequate quality unit and the responsibilities and procedures applicable to the quality control unit are not in writing and fully followed (21 CFR 211.22 (a) and 211.22 (d)).

4. 你公司未能建立适当的质量部门，适用于质量部门的责任和程序未以书面形式呈现且未得到完全遵守 [21 CFR 211.22 (a) 和 (d)]。

Your quality unit (QU) did not provide adequate oversight for the manufacture of your drug products. For example, your QU failed to ensure：

你公司的质量部门（QU）没有对药品的生产提供充分的监督。例如，你公司的 QU 未能确保：

● Adequate procedures for that are designed to prevent microbiological contamination of drug products purporting to be sterile (21 CFR 211.113 (b)).

● 适当的程序，以防止声称无菌的药品受到微生物污染 [21 CFR 211.113 (b)]。

● Adequate procedures to establish laboratory controls that include scientifically sound and appropriate specifications, standards, and sampling plans sampling plans, and test procedures designed to assure that drug products conform to appropriate standards of identity, strength, quality, and purity (21 CFR 211.160 (b)).

● 建立实验室控制的充分程序，包括科学合理且相应的质量规范、标准和取样计划，以及旨在确保药品符合适当的鉴别、规格、质量和纯度标准的检验程序 [21 CFR 211.160 (b)]。

● Adequate procedures to ensure that laboratory records included complete data (21 CFR 211.194 (a)).

● 确保实验室记录包含完整数据的适当程序 [21 CFR 211.194 (a)]。

● Adequate QU oversight to ensure the use of harmless components in your drug products.

● 充分的 QU 监督以确保你公司的药品中使用无害原辅料。

Your firm's quality systems are inadequate. You may refer to FDA's guidance document

Quality Systems Approach to Pharmaceutical cGMP Regulations for help implementing quality systems and risk management approaches to meet the requirements of cGMP regulations 21 CFR, parts 210 and 211 at https://www.fda.gov/media/71023/download.

你公司的质量体系不完善。请参阅 FDA 指南，药品 cGMP 法规的质量体系方法，帮助实施质量体系和风险管理方法，以满足 cGMP 法规 21 CFR 第 210 和 211 部分的要求，网址（略，见上）。

In response to this letter, provide:

在回复本函时，请提供：

（略）

此处与 FDA 发给 Cosmobeauti Laboratories & Manufacturing Inc. 的警告信（编号：MARCS-CMS 657682，即"12 批生产记录存在倒记问题"）中有关 QU 的回应要求部分的内容类似，故略去。

○ Take prompt and appropriate actions for all batches of drug products that contain unacceptable levels of ingredients that could cause them to be harmful, including customer notifications and other applicable market actions for any batches containing harmful ingredients. Detail these actions in your response to this letter.

○ 针对所有含有可能导致有害物料含量不可接受的药品批次，采取迅速和适当的行动，包括对任何含有有害原辅料的批次进行客户通知和其他适用的市场行动。在你公司对本函的回复中详细说明这些行动。

Products Containing Glycerin and Sorbitol Solution
含有甘油和山梨醇溶液的产品

You manufacture multiple drugs that contain glycerin or sorbitol solution. Identity testing for these and certain other high-risk drug components includes a limit test in the United States Pharmacopeia (USP) to ensure that the component meets the relevant safety limits for levels of diethylene glycol (DEG) or ethylene glycol (EG).

你公司生产多种含有甘油或山梨醇溶液的药品。就这些和某些其他高风险药品原辅料的鉴别检验，应包括 USP 中的限度检验，以确保该原辅料符合二甘醇（DEG）或乙二醇（EG）含量的相关安全限度。

The use of ingredients contaminated with DEG or EG has resulted in various lethal poisoning incidents in humans worldwide. See FDA's guidance document *Testing of Glycerin*, *Propylene Glycol*, *Maltitol Solution*, *Hydrogenated Starch Hydrolysate*, *Sorbitol Solution*,

and Other High-Risk Drug Components for Diethylene Glycol and Ethylene Glycol at https://
www.fda.gov/media/167974/download，to help you meet the cGMP requirements when
manufacturing drugs containing ingredients at high–risk for DEG or EG contamination.

　　在全球范围内，使用受 DEG 或 EG 污染的原辅料已导致多起人类致命中毒事件。
请参阅 FDA 指南，甘油、丙二醇、麦芽糖醇溶液、氢化淀粉水解物、山梨醇溶液和其
他高风险药品原辅料中二甘醇和乙二醇的检验，以帮助你公司在生产含有 DEG 或 EG
污染风险原辅料的药品时，满足 cGMP 要求，请访问网址（略，见上）。

6 无菌操作技术存在问题

警告信编号： MARCS-CMS 636199

签发时间： 2023-10-16；**公示时间：** 2023-10-16

签发机构： 药物审评与研究中心 | CDER（Center for Drug Evaluation and Research | CDER）

公　　司： Sun Pharmaceutical Industries Ltd.

所在国家 / 地区： 印度

主　　题： cGMP/ 原 料 药（API）/ 掺 假［cGMP/Active Pharmaceutical Ingredient（API）/Adulterated］

简　　介： 太阳制药是一家总部位于印度孟买的跨国制药公司，主要在印度和美国生产销售各种制剂和原料药。公司成立于 1983 年，并在 2014 年收购了兰伯西，因此成为印度最大的制药公司。其市场的 72% 位于国外，其中美国是最大的市场，公司一半的营业额来自于美国。在 2022 年 4 月至 5 月期间，FDA 对其位于印度的药品生产设施进行了检查。在检查中，FDA 观察到操作员的无菌操作技术存在较大问题。举例来说，操作员用戴手套的手将器具插入无菌容器内；操作员在关键区域的动作并不总是缓慢而谨慎的；操作员在各种活动期间阻挡气流，伸手越过敞开的无菌容器，并且倾斜身体以观察其内部。为此，FDA 要求企业进行彻底的回顾性审查和风险评估，评估不良的无菌技术和洁净室行为可能如何影响药品的质量和无菌性。

本警告信以下部分与本书此前其他警告信内容类似，故略去：前言、质量体系失效（Ineffective Quality Systems）、cGMP 顾问推荐（cGMP Consultant Recommended）、结论（Conclusion）。

无菌和灭菌工艺验证

1. Your firm failed to establish and follow appropriate written procedures that are designed to prevent microbiological contamination of drug products purporting to be sterile, and that include validation of all aseptic and sterilization processes（21 CFR 211.113（b））.

1. 你公司未能建立并遵循适当的书面程序，包括验证所有无菌和灭菌工艺的程序，以防止声称无菌的药品受到微生物污染 ［21 CFR 211.113（b）］。

■ Inadequate Media Fills ｜ 培养基灌装不充分

Your media fills failed to accurately simulate commercial operations. Our inspection found the aseptic operations simulated during your media fills were not sufficiently representative of commercial aseptic manufacturing operations for medroxyprogesterone acetate injectable suspension USP, 150mg/mL, 1ml prefilled syringes and vials. For example, data from the inspection indicated：

你公司的培养基模拟灌装未能准确模拟商业批操作。我们的检查发现，在你公司的培养基模拟灌装过程中模拟了无菌操作，其不足以代表醋酸甲羟孕酮注射混悬剂 USP（150mg/ml，1ml 预装注射器和西林瓶）的商业无菌生产操作。例如，检查数据表明：

A. Personnel simulated the manual addition of approximately（b）（4）grams of sterile（b）（4）to the compounding tank for up to（b）（4）. However, for commercial manufacturing, approximately（b）（4）grams of sterile active pharmaceutical ingredient（API）was added to the compounding tank. This hand（b）（4）operation took up to（b）（4）and included a（b）（4）change during routine commercial manufacturing.

A. 人员模拟人工添加大约（b）（4）g 无菌（b）（4）到混合罐中，最多占用（b）（4）时间。然而，对于商业生产，大约（b）（4）g 无菌原料药（API）被添加到混合罐中。此人工（b）（4）操作占用了（b）（4）时间，并包括了常规商业生产期间的（b）（4）变化。

B. Approximately（b）（4）grams of sterile（b）（4）was hand-（b）（4）from（b）（4）sealed（b）（4）container into（b）（4）or more（b）（4）. This process was not consistent with commercial manufacturing, where approximately（b）（4）grams of sterile API was hand-（b）（4）from（b）（4）different（b）（4）pouches into（b）（4）. Pouches used in commercial manufacturing may also have been previously opened and re-sealed.

B. 将约（b）（4）g 无菌（b）（4）从（b）（4）密封（b）（4）容器中，手工（b）（4）

放入（b）（4）或更多（b）（4）。该工艺与商业生产不一致，其中大约（b）（4）g 无菌 API 是从（b）（4）不同的（b）（4）袋手工（b）（4）装入（b）（4）。用于商业生产的袋子也可能之前已打开并重新密封。

The dispensing and compounding steps were high-risk steps, and there were no additional sterilization steps following these operations.

称量和混合步骤是高风险步骤，并且这些操作之后没有额外的灭菌步骤。

Your operators performed lengthy, highly manually intensive aseptic operations. As such, the duration of process simulation should closely resemble the actual manufacturing process. If a media fill program fails to incorporate contamination risk factors and closely simulate actual drug product exposure, the state of process control and sterility assurance cannot be accurately assessed.

你公司的操作员执行了耗时、高度人工密集的无菌操作。因此，工艺模拟的持续时间应该与实际生产工艺非常相似。如果培养基模拟灌装程序未能纳入污染风险因素，并且未能密切模拟实际药品暴露，则无法准确评估过程控制和无菌保证的状态。

■ Poor Aseptic Behavior ｜ 无菌行为不良

Media fill and smoke studies of your manually intensive aseptic operations, such as dispensing of sterile API, and addition of sterile API to the compounding tank, revealed poor aseptic techniques by your operators. Examples include, but are not limited to：

对人工密集型无菌操作（例如无菌 API 的称量以及将无菌 API 添加到配制罐中）进行的培养基模拟灌装和烟雾研究表明，操作员的无菌技术较差。示例包括但不限于：

● An operator inserted his gloved hand inside the（b）（4）to（b）（4）out sterile（b）（4）with a（b）（4）utensil.

● 操作员用戴手套的手，将（b）（4）器具插入无菌（b）（4）内的（b）（4）至（b）（4）内。

● An operator touched the product contact surface of the（b）（4）stopper prior to placing it back on the（b）（4）.

● 在将（b）（4）胶塞放回（b）（4）上之前，操作员触摸其产品接触表面。

● Operator movements in the critical areas were not always slow and deliberate.

● 操作员在关键区域的动作并不总是缓慢而谨慎的。

● An operator blocked（b）（4）air during various activities, including but not limited to, reaching over the open sterile（b）（4）container multiple times, and tilting the（b）（4）towards his body to visualize its interior while（b）（4）out the sterile（b）（4）.

● 操作员在各种活动期间阻挡（b）（4）空气，包括但不限于：多次伸手越过敞开的无菌（b）（4）容器，并将向他的身体倾斜（b）（4）以观察其内部，而（b）（4）处于无菌状态（b）（4）。

Your response is inadequate. You experienced a significant media fill failure in November 2021, which revealed serious flaws and risks in your operation. You failed to perform a timely risk assessment to evaluate if the quality and sterility of your distributed drug products were affected by these deficiencies. You waited over five months to initiate a recall of the affected batches. The failure to proactively identify deficiencies and implement timely and sustainable corrective actions and preventive actions（CAPA）is unacceptable because it puts patients at risk.

你公司的回应不够充分。在 2021 年 11 月经历了培养基模拟灌装的显著不合格，这暴露了你公司运营中的严重缺陷和风险。你公司未能及时进行风险评估，以评估你们流通的药品的质量和无菌性是否受到这些缺陷的影响。你公司等了五个多月，才开始召回受影响批次。未能主动识别缺陷并及时实施可持续的纠正和预防措施（CAPA）是不可接受的，因为这会将患者置于危险之中。

We acknowledge you discontinued medroxyprogesterone acetate injectable suspension pre-filled syringe and vial manufacturing operations in Block（b）（4）as of November 30, 2021. This decision was based on the risks identified through your media fill failure investigation. You recalled all batches of the drug product following the FDA inspection. We also acknowledge that you intend to move the manufacturing operations to a new block equipped with（b）（4）.

我们知晓，自 2021 年 11 月 30 日起，你公司已停止在厂区（b）（4）中进行醋酸甲羟孕酮注射混悬液预充针和西林瓶的生产业务。该决定是基于你公司的培养基模拟灌装不合格调查发现的风险。你公司在 FDA 检查后召回了所有批次的药品。我们还知晓，你公司打算将生产业务转移到配备（b）（4）的新厂区。

See FDA's guidance document *Sterile Drug Products Produced by Aseptic Processing-Current Good Manufacturing Practice* to help you meet the cGMP requirements when manufacturing sterile drugs using aseptic processing, at https://www.fda.gov/media/71026/download.

请参阅 FDA 的指南，通过无菌工艺生产的无菌药品 - 现行药品生产质量管理规范，以帮助你公司在使用无菌工艺生产无菌药品时满足 cGMP 要求，网址（略，见上）。

In response to this letter, provide the following:

在回复本函时,请提供以下信息:

● Your plan to ensure appropriate aseptic practices and cleanroom behavior during production. Include steps to ensure routine and effective supervisory oversight for all production batches. Also describe the frequency of quality unit (QU) oversight (e.g., audit) during aseptic processing and its support operations.

● 你公司确保生产工艺中采取适当的无菌操作和洁净室行为的计划。包括确保对所有生产批次进行常规和有效监督的步骤。另外,描述无菌工艺操作和支持操作期间质量部门监督(例如审计)的频率。

● A thorough retrospective review and risk assessment that evaluates how poor aseptic technique and cleanroom behavior may have affected the quality and sterility of your drug products.

● 彻底的回顾性审查和风险评估,评估不良的无菌技术和洁净室行为可能如何影响药品的质量和无菌性。

● A comprehensive review of your media fill program, and CAPA to ensure an accurate simulation, including appropriately incorporating the worst-case conditions of commercial manufacturing.

● 对你公司的培养基模拟灌装程序和CAPA进行全面审查,以确保准确的模拟,包括适当地纳入商业生产中的最差情况。

● A list of the third parties performing consulting functions for your firm. Include their responsibilities and an estimated time frame for completion of their activities.

● 为你公司履行咨询职能的第三方清单。包括他们的职责和完成其活动的预期时间范围。

无菌工艺操作设计

2. Your firm failed to perform operations within specifically defined areas of adequate size and to have separate or defined areas or such other control systems necessary to prevent contamination or mix-ups in aseptic processing areas(21 CFR 211.42(c)(10)).

2. 你公司未能在足够大小的明确界定区域内进行操作,也未能拥有单独或界定的区域,或其他必要的控制系统,来防止无菌工艺区的污染或混淆 [21 CFR 211.42(c)(10)]。

Cleanroom Design ｜洁净室设计

Your ISO 5 cleanroom areas used for aseptic compounding and filling were poorly designed and lacked adequate protection. For example, your ISO 5 area in Room（b）（4） lacked physical barriers to prevent potential contamination of your sterile components, including the sterile API, during manually intensive dispensing and compounding operations. Operators' bodies and hands were in immediate proximity to the sterile API during dispensing, compounding, and syringe-loading in the filling station. Additionally, operators hand-（b）（4）sterile components into a compounding tank through a large funnel with a wide opening. Your smoke studies demonstrated non-unidirectional, recirculating airflow on and around the funnel.

你公司用于无菌混合和灌装的 ISO 5 洁净室区域设计不当，且缺乏充分的保护。例如，位于（b）（4）室的 ISO 5 区域缺乏物理屏障，无法防止在人工密集操作的配料和配液操作期间对无菌物料（包括无菌 API）造成潜在污染。在灌装站进行称量、配制和注射器装载期间，操作员的身体和手紧邻无菌原料药。此外，通过具有宽开口的大漏斗，操作员将（b）（4）无菌原辅料人工放入混合罐中。你公司的烟雾研究表明，漏斗上及其周围存在非单向再循环气流。

The ISO 5 area is critical because sterile drug products are exposed and therefore vulnerable to contamination. Your aseptic manufacturing process should be designed and operations should be executed to minimize contamination hazards to your sterile drug product. Basic design deficiencies and manually intensive interventions in your operation undermine the ability to maintain asepsis.

ISO 5 区域至关重要，因为无菌药品暴露在外，因此容易受到污染。你公司的无菌生产工艺的设计和操作的执行应尽量减少对无菌药品的污染危害。基本设计缺陷和操作中的人工密集干预会削弱维持无菌的能力。

Environmental Monitoring ｜环境监测

You failed to establish an adequate system for monitoring environmental conditions. For example, you did not perform viable（surface and air）environmental monitoring in close proximity to aseptic dispensing operations in Room（b）（4）. Likewise, no environmental monitoring was performed where sterile API was manually added to the compounding tank. Data reviewed during the inspection noted this aseptic operation lasted up to（b）（4）. Your protocol failed to identify these locations as "high-risk" sampling points for environmental monitoring. Furthermore, personnel monitoring data was not captured appropriately.

你公司未能建立适当的环境条件监测系统。例如，没有在（b）（4）室的无菌称量操作附近进行微生物（表面和空气）环境监测。同样，当人工将无菌API添加到配制罐时，也没有进行环境监测。检查期间审查的数据表明，这种无菌操作持续到（b）（4）。你公司的方案未能将这些位置识别为环境监测的"高风险"取样点。此外，人员监测数据未得到适当留存。

Vigilant and responsive environmental and personnel monitoring programs should be designed to provide meaningful information on the state of control of your aseptic processing environment. Operations that include highly manually intensive aseptic activities warrant a more extensive environmental and personnel monitoring program, including but not limited to emphasis on well-timed sampling that appropriately monitors batch manufacturing conditions.

应设计具有警戒性且反应灵敏的环境和人员监控计划，以提供有关无菌工艺操作环境控制状态的有意义的信息。对于诸如高度人工密集型无菌活动的操作，其需要更广泛的环境和人员监测计划，包括但不限于强调适时取样，以适当监测批生产条件。

In your response you acknowledge the inadequacies of your environmental and personnel monitoring program. You state the drug products impacted by the observation are being recalled, and the specific filling line ((b)(4)) involved in the observation is no longer in use. You provide a high-level overview of an action plan with assurance to map the manufacturing process from a contamination prevention perspective.

在你公司的回复中，你们承认你公司的环境和人员监测计划存在不充分。你公司声称受观察项影响的药品正在被召回，并且观察项涉及的特定灌装线［(b)(4)］不再使用。你公司提供了行动计划的总览概述，并确保从污染预防的角度详细规划生产工艺。

You fail to adequately explain how your quality and operations management will ensure appropriate cleanroom design, control, aseptic practices, and cleanroom behavior during production.

就你公司的质量和运营管理将如何确保生产过程中适当的洁净室设计、控制、无菌操作和洁净室行为，你公司未能充分解释。

In response to this letter, provide the following:

在回复本函时，请提供以下信息：

（略）

此处与FDA发给Iso-Tex Diagnostics, Inc.的警告信（编号：MARCS-CMS 655666，即"2 无菌洁净室的压差问题"）中有关无菌药品的污染风险部分的内容类似，故略去。

设备问题

3. Your firm failed to use equipment in the manufacture, processing, packing, or holding of drug products that is of appropriate design, adequate size, and suitably located to facilitate operations for its intended use and for its cleaning and maintenance（21 CFR 211.63）.

3. 在药品的生产、加工、包装或储存中，你公司未能使用设计合理、尺寸足够且位置适当的设备，以实现预期用途及清洁和维护操作（21 CFR 211.63）。

You failed to identify and use equipment suitable for the filling of your viscous parenteral drug product. Inappropriately designed vial filling equipment led to substantial extraneous matter contamination in testosterone cypionate injection 200mg/mL, 1ml vials. Further, your production department failed to establish adequate personnel practices and supervisory oversight to prevent the use of damaged equipment.

你公司未能识别并使用适合黏性注射剂药品灌装的设备。西林瓶灌装设备设计不当，导致环丙酸睾酮注射液（200mg/ml，1ml 西林瓶）中存在大量异物污染。此外，你公司的生产部门未能建立充分的人员实践和监督机制，来防止使用损坏的设备。

You determined the design of the filling equipment（(b)(4)）in combination with the viscous nature of your drug product generated friction. This friction caused an abrasive effect on the surface of (b)(4) during (b)(4) movement which introduced blackish fine metallic particles into your vial during filling. You explained that these (b)(4) could not be fixed once damaged. Although reportedly removed from service, the damaged (b)(4) were listed as approved equipment in your master manufacturing batch record approved on April 5, 2022, approximately two years after they were identified as the root cause for cross-contamination.

结合药品产生摩擦的黏性性质，你公司确定了灌装设备［(b)(4)］的设计。在（b)(4) 运行过程中，这种摩擦会对（b)(4) 表面造成磨损，从而在灌装过程中将黑色细小金属颗粒带入西林瓶中。你公司解释说这些（b)(4) 一旦损坏就无法修复。尽管据称损坏的（b)(4) 已停止使用，但其在 2022 年 4 月 5 日批准的主生产批记录中被列为批准设备，大约是在它们被确定为交叉污染的根本原因的两年后。

Notably, one of the damaged (b)(4)（H102）was used to fill numerous batches of testosterone cypionate injection.

值得注意的是，受损的（b)(4)（H102）之一被用来灌装多批环丙酸睾酮注射液。

It is your responsibility to ensure that only appropriately designed and maintained equipment are used in the manufacture of your drug products.

你公司有责任确保，在药品生产中仅使用经过适当设计和维护的设备。

We acknowledge that after our inspection you voluntarily recalled five marketed testosterone cypionate injection lots associated with the（b）（4）investigations.

我们知晓，在检查后，你公司自愿召回了与（b）（4）调查相关的五个已上市的环丙酸睾酮注射液批次。

Your response is inadequate. Your response fails to address the flaws in your change management system that permitted continued use of damaged and inappropriately designed （b）（4）. Your response states that damaged（b）（4）were isolated and not used in filling testosterone cypionate injection but were inadvertently not removed from the manufacturing batch record. You also state that an associated（b）（4）（H102）was reconditioned and was acceptable for use. However, your firm indicated during the inspection that these damaged （b）（4）could not be reconditioned and acknowledged that they were not suitably designed. Your response also did not include a risk assessment that thoroughly evaluates the design and lifecycle control of manufacturing equipment including（b）（4）and（b）（4）.

你公司的回应不够充分。回复中未能解决变更管理系统中的缺陷，这些缺陷允许继续使用损坏的和设计不当的（b）（4）。你公司在回复中指出，损坏的（b）（4）已被隔离，未用于灌装环丙酸睾酮注射液，但无意中未从生产批记录删除。你公司还声称相关的（b）（4）（H102）已整改并且可以使用。然而，你公司在检查期间表示，这些损坏的（b）（4）无法修复，并承认它们设计不合适。你公司的回复也没有包括彻底评估生产设备的设计和生命周期控制的风险评估，包括（b）（4）和（b）（4）。

In response to this letter, provide：

在回复本函时，请提供：

● Your CAPA plan to implement routine, vigilant operations management oversight （corporate and local）of facilities and equipment. This plan should ensure, among other things, prompt detection of equipment/facilities performance issues, effective execution of repairs, adherence to appropriate preventive maintenance schedules, timely technological upgrades to the equipment/facility infrastructure, appropriately qualified production management personnel, and improved systems for ongoing management review. Your plan should also ensure that appropriate actions are taken throughout the company network.

● 你公司的 CAPA 计划，以便对设施和设备实施日常、警戒性的运营管理监督（集团和本地公司层面）。至少，该计划应确保及时发现设备 / 设施性能问题，有效执行维修，遵守适当的预防性维护计划，及时对设备 / 设施进行技术升级，配备相应有资质的生产管理人员，并改进持续管理评审系统。你公司的计划还应确保在整个公司网络中采取适当的措施。

● A thorough evaluation and risk assessment that addresses the suitability of your equipment for its intended use. You should include a determination of whether equipment is of appropriate design and a robust program for ongoing control and maintenance. Also describe how Quality Assurance will oversee the efficacy of systems used by operations to accomplish these critical objectives.

● 彻底的评估和风险评估，确定你公司的设备是否适合其预期用途。你公司应该确定设备是否具有适当的设计以及用于持续控制和维护的可靠程序。并说明质量保证将如何监督运营所使用的系统的有效性，以实现这些关键目标。

● An independent retrospective review of your manufacturing batch records to ensure that defective（b）（4）manufactured by（b）（4）or（b）（4）were not used during filling operations.

● 对你公司的生产批记录进行独立的回顾性审查，以确保在灌装操作期间不会使用（b）（4）或（b）（4）生产的有缺陷的（b）（4）。

● An independent retrospective review of all complaints, including the associated investigations, for discoloration and particulates, for sterile drug products within expiry as of the date of this letter. Include the drug product name, batch number, and date of manufacture, line number, along with a summary of the complaint, description of likely root cause（s）, CAPA plan, and status of CAPA.

● 对截至本函日期有效的无菌药品的所有投诉（包括相关调查）进行独立回顾性审查，包括变色和颗粒问题。包括药品名称、批号、生产日期、行号以及投诉汇总、可能的根本原因的描述、CAPA 计划和 CAPA 状态。

● An independent, comprehensive review of your complaint system that identifies deficiencies in the system and corresponding CAPA that are needed.

● 对你公司的投诉系统进行独立、全面的审查，确定系统中的缺陷以及所需的相应 CAPA。

● A comprehensive, independent assessment of your change management system. This assessment should include, but not be limited to, your procedure（s）to ensure changes are appropriately justified, evaluated, and reviewed to a final determination of acceptability by your QU. Your change management program should include provisions for determining change effectiveness.

● 对你公司的变更管理系统进行全面、独立的评估。该评估应包括但不限于确保变更合理、经过质量部门审查和批准的程序。你公司的变更管理计划还应包括确定变更有效性的规定。

偏差调查

4. Your firm failed to thoroughly investigate any unexplained discrepancy or failure of a batch or any of its components to meet any of its specifications, whether or not the batch has already been distributed(21 CFR 211.192).

4. 无论批次是否已经流通，对于该批次或其原辅料不满足其质量标准、存在无法解释的差异或不合格，你公司未能进行彻底调查（21 CFR 211.192）。

Your investigations into water leaks in your cleanroom were inadequate because they lacked appropriate CAPA and failed to extend to other potentially affected batches.

你公司对洁净室漏水问题的调查不够充分，因为缺乏适当的 CAPA，并且未能扩展到其他可能受影响的批次。

For example, water leaked from the service floor through the heating, ventilation, and air conditioning(HVAC) duct floor and into the ceiling directly above the ISO 5 filling area. Your investigation report noted water accumulated on the service floor due to a leak from an old, punctured (b)(4). Water then collected over the (b)(4) partition ceiling prior to entering the aseptic filling room where medroxyprogesterone acetate injectable suspension USP, was manufactured. Your personnel confirmed there was substantial water accumulation on the service floor.

例如，从技术夹层通过采暖、通风和空调（HVAC）管道地板，水泄漏到 ISO 5 灌装区域正上方的天花板。你公司的调查报告指出，由于旧的、刺破的（b）（4）漏水，技术夹层积水。然后在进入生产醋酸甲羟孕酮注射混悬剂 USP 的无菌灌装室之前，在（b）（4）隔板天花板上积存了水。你公司的工作人员确认技术夹层有大量积水。

Although you sealed gaps in the ceiling, you did not sufficiently inspect the service floor, (b)(4) LAF ceiling, and HVAC duct floor for mold growth and water damage after the repairs were made. You also failed to extend the scope of your investigation to potentially impacted batches of medroxyprogesterone acetate injectable suspension USP manufactured in this room since the last preventive maintenance of the (b)(4), approximately two months before the leak was observed.

尽管你公司密封了天花板上的间隙，但在维修后，你们没有充分检查服务楼层的地板、（b）（4）LAF 天花板和 HVAC 管道地板，确定是否有霉菌生长和由积水引起的损害。你公司也未能将调查范围扩大到自上次（b）（4）预防性维护（即观察到泄漏前大约两个月）以来，在该房间生产的可能受影响的醋酸甲羟孕酮注射混悬液 USP 批次。

In your response, you state the leak was isolated to the day it was observed. You acknowledge that your investigation did not evaluate the impact of the leak to other batches. You initiated a recall on May 17, 2022, for all marketed batches of medroxyprogesterone acetate injectable suspension USP, 150mg/mL, 1 mL vials manufactured on this line, for events unrelated to this investigation.

在你公司的回复中，声明泄漏自观察到之日起就已被隔离。你公司承认你们的调查并未评估泄漏对其他批次的影响。针对与本次调查无关的事件，你公司于 2022 年 5 月 17 日，对该生产线生产的所有上市批次的醋酸甲羟孕酮注射混悬液 USP（150mg/ml，1ml 西林瓶）发起召回。

Your response is inadequate. While we acknowledge you initiated actions to address this specific leak, your investigation failed to sufficiently address facility damage and the potential for microbial（i.e., particularly fungal）contamination that could persist in the facility due to water leaks and moisture.

你公司的回应不够充分。虽然我们知晓，你们已采取行动来解决此特定泄漏问题，但就设施损坏以及由于漏水和潮湿而可能在设施中持续存在的微生物（即特别是真菌）污染的可能性，你公司的调查未能充分解决。

In response to this letter, provide a comprehensive, independent assessment of your overall system for investigating deviations, discrepancies, complaints, OOS results, and failures. Provide a detailed action plan to remediate this system. Your action plan should include, but not be limited to, significant improvements in investigation competencies, scope determination, root cause evaluation, CAPA effectiveness, quality assurance unit oversight, and written procedures. Address how your firm will ensure all phases of investigations are appropriately conducted.

作为对本函的回应，请对你公司的整个系统进行全面、独立的评估，以调查偏差、差异、投诉、OOS 结果和不合格。提供详细的行动计划来整改该系统。你公司的行动计划应包括但不限于调查能力、范围确定、根本原因评估、CAPA 有效性、质量保证部门监督和书面程序方面的显著提高。说明你公司将如何确保所有阶段的调查都被适当执行。

设备清洁

5. Your firm failed to clean, maintain, and, as appropriate for the nature of the drug, sanitize and/or sterilize equipment and utensils at appropriate intervals to prevent malfunctions or contamination that would alter the safety, identity, strength, quality, or purity of the drug product beyond the official or other established requirements（21 CFR 211.67（a））.

5. 你公司未能根据药品的性质，按照适当的时间间隔对设备和器具进行消毒和（或）灭菌，以防止出现故障或污染，从而改变药品安全性、鉴别、规格、质量或纯度，超过 USP 或其他既定要求［21 CFR 211.67（a）］。

You failed to adequately clean and maintain your equipment used for drug product manufacturing. For example：

你公司未能充分清洁和维护用于药品生产的设备。例如：

A. Our investigators observed visible residue on（b）（4）after it was identified as clean. Also, colored particles and pellets were observed inside a crevice where the（b）（4）was attached to（b）（4）. During the inspection your analytical testing identified that the pellets contained（b）（4）API.

A.（b）（4）被标识为干净，我们的调查员观察到了其有可见的残留物。此外，在（b）（4）附着于（b）（4）的缝隙内观察到有色颗粒和药丸。在检查过程中，你公司的分析检验发现药丸含有（b）（4）原料药。

The equipment cleaning record indicated a Type-B cleaning was performed on（b）（4）, which is defined as complete removal of previous drug product and involves dismantling of（b）（4）.

设备清洁记录表明对（b）（4）进行了 B 型清洁，其定义为完全去除先前的药品，并涉及拆除（b）（4）。

B. Our investigators observed numerous scratches and dents on product contact surfaces of the（b）（4）bowl-Ⅱ. Additionally, shiny metal fragments were observed on the top of the（b）（4）gaskets that connected the（b）（4）in（b）（4）.

B. 我们的调查员在（b）（4）锅-Ⅱ的产品接触表面上，观察到很多划痕和凹痕。此外，在（b）（4）中连接（b）（4）的（b）（4）垫圈顶部观察到闪亮的金属碎片。

Inadequately cleaned and maintained equipment can lead to cross contamination and poor quality drug products.

设备清洁和维护不当，可能导致交叉污染和药品质量低劣。

Your response states that the（b）（4）was not disassembled during the cleaning process because engineering staff was not available. The residue and powder were from the previously manufactured drug product（which was the same drug）. You also confirm the shiny fragments on the（b）（4）gaskets are（b）（4）and stated that the shedding of metal fragments most likely occurred during the assembly and disassembly process. You state that your protocol-based visual inspection of（b）（4）performed in response to this observation did not result in any similar findings.

你公司的回复指出，（b）（4）在清洁过程中没有被拆卸，因为工程人员不在场。残留物和粉末来自先前生产的药品（是同一种药品）。你公司还确认（b）（4）垫圈上的闪亮碎片是（b）（4），并指出金属碎片的脱落很可能发生在组装和拆卸过程中。你公司声称针对这一观察项，对（b）（4）进行了基于协议的目检，其并未得出任何类似的结果。

Your response is inadequate. You state that your impact assessment is ongoing, and the batches manufactured since the last campaign are on hold. However, you do not provide information on how long the damaged and inadequately cleaned equipment has been used. You also do not provide a risk assessment for drug products manufactured and distributed using such equipment.

你公司的回应不够充分。你们声称对影响的评估正在进行中，并且自上次活动以来生产的批次已处于暂缓状态。但是，你公司没有提供有关损坏和未充分清洁的设备已使用多长时间的信息。你公司也未对使用此类设备生产和流通的药品提供风险评估。

Your response fails to sufficiently address the confirmed complaints you received since January 2020 pertaining to stains, specks, and spots in your（b）（4）tablets,（b）（4）mg, and（b）（4）tablets（b）（4）mg drug products.

自 2020 年 1 月以来，你公司收到的有关（b）（4）片剂（b）（4）mg 和（b）（4）片剂（b）（4）mg 药品中污渍、斑点和污点的已确认投诉，你公司的回复未能充分解决这些问题。

In response to this letter, provide：

在回复本函时，请提供：

（略）

此处与 FDA 发给 Baxter Healthcare Corporation 的警告信（编号：MARCS–CMS 654136，即 "3 注射剂药品的颗粒物检查存在缺陷"）中有关设备清洁回应要求部分的内容类似，故略去。

● An independent review of your investigations and complaints of foreign matter contamination in your products. The review should comprehensively assess your program, including but not limited to sources of foreign matter, risks associated with the product, and appropriate investigations and CAPA.

● 对你公司的产品中异物污染的调查和投诉进行独立审查。审查应全面评估你们的计划，包括但不限于异物来源、与产品相关的风险以及适当的调查和 CAPA。

● Your protocol to test any drug product, within expiry and manufactured on non–

dedicated（b）（4）equipment，for contamination.

● 你公司对任何在有效期内且在非专用（b）（4）设备上生产的药品进行污染检验的方案。

（略）

此处与 FDA 发给 Cosmobeauti Laboratories & Manufacturing Inc. 的警告信（编号：MARCS–CMS 657682，即 "12 批生产记录存在倒记问题"）中有关 QU 的回应要求部分的内容类似，故略去。

7 美国多州暴发细菌感染，触发 FDA 检查

警告信编号: MARCS-CMS 657325

签发时间: 2023-10-20; **公示时间:** 2023-11-14

签发机构: 药物审评与研究中心 | CDER (Center for Drug Evaluation and Research | CDER)

公　　司: Global Pharma Healthcare Private Limited

所在国家 / 地区: 印度

主　　题: cGMP/ 成品制剂 / 掺假 / 标识错误 (cGMP/Finished Pharmaceuticals/Adulterated/Misbranded)

简　　介: 2023 年 2 月至 3 月，FDA 检查了该药品生产设施，起因是 2022 年 12 月 FDA 与 CDC 开始调查美国多州暴发的铜绿假单胞菌感染，该事件造成 80 多名患者受影响，其中 4 人死亡，至少 14 人视力丧失。作为调查的一部分，FDA 收集了该公司的人工泪液和人工眼膏成品样品，发现 18 批次人工泪液和一批人工眼膏均非无菌。通过全基因组测序分析，发现从三个不同批次的人工泪液中分离出的铜绿假单胞菌与超过 85 个与疫情相关的临床分离株基因相符。在检查中，FDA 发现该公司未能验证眼科药品无菌方法，缺乏证明其人工泪液灭菌效果的研究。该公司提到 2023 年 1 月采集的环境样品未发现铜绿假单胞菌，但 FDA 认为这一回应不够充分。根据记录显示，最后一批运往美国的人工泪液是在该公司进行有限取样之前数月生产的，因此数月后进行的环境检验缺乏意义。

本警告信以下部分与本书此前其他警告信内容类似，故略去：数据可靠性整改（Data Integrity Remediation）、标识错误的药品违法行为（Misbranded Drug Violations）、作为合同商的责任（Responsibilities as a Contractor）、质量体系失效（Ineffective Quality System）、结论（Conclusion）。

The U.S. Food and Drug Administration（FDA）inspected your drug manufacturing facility, Global Pharma Healthcare Private Limited, FEI 3012323885, at A-9 SIDCO Pharmaceutical Complex, Thiruporur, from February 20 to March 2, 2023.

2023 年 2 月 20 日至 3 月 2 日，美国食品药品管理局（FDA）检查了 Global Pharma Healthcare Private Limited（FEI 3012323885）的药品生产设施，其位于印度 Thiruporur A-9 SIDCO 制药园区。

This warning letter summarizes significant violations of current Good Manufacturing Practice（cGMP）regulations for finished pharmaceuticals. See Title 21 Code of Federal Regulations（CFR）, parts 210 and 211（21 CFR parts 210 and 211）.

本警告信总结了对成品制剂现行药品生产质量管理规范（cGMP）法规的严重违反情况。请参见美国联邦法规（CFR）第 21 篇第 210 和 211 部分（21 CFR 第 210 和 211 部分）。

Because your methods, facilities, or controls for manufacturing, processing, packing, or holding do not conform to cGMP, your drug products are adulterated within the meaning of section 501（a）（2）（B）of the Federal Food, Drug, and Cosmetic Act（FD&C Act）, 21 U.S.C. 351（a）（2）（B）.

由于你公司用于生产、加工、包装或储存的方法、设施或控制措施不符合 cGMP，因此根据 FD&C 法案 501（a）（2）（B）条、21 U.S.C.351（a）（2）（B）的规定，你公司的药品被认为是掺假。

Because your drug products were prepared, packed, or held under insanitary conditions, whereby they may have become contaminated with filth or rendered injurious to health, your drug products are also adulterated within the meaning of section 501（a）（2）（A）of the FD&C Act, 21 U.S.C. 351（a）（2）（A）.

由于你公司的药品是在不卫生的条件下制备、包装或储存的，因此它们可能已被污物污染或对健康有害，导致你公司的药品根据 FD&C 法案第 501（a）（2）（A）条、21 U.S.C. 351（a）（2）（A）被视为掺假。

In addition, EZRICARE Artificial Tears, Delsam Pharma's ARTIFICIAL TEARS, and Delsam Pharma's ARTIFICIAL EYE OINTMENT are misbranded under section 502（j）of the FD&C Act, 21 U.S.C. 352（j）, and Delsam Pharma's ARTIFICIAL EYE OINTMENT is further misbranded under section 502（a）of the FD&C Act, 21 U.S.C. 352（a）. Introduction or delivery for introduction of misbranded products into interstate commerce is prohibited under section 301（a）of the FD&C Act, 21 U.S.C. 331（a）. These violations are described in more detail below.

此外，根据 FD&C 法案第 502（j）条、21 U.S.C. 352（j），EZRICARE 人工泪液、Delsam Pharma 的人工泪液和 Delsam Pharma 的人工眼膏为标识错误，并且 Delsam Pharma 的人工眼膏根据 FD&C 法案第 502（a）条、21 U.S.C. 352（a），被进一步认为是标识错误。FD&C 法案第 301（a）条，也即 21 U.S.C. 331（a），禁止将这些标识错误的产品引入或交付州际贸易。下面将更详细地描述这些违规情况。

Pseudomonas aeruginosa Outbreak and FDA Testing of Samples
铜绿假单胞菌暴发和 FDA 样品检测

In December 2022, FDA began collaborating with the Center for Disease Control and Prevention（CDC）on an investigation into the multistate outbreak of antibiotic-resistant *Pseudomonas aeruginosa* infections that ultimately affected more than 80 patients and led to 4 patient deaths and at least 14 cases of vision loss. As part of this investigation, FDA collected finished product samples of Artificial Tears and Artificial Eye Ointment batches that were manufactured by your facility, and we sent the samples for sterility testing at FDA laboratories. Our analysis of intact（unopened）units found that 18 batches of Artificial Tears were non-sterile. In addition, we also sampled a batch of your Artificial Eye Ointment product, and this batch was also found to be non-sterile. The testing of these intact units revealed that your ophthalmic drug products were intrinsically contaminated with microorganisms. Microbiological isolates from the non-sterile samples were further characterized using whole genome sequencing and compared to isolates in a national database. *Pseudomonas aeruginosa* isolates from three different batches of intact Artificial Tears samples collected by FDA were found to be close genetic matches to more than 85 clinical isolates associated with this outbreak. These test results demonstrate that these lots are adulterated under section 501（a）（1）of the FD&C Act, in that they have been contaminated with filth, and rendered injurious to health.

2022 年 12 月，FDA 开始与美国疾病控制预防中心（CDC）合作，对多州暴发的抗生素耐药性铜绿假单胞菌感染进行调查，该感染最终影响了 80 多名患者，并导致 4 名患者死亡和至少 14 例病例视力丧失。作为本次调查的一部分，FDA 收集了你公司设施生产的人工泪液和人工眼膏批次的成品样品，并将样品送往 FDA 实验室进行无菌检验。我们对完整（未开封）产品的分析发现，18 批次人工泪液非无菌。此外，我们还对你公司的一批人工眼膏产品进行了取样，发现该批次产品也非无菌。对这些完整产品的检验表明，你公司的眼科药品总体上受到微生物污染。使用全基因组测序进一步表征来自非无菌样品的微生物分离株，并与国家数据库中的分离株进行比较。从 FDA 收集三个不同批次的完整人工泪液样品中分离出了铜绿假单胞菌，发现其与本次疫情相关的超过 85 个临床分离株具有密切的基因匹配。检验结果表明，根据 FD&C 法案第 501（a）（1）条，这些批次的产品已被污物污染，对健康有害。

Significantly, the pervasive contamination of your drug products, as indicated by FDA sample results, also demonstrates that all drugs made at your facility are adulterated under section 501(a)(2)(A)of the FD&C Act as they have been manufactured under insanitary conditions.

值得注意的是，FDA 样品结果表明，你公司的药品普遍受到污染，这也表明根据 FD&C 法案第 501（a）（2）（A）条，你公司设施生产的所有药品根据 FD&C 法案均涉及掺假，因为它们是在不卫生条件下生产的。

In addition, two intact samples of Artificial Tears from different batches were found to contain visible, foreign particles.

此外，两个不同批次的完整人工泪液样品被发现含有可见的异物颗粒。

cGMP Violations ｜ cGMP 违规

We reviewed your March 22, 2023, response to our Form FDA 483 in detail. During our inspection, our investigators observed specific violations including, but not limited to, the following.

我们详细审查了你公司于 2023 年 3 月 22 日对我们的 FDA 483 表格的回复。在检查过程中，我们的调查员发现了具体的违规情况，包括但不限于以下内容。

无菌和灭菌工艺验证

1. Your firm failed to establish and follow appropriate written procedures that are designed to prevent microbiological contamination of drug products purporting to be sterile, and that include validation of all aseptic and sterilization processes(21 CFR 211.113(b)).

1. 你公司未能建立并遵循适当的书面程序，包括验证所有无菌和灭菌工艺的程序，以防止声称无菌的药品受到微生物污染〔21 CFR 211.113（b）〕。

Inadequate Equipment and Processes ｜设备和工艺不足

A. You lacked adequate scientific evidence that the aseptic filling machine used for manufacture of Artificial Tears was suitable for its intended use. Your qualification report was inadequate, including a lack of data on any batches filled as part of the qualification study. Further, all batches of Artificial Tears distributed to the U.S. market were manufactured using filling machine parameters that were outside the design specifications of the equipment.

A. 你公司缺乏充分的科学证据，来证明用于生产人工泪液的无菌灌装机适合其预期用途。你公司的确认报告不充分，包括缺乏作为确认研究一部分的所有批次的数据。此外，对于销往美国市场的所有批次人工泪液，其均使用超出设备设计规格的灌装机参数进行生产。

B. You lacked validation of the processes used to manufacture your aseptically filled Artificial Tears, for example：

B. 你公司缺乏对用于生产无菌灌装人工泪液的工艺的验证，例如：

● You failed to validate methods that were intended to render your ophthalmic drug products sterile. Specifically, you lacked a study to show the（b）（4）performed on your Artificial Tears product using a（b）（4）can reliably achieve sterilization.

● 你公司未能验证旨在使眼科药品达到无菌的方法。具体来说，你公司缺乏一项研究，来证明使用（b）（4）对人工泪液产品执行（b）（4），可以可靠地实现灭菌。

● Your media fill program lacked assurance that aseptic processing operations are appropriately performed to prevent microbial contamination. Our inspection found that you failed to perform appropriate and sufficient media fills studies, for example：

● 你公司的培养基模拟灌装程序无法确保正确执行无菌工艺操作，以防止微生物污染。我们的检查发现，你公司未能执行适当且充分的培养基模拟灌装研究，例如：

○ Your media fills failed to adequately simulate the commercial aseptic manufacturing operation. Interventions were not simulated sufficiently or accurately. In addition, you have a manually intensive line with minimal barrier protection where the possibility of contamination is greater. Despite this, you filled（b）（4）–（b）（4）% of the production batch size during media fills.

○ 你公司的培养基模拟灌装未能充分模拟商业无菌生产操作。干预措施的模拟不够充分或准确。此外，你公司还有一条人工密集型生产线，其屏障保护程度非常低，污染的可能性更大。尽管如此，你公司在培养基灌装期间灌装了（b）（4）%–（b）（4）%的生产批量。

○ Manufacturing lines used to produce the Artificial Tears and Artificial Eye Ointment products were not qualified by three successful media fills.

○ 用于生产人工泪液和人工眼膏产品的生产线未通过三个成功的培养基模拟灌装批次的确认。

○ You removed integral units（i.e., units with intact container-closure systems）from media fills without adequate justification and failed to incubate all integral units for the full（b）（4）period.

○ 你公司在没有充分论证的情况下，从培养基灌装中取出了完整单元（即具有完整容器封闭系统的产品单元），并且未能在整个（b）（4）期间培养所有完整单元。

○ The personnel responsible for visual inspection of media-filled units lacked appropriate training and qualification.

○ 负责对灌装培养基的单元进行目检的人员缺乏适当的培训和资质确认。

C. You lacked meaningful airflow pattern studies for your aseptic processing lines. The studies were not performed under dynamic conditions and lacked simulation of interventions and other routine activities that occur during aseptic manufacturing operations.

C. 你公司的无菌生产线缺乏有意义的气流模式研究。这些研究不是在动态条件下进行的，并且缺乏对无菌生产操作期间发生的干预措施和其他常规活动的模拟。

D. Your firm also shipped an ointment product to the United States that was manufactured using a（b）（4）sterilization process. You failed to ensure the（b）（4）process employed by your contractor to sterilize your Artificial Eye Ointment was validated.

D. 你公司还向美国流通了一种采用（b）（4）灭菌工艺生产的软膏产品。你公司未能确保你们的合同商采用（b）（4）工艺对你们的人工眼膏进行消毒。

Your response is inadequate, including the following：

你公司的回复不充分，包括以下内容：

● You lack details of your internal investigation into the product contamination. Your investigation is not comprehensive, including but not limited to, a lack of descriptions of the activities performed and root cause analysis. You also lack details on sampling and laboratory methods used for environmental and other tests.

● 缺乏对产品污染进行内部调查的详细信息。你公司的调查并不全面，包括但不限于：缺乏对所执行活动的描述和根本原因分析。你公司还缺乏用于环境和其他检验的取样和实验室方法的详细信息。

● There is a lack of detail relating to future dynamic airflow pattern studies；heating, ventilation, and air conditioning（HVAC）system qualification；or media fill procedural revisions.

● 缺乏与未来动态气流模式研究相关的细节；采暖、通风和空调（HVAC）系统确认；或培养基模拟灌装程序修订。

● You also fail to include a commitment to validate the（b）（4）sterilization process and sterility test methods for the Artificial Eye Ointment products.

● 你公司未能承诺验证人工眼膏产品的（b）（4）灭菌工艺和无菌检验方法。

■ Lack of Container Closure Integrity ｜ 容器封闭完整性缺失

You lacked evidence of reliable container closure integrity for your multi-use ophthalmic products that purport to be sterile. While visual inspections revealed leakers during batch manufacture, there was no assurance that your visual inspection procedure was adequate.

对于声称无菌的多剂量眼科产品，你公司缺乏可靠的容器密封完整性的证据。虽然目检在批生产过程中识别了泄漏，但不能保证你公司的目检程序是充分的。

Your product distributors received complaints of leaking Artificial Tears and Artificial Eye Ointment units. FDA's laboratory performed container closure integrity testing of Artificial Eye Ointment, batch H29, manufactured at your facility. FDA tested 20 units, and 1 unit was found to allow microbiological ingress, which further confirmed that your container-closure system lacks integrity and is insufficient for maintaining sterility. Notably, batch H29 was also found to be non-sterile through FDA testing.

你公司的产品经销商收到了关于人工泪液和人工眼膏装置泄漏的投诉。FDA 实验室对你公司设施生产的批次 H29 人工眼膏进行了容器密封完整性检验。FDA 检验了 20 个样品，发现其中 1 个允许微生物进入，这进一步证实你们的容器封闭系统缺乏完整性，不足以保持无菌性。值得注意的是，通过 FDA 检测，H29 批次也被发现是非无菌的。

All sterile drugs must be packaged using a container-closure system that protects product integrity for the duration of its shelf-life. Maintenance of product integrity throughout stresses of its manufacture, storage, distribution, and consumer use is critical to product quality and safety. Loss of container-closure integrity is a direct cause of non-sterility of medicines.

所有无菌药品必须使用容器封闭系统进行包装，以在有效期内保护产品的完整性。在生产、储存、流通和消费者使用的整个过程中，保持产品完整性对于产品质量和安全至关重要。容器密封完整性的丧失是药品非无菌的直接原因。

In your response, you state you will perform container-closure integrity testing using a dye ingress method for your Artificial Tears product and a comprehensive sterility assessment. Your response is inadequate because your container-closure integrity testing protocol does not extend to Artificial Eye Ointment. In addition, you do not sufficiently address the sensitivity of your dye ingress method. The sensitivity of the method to be employed for your study is unclear, and you do not indicate whether it is capable of correlating with detection of bacteria comparable in size to *Pseudomonas aeruginosa*. Furthermore, your response does not include details on the comprehensive sterility assessment.

在你公司的回复中，你们声称将使用色水法，对你公司的人工泪液产品进行容器密封件完整性检验以及全面的无菌评估。你公司的回复不充分，因为你们的容器封闭完整性检验方案未扩展到人工眼膏。此外，你公司没有充分解决色水法的灵敏度问题。你公司的研究所采用的方法的灵敏度尚不清楚，并且没有表明它是否能够与跟铜绿假单胞菌大小相当的细菌的检测相关联。此外，你公司的回复不包括全面无菌评估的详细信息。

Inadequate Formulation for Artificial Tears and Artificial Eye Ointment
人工泪液和人工眼膏配方不当

You manufactured multi-dose, over-the-counter (OTC) ophthalmic drug products for the product owners, EzriCare LLC, and Delsam Pharma LLC. These products lacked antimicrobial properties to preserve the formulation. Significantly, your firm also marketed this multi-dose product without performing antimicrobial effectiveness studies. It is essential that multi-dose ophthalmic drug products contain one or more suitable substances that will preserve the product and minimize the hazard of injury resulting from incidental contamination during use.

你公司为产品所有者 EzriCare LLC 和 Delsam Pharma LLC 生产多剂量非处方（OTC）眼科药品。这些产品缺乏抗菌特性来保存处方。值得注意的是，你公司还上市了这种多剂量产品，但没有进行抗菌效能研究。多剂量眼科药品必须含有一种或多种合适的物质，以保护产品并最大限度地减少使用过程中偶然污染造成的危害。

In your response, you state that antimicrobial effectiveness testing (AET) will be initiated for your Artificial Tears product, and you will use these studies to determine if a suitable preservative will be added to the formulation. Your response is inadequate because you do not explain why you failed to perform AET studies prior to launch of your drug product, and how you will correct such fundamental flaws in your product development program. You also make no commitment to conduct AET for the Artificial Eye Ointment formulation. In addition, although your protocol indicates that you follow the United States Pharmacopeia (USP), the acceptance criteria in the Artificial Tears protocol is less stringent and not in alignment with USP <51> Antimicrobial Effectiveness Testing.

在回复中，你公司声称将对你们的人工泪液产品启动抗菌效能检验（AET），并且使用这些研究来确定是否会将合适的防腐剂添加到处方中。你公司的回应是不充分的，因为没有解释为什么你们在药品上市之前未能进行 AET 研究，以及你公司将如何纠正产品开发计划中的这些根本缺陷。你公司也未承诺对人工眼膏处方进行 AET。此外，虽然你公司的方案表明遵循 USP，但人工泪液方案中的可接受标准不太严格，并且与 USP <51> 抗菌效能检验不符。

■ Inadequate Gowning Practices & Operator Qualification
更衣实践和操作员资质确认不充分

Cleanroom operators lacked adequate gowning and qualification for performing aseptic operations. Your deficient practices and procedures placed products at high risk for contamination, for example:

洁净室操作员缺乏充分的更衣实践和执行无菌操作的资质确认。你公司的实践和程序存在缺陷，导致产品面临很高的污染风险，例如：

A. A gowning demonstration revealed that cleanroom operators do not don sterile goggles and therefore have exposed skin around their eyes during aseptic operations.

A. 更衣演示显示，洁净室操作员没有戴无菌护目镜，因此在无菌操作期间眼睛周围的皮肤暴露在外。

B. Cleanroom garments were not suitable for their intended use. For example, garments indicated to be clean were observed to be stained, worn out, and stored improperly. In addition, your firm re-used cleanroom garments for an unspecified number of times without tracking or validation.

B. 洁净室服装不适合其预期用途。例如，标明干净的衣服被发现有污渍、磨损和存放不当。此外，你公司在未进行跟踪或验证的情况下，重复使用了洁净室服装，次数不详。

C. You lacked written procedures and a training program on proper aseptic behavior and gowning for cleanroom operators. You also lacked evidence that all cleanroom operators are qualified through participation in a media fill, and the microbiological limit set in your gowning validation procedure is unsuitable for aseptic operations.

C. 你公司缺乏关于洁净室操作员正确无菌行为和更衣的书面程序和培训计划。还缺乏证据来证明所有洁净室操作员都通过参与培养基模拟灌装而获得资质确认，并且你公司的更衣验证程序中设定的微生物限度不适合无菌操作。

D. You lacked written procedures and a training program on proper aseptic behavior and gowning for cleanroom operators. You also lacked evidence that all cleanroom operators were qualified through participation in a media fill and justification for the microbiological limits used in your aseptic processing operator gowning qualification procedure (i.e., no more than (NMT)(b)(4) colony forming units (cfu) for each gowning location). You also lacked a commitment to systematically review staff qualifications and competencies throughout your operation, including but not limited to, ensuring an effective cGMP training program.

D. 你公司缺乏关于洁净室操作员正确无菌行为和更衣的书面程序和培训计划。还缺乏证据来证明所有洁净室操作员通过参加培养基灌装而获得资质确认，以及对无菌工艺操作员更衣资质确认程序中使用的微生物限度的合理性进行论证［即对于每个洁净服位置，不超过（NMT）（b）（4）菌落形成单位（cfu）］。你公司还缺乏在整个运营过程中系统地审查员工资质和能力的承诺，包括但不限于确保有效的 cGMP 培训计划。

In your response, you state that gowning qualification will be performed through media fills, and an in-house study will evaluate the impact of repeated sterilization cycles on cleanroom garments to establish an acceptable number of sterilizarion cycles. Your response is inadequate. You lack a comprehensive review of all aspects of personnel gowning, the qualification program, aseptic technique, cleanroom behavior, and an examination of the role of people as a contamination hazard in your processes. To further illustrate, you continue to lack substantive actions to implement sterile goggles, enhance practices to prevent sterile gown contamination, gowning qualification criteria (e.g., sampling requirements, location descriptions, acceptance limits with justifications), and many other basic elements of a compliant sterile facility. Your response also fails to address how your inadequate gowning practices impacted your sterile drug products.

在回复中，你公司声称将通过培养基模拟灌装来进行更衣确认，并且内部研究将评估重复灭菌周期对洁净室服装的影响，以确定可接受的灭菌周期数。你公司的回应不够充分。缺乏对人员更衣、资质确认计划、无菌技术、洁净室行为的所有方面的全面审查，以及对人员在工艺中作为污染隐患的检查。进一步来说，你公司仍然缺乏实质性行动，来实施无菌护目镜、加强防止无菌洁净服污染的实践、更衣资质确认标准（例如，取样要求、位置描述、带有论证的可接受限度），以及合规无菌设施的很多其他基本要素。就你公司不适当的更衣实践如何影响无菌药品，你公司的回复也未能解决。

See FDA's guidance document *Sterile Drug Products Produced by Aseptic Processing—Current Good Manufacturing Practice* to help you meet the cGMP requirements when manufacturing sterile drugs using aseptic processing at https://www.fda.gov/media/71026/download.

请参阅 FDA 指南，通过无菌工艺生产的无菌药品 – 现行药品生产质量管理规范，以帮助你公司在使用无菌工艺生产无菌药品时满足 cGMP 要求，网址（略，见上）。

In response to this letter, provide the following:

在回复本函时，请提供以下信息：

● Comprehensive risk assessment of all contamination hazards with respect to your aseptic processes, equipment, and facilities, including an independent assessment that

267

includes, but is not limited to:

● 就你公司的无菌工艺、设备和设施的所有污染隐患，进行全面的风险评估，包含独立评估，这包括但不限于：

○ All human interactions within the ISO 5 area

○ ISO 5 区域内的所有人员交互

○ Equipment placement and ergonomics

○ 设备放置和人体工程学

○ Air quality in the ISO 5 area and surrounding room

○ ISO 5 区域和周围房间的空气质量

○ Facility layout

○ 设施布局

○ Personnel Flows and Material Flows（throughout all rooms used to conduct and support sterile operations）

○ 人流和物流（用于执行和支持无菌操作的所有房间）

● A detailed remediation plan with timelines to address the findings of the independent contamination hazards risk assessment. Describe specific tangible improvements to be made to aseptic processing operation design and control at your facility. Explain how your corrective action and preventive action（CAPA）will robustly remediate your deficient sterile manufacturing operation. Also describe your plans for qualification and validation of your comprehensively remediated facility, processes and equipment.

● 详细的整改计划和时间表，以解决独立污染危害风险评估所发现的问题。描述要在你公司的设施中对无菌工艺操作设计和控制进行的具体切实改进，解释你公司的纠正和预防措施（CAPA）将如何有力地整改无菌生产操作缺陷。对全面整改后的设施、工艺和设备，描述你公司对其进行确认和验证的计划。

● A remediation plan that better assures ongoing management oversight throughout the manufacturing lifecycle of all drug products. Provide a more data-driven and scientifically sound program that identifies sources of process variability and assures that manufacturing（including both production and packaging）operations meet appropriate parameters and quality standards. This includes, but is not limited to, evaluating suitability of equipment for its intended use, ensuring quality of input materials, determining the capability and reliability of each manufacturing process step and its controls, and vigilant ongoing monitoring of process performance and product quality.

● 一项整改计划，可以更好地确保在所有药品的整个生产生命周期中进行持续的管理监督。提供更加数据驱动且科学合理的程序，识别工艺波动的来源，并确保生产（包括生产和包装）操作满足适当的参数和质量标准。这包括但不限于评估设备对其预期用途的适用性，确保输入物料的质量，确定每个生产工艺步骤及其控制的能力和可靠性，以及对工艺性能和产品质量进行警戒性的持续监控。

● Your CAPA plan to implement routine, vigilant operations management oversight of facilities and equipment. This plan should ensure, among other things, prompt detection of equipment/facilities performance issues, effective execution of repairs, adherence to appropriate preventive maintenance schedules, timely technological upgrades to the equipment/facility infrastructure, and improved systems for ongoing management review.

● 你公司的 CAPA 计划，对设施和设备实施日常、警戒性的运营管理监督。至少，该计划应确保及时发现设备 / 设施性能问题，有效执行维修，遵守适当的预防性维护计划，及时对设备 / 设施进行技术升级，并对持续管理评审的系统进行改进。

● Your plan to ensure that inspection and other quality control methods for container-closure systems, including but not limited to opaque bottles and ointment tubes, can robustly detect integrity breaches.

● 你公司的计划，来确保容器封闭系统（包括但不限于不透明瓶子和软膏管）的检查和其他能够可靠地检测完整性被破坏的情况的质量控制方法。

● A comprehensive, independent assessment of the qualifications and competencies of staff to conduct their job duties throughout your operations, including:

● 对员工在整个运营过程中履行工作职责的资质确认和能力进行全面、独立的评估，包括：

○ a system that ensures each staff member receives training to enable them to properly perform each of their job duties in advance of performing job tasks

○ 一项系统，确保每位员工接受培训，使他们能够在执行工作任务之前正确履行每项工作职责

○ a review of your training curriculum, including courses, timing, frequency, and training effectiveness

○ 审查你公司的培训课程，包括科目、时间安排、频率和培训效果

○ supervision to determine ongoing adherence of staff to procedures and proper practices

○ 进行监督，以确定员工是否持续遵守程序和正确实践

○ provisions for retraining in response to deficient performance or, when appropriate, re-evaluating whether the individual has the appropriate qualifications and expertise（training, education, skills）for the type and complexity of their assigned work

○ 制定针对有缺陷表现的再培训规定，或者在适当的情况下，重新评估个人是否拥有适合其所分配工作的类型和复杂性的资质确认和专业知识（培训、教育、技能）

○ training of supervisors and managers in cGMPs

○ 对主管和经理进行 cGMP 培训

物料检验

2. Your firm failed to test samples of each component for identity and conformity with all appropriate written specifications for purity, strength, and quality. Your firm also failed to validate and establish the reliability of your component supplier's test analyses at appropriate intervals（21 CFR 211.84（d）（1）and 211.84（d）（2））.

2. 你公司未进行至少一项检验来确认药品中每种原辅料的鉴别，并使其符合所有适当的纯度、规格和质量的书面质量标准。你公司也未能在适当的时间间隔内，验证和确定物料供应商检验分析的可靠性［21 CFR 211.84（d）（1）和（2）］。

You did not ensure that incoming lots of active pharmaceutical ingredient（API）and packaging materials were suitable for use in manufacturing.

你公司没有确保进场批次的原料药（API）和包装材料适合用于生产。

Your firm released API for use in drug manufacturing based on a component supplier's certificate of analysis（COA）, although you neither established the reliability of the analysis through appropriate validation nor performed identity testing. Notably, examples included two lots of carboxy methyl cellulose sodium API used to manufacture Artificial Tears batches distributed to the U.S. market.

基于原辅料供应商的分析证书（COA），你公司放行了用于药品生产的 API，即使你们既没有通过适当的验证来确定分析的可靠性，也没有进行鉴别检验。值得注意的是，例子包括两批用于生产销往美国市场的人工泪液的羧甲基纤维素钠原料药。

You also failed to adequately test primary packaging materials, including caps and plugs, used in the Artificial Tears container-closure system. For example, between 2019 and 2022, you received（b）（4）shipments of caps and plugs supplied as sterile from a vendor and released them for use based on the supplier's COA without adequate testing.

你公司还未能充分检验人工泪液容器封闭系统中使用的主要包装材料，包括盖子和塞子。例如，在 2019 年至 2022 年间，你公司收到了供应商以无菌状态提供的（b）（4）批瓶盖和塞子，并根据供应商的 COA 未经充分检验就将其放行以供使用。

Identity testing for each component lot used in drug product manufacturing is required, and you may only rely on COA for other component attributes if you validate the supplier's test results to ensure their reliability at appropriate intervals.

需要对药品生产中使用的每个原辅料批次进行鉴别检验，并且只能在以适当时间间隔验证供应商的检验结果以确保其可靠性后，才能仅依赖 COA 来确认其他原辅料的属性。

A drug product produced by aseptic processing can become contaminated not only by unacceptable practices in the manufacturing operation, but also due to the use of one or more defective components, containers, or closures.

对于通过无菌工艺生产的药品，其不仅可能因生产操作中不可接受的实践而受到污染，还可能由于使用一个或多个有缺陷的物料、容器或密封件而受到污染。

Your response is inadequate for reasons that include, but are not limited to, the following:

你公司的回复不充分，原因包括但不限于以下内容：

- You fail to indicate that all existing and new suppliers will be qualified.

- 你公司未能表明所有现有和新的供应商均得到资质确认。

- It lacks details on procedural revisions to be made, including how you intend to establish and maintain assurance of the reliability of your supplier's COA.

- 缺乏有关程序修订的详细信息，包括你公司打算如何建立和维持对供应商 COA 可靠性的保证。

- It also lacks details on your retrospective testing, including the scope of materials to be tested, sampling and testing methods, and how you intend to ensure that incoming materials are suitable for their intended use.

- 还缺乏有关你公司的回顾性检验的详细信息，包括待检物料的范围、取样和检验方法，以及你们打算如何确保进场的物料适合其预期用途。

We also note that you listed drug products with FDA as being manufactured at your facility and intended for distribution in the United States, including paracetamol syrup, clotrimazole 1%, and Diaprene Children Maximum Topical Creams, that contain components with a high risk of diethylene glycol（DEG）or ethylene glycol（EG）contamination, such as glycerin and propylene glycol. The use of ingredients contaminated with DEG or EG has resulted in various lethal poisoning incidents in humans worldwide. See FDA's guidance document *Testing of Glycerin, Propylene Glycol, Maltitol Solution, Hydrogenated Starch Hydrolysate, Sorbitol Solution, and Other High-Risk Drug Components for Diethylene Glycol and Ethylene Glycol* to help you meet the cGMP requirements when manufacturing drugs containing ingredients at high-risk for DEG or EG contamination（"high-risk drug components"）, at https://www.fda.gov/media/167974/download.

我们还注意到，你公司向 FDA 列出了在你们的设施生产并打算在美国流通的药品，包括对乙酰氨基酚糖浆、克霉唑 1% 和 Diaprene Children Maximum 外用乳膏，这些产品中包括例如甘油和丙二醇等原辅料，具有二甘醇（DEG）或乙二醇（EG）高风险污染。在全球范围内，使用受 DEG 或 EG 污染的原辅料已导致多起人类致命中毒事件。请参阅 FDA 指南，甘油、丙二醇、麦芽糖醇溶液、氢化淀粉水解物、山梨醇溶液和其他高风险药品原辅料中二甘醇和乙二醇的检验，以帮助你公司在生产含有 DEG 或 EG 污染风险原辅料的药品时，满足 cGMP 要求，请访问网址（略，见上）。

In response to this letter, provide the following:

作为对本函的回应，请提供以下信息：

● A comprehensive, independent review of your material system to determine whether all suppliers of components, containers, and closures, are each qualified and the materials are assigned appropriate expiration or retest dates. The review should also determine whether incoming material controls are adequate to prevent use of unsuitable components, containers, and closures.

● 对你公司的物料系统进行全面、独立的审查，以确定所有物料、容器和密封件的供应商是否均合格，并为物料指定适当的有效期或复验日期。审查还应确定进场物料控制是否足以防止使用不合适的物料、容器和密封件。

● The chemical and microbiological quality control specifications you use to test and release each incoming lot of components for use in manufacturing.

● 针对每批生产目的的进场物料，用于检验和放行的化学和微生物质控标准。

● A summary of results obtained from testing all components to evaluate the reliability of the COA from each component manufacturer. Include your standard operating procedure（SOP）that describes this COA validation program.

● 对所有物料进行检验的结果汇总，以评估每个物料生产商的 COA 可靠性。包括描述此 COA 验证计划的标准操作程序（SOP）。

● A summary of your program for qualifying and overseeing contract facilities that test the drug products you manufacture.

● 对检验你公司生产的药品的外包设施，进行资质审查和监督计划的汇总。

● A commitment to provide DEG and EG test results, no later than 30 calendar days from the date of this letter, from testing retains for all lots of high-risk drug components used in the manufacture of drug products. Alternatively, if a retain of a component lot is unavailable, perform retain sample testing of all potentially affected finished drug product batches for the presence of DEG and EG.

● 承诺在自本函之日起 30 个日历日内，针对用于所有批次药品生产中高风险药品原辅料，提供 DEG 和 EG 检验结果。或者，如果没有某个原辅料批次的留样，则对所有可能受影响的成品制剂批次进行留样检验，以确定 DEG 和 EG 的存在。

● A full risk assessment for drug products that are within expiry which contain any ingredient at risk for DEG or EG contamination (including but not limited to glycerin). Take prompt and appropriate actions to determine the safety of all lots of the component (s) and any related drug product that could contain DEG or EG, including customer notifications and product recalls for any contaminated lots. Identify additional appropriate corrective actions and preventive actions that secure supply chains in the future, including but not limited to ensuring that all incoming raw material lots are from fully qualified manufacturers and free from unsafe impurities. Detail these actions in your response to this letter.

● 就含有任何有 DEG 或 EG 污染风险的原辅料（包括但不限于甘油）且在效期内的药品，提供全面的风险评估。立即采取适当的措施，就任何可能含有 DEG 或 EG 的原辅料或相关药品批次，确定其安全性，包括通知客户和召回任何受污染批次的产品。确定其他适当的 CAPA，以确保未来的供应链安全，包括但不限于：确保所有进场原料批次均来自有充分资质的生产商，且不含不安全的杂质。在你公司对本函的回复中详细说明这些行动。

● A description of how you will test each component lot for conformity with all appropriate specifications for identity, strength, quality, and purity. If you intend to accept any results from your supplier's COA instead of testing each component lot for strength, quality, and purity, specify how you will robustly establish the reliability of your supplier's results through initial validation as well as periodic revalidation. In addition, include a commitment to always conduct at least one specific identity test for each incoming component lot. In the case of glycerin, propylene glycol, and certain additional high-risk components we note that this includes the performance of parts A, B, and C of the United States

Pharmacopeia（USP）monograph.

● 说明如何检验每个批次，确定是否符合有关鉴别、规格、质量和纯度质量标准。如果你公司打算接受供应商 COA 的结果，而不是检验每个物料批次的规格、质量和纯度，请说明如何进行初始验证和定期再验证，从而稳健地确定供应商结果的可靠性。此外，还应承诺：对于每个进场原辅料批次，至少进行一个专属鉴别检验。就甘油、丙二醇以及其他高风险原辅料而言，我们注意到这包括 USP 专论 A、B 和 C 部分的性能表现。

无菌环境

3. Your firm failed to establish a system for monitoring environmental conditions in aseptic processing areas and an adequate system for cleaning and disinfecting the room to produce aseptic conditions（21 CFR 211.42（c）（10）（iv）and 211.42（c）（10）（v））.

3. 你公司未能建立系统，来监测无菌工艺区的环境条件，以及适当的系统来清洁和消毒房间和设备，以产生无菌条件［21 CFR 211.42（c）（10）（iv）和 211.42（c）（10）（v）］。

■ Sterilization and Cleaning｜灭菌和清洁

You failed to adequately sterilize and clean your equipment used for drug product manufacturing, for example：

你公司未能对用于药品生产的设备进行充分灭菌和清洁，例如：

A. You failed to ensure that all equipment with direct product contact was sterilized. During the inspection, you were not able to provide records showing sterilization of product contact equipment on the "（b）（4）Line", including the filling（b）（4）,（b）（4）tubing, and（b）（4）bowls. Review of sterilization records revealed that you only documented that garments and tools were sterilized. You also lacked written procedures describing sterilization of the manufacturing equipment.

A. 你公司未能确保所有直接接触产品的设备都经过灭菌。在检查期间，你公司无法提供记录显示"（b）（4）生产线"上产品接触设备的灭菌情况，包括灌装（b）（4）、（b）（4）管道和（b）（4）锅。灭菌记录审查显示，你公司仅记录了服装和工具的灭菌情况。此外，还缺乏描述生产设备灭菌的书面程序。

B. You failed to adequately clean the equipment used to aseptically produce Artificial Tears. Significantly, our investigators observed visible grease-like residue on product contact surfaces of your filling machine after they had been cleaned.

B. 你公司未能充分清洁用于无菌生产人工泪液的设备。值得注意的是，在清洁后的灌装机产品接触表面上，我们的调查员发现了明显的油脂状残留物。

You also lacked written procedures and other documentation describing cleaning of the manufacturing equipment.

你公司还缺乏描述生产设备清洁的书面程序和其他文件。

C. You lacked cleaning validation studies for the shared manufacturing equipment on the "(b)(4)Line."

C. 你公司缺乏对"（b）（4）生产线"上共享生产设备的清洁验证研究。

Inadequately cleaned and maintained equipment can lead to cross-contamination and poor quality drug products.

设备清洁和维护不当，这可能会导致交叉污染和药品质量低劣。

Your response is inadequate for reasons that include, but are not limited to, the following:

你公司的回复不充分，原因包括但不限于以下内容：

● You fail to provide cleaning procedures or cleaning validation protocols. In addition, no commitment is made to comprehensively evaluate the suitability of your filling machine and other equipment for the manufacture of sterile drug products.

● 你公司未能提供清洁程序或清洁验证方案。此外，未承诺全面评估你公司的灌装机和其他设备是否适合生产无菌药品。

● You fail to provide details of your proposed testing of retain samples.

● 你公司未能提供所提出的留样检验的详细信息。

● You fail to provide explanations for the conflicting information provided to FDA investigators during the inspection. For example, investigators were initially told that(b)(4) bowls on the filling line were not cleaned or sterilized. These statements were later retracted; however, you were unable to provide sufficient information to support claims that (b)(4) bowls were cleaned and sterilized.

● 检查期间，你公司向 FDA 调查员提供相互矛盾的信息，对此未能作出解释。例如，调查员最初被告知灌装线上的（b）（4）锅没有清洁或消毒。这些声明后来被否认；然而，你公司无法提供充分的信息来支持（b）（4）锅已清洁和消毒的说法。

▣ Monitoring Environmental Conditions ｜环境条件的监测

Your environmental monitoring（EM）program（including personnel monitoring（PM））was inadequate for classified areas used to produce sterile ophthalmic drug products. For example, non-viable air samples were not collected inside the Grade A filling zone or the Grade B surrounding areas during active filling, you lacked studies to demonstrate that residual disinfectant would not interfere with the swabs used for viable surface monitoring, and you lacked identification data on isolates recovered from EM and PM sampling.

对于用于生产无菌眼科药品的洁净级别区域来说，你公司的环境监测（EM）计划［包括人员监测（PM）］是不够的。例如，在灌装过程中，未在 A 级灌装区域内或 B 级周围区域采集空气悬浮粒子样品；缺乏研究，来证明残留消毒剂不会干扰用于表面微生物监测的拭子；针对从 EM 和 PM 取样中回收的分离株，缺乏鉴别数据。

Vigilant and responsive environmental and personnel monitoring programs should be designed to provide meaningful information on the state of control of your aseptic processing environment. Operations that include highly manually intensive aseptic activities warrant a more extensive environmental and personnel monitoring program, including but not limited to, heightened emphasis on well-timed sampling to appropriately monitor batch manufacturing conditions.

应设计具有警戒性且反应灵敏的环境和人员监控计划，以提供有关无菌工艺操作环境控制状态的有意义信息。无菌操作涉及高度密集人工活动时，需要更广泛的环境和人员监测计划，包括但不限于高度重视适时的取样，以便适当地监测批生产条件。

In your response, you mention a limited number of environmental samples taken in January 2023 were sent to a third-party laboratory and these samples did not reveal *Pseudomonas aeruginosa* in your environment. This response is inadequate. The last batches of Artificial Tears shipped to the United States had been manufactured many months before（in April 2022）your limited sampling was conducted, according to records provided by your firm. Environmental sampling that occurs several months after batch manufacture is of little temporal significance. There is also minimal scientific value in testing sterile drug manufacturing areas solely for the presence of a single microbial species. You also had batch retain samples tested by a third-party laboratory and you reported in your response that these samples did not fail sterility testing. However, it is not unexpected that sterility testing of retains of otherwise contaminated batches may pass sterility testing because of the non-uniform nature of microbiological contamination. As noted above, many of your firm's batches were found to be non-sterile upon FDA testing and were associated with grave adverse events.

在你公司的回复中，提到 2023 年 1 月采集的有限数量的环境样品被送往第三方实验室，这些样品没有显示出你公司的环境中存在铜绿假单胞菌。这种回应是不充分的。根据你公司提供的记录，运往美国的最后一批人工泪液是在你们进行有限取样之前数月（2022 年 4 月）生产的。批生产几个月后进行的环境取样没有什么时间上的意义。仅针对单一微生物物种的存在来检验无菌药品生产区域，其科学价值也很小。你公司还让第三方实验室对批次留样进行了检验，并且你公司在回复中报告称这些样品通过无菌检验。然而，由于微生物污染的不均匀性，被污染批次留样可能会通过无菌检验，这并不令人意外。如上所述，FDA 检测发现你公司的很多批次产品是非无菌的，并且与严重的不良事件有关。

In response to this letter, provide the following:

在回复本函时，请提供以下信息：

● A comprehensive, independent assessment of the design and control of your firm's manufacturing operations, with a detailed and thorough review of all microbiological hazards.

● 对你公司生产操作的设计和控制进行全面、独立的评估，并对所有微生物危害进行详细、彻底的审查。

● A comprehensive, independent retrospective assessment of your cleaning effectiveness to evaluate the scope of cross-contamination hazards. Include the identity of residues, other manufacturing equipment that may have been improperly cleaned, and an assessment whether cross-contaminated products may have been released for distribution. The assessment should identify any inadequacies of cleaning procedures and practices and encompass each piece of manufacturing equipment used to manufacture more than one product.

● 对清洁效果进行全面、独立的回顾性评估，以评估交叉污染危害的范围。包括残留物的鉴别、其他可能未正确清洁的生产设备，以及对交叉污染的药品是否可能已被放行以供流通的评估。评估应确定清洁程序和实践的任何不足之处，并涵盖用于生产多个产品的每台生产设备。

● A CAPA plan, based on the retrospective assessment of your cleaning and disinfection program, that includes appropriate remediations to your cleaning and disinfection processes and practices, and timelines for completion. Provide a detailed summary of vulnerabilities in your process for lifecycle management of equipment cleaning and disinfection. Describe improvements to your cleaning and disinfection program, including enhancements to cleaning effectiveness; improved ongoing verification of proper cleaning and disinfection execution for all products and equipment; and all other needed remediations.

● 一项 CAPA 计划，基于对清洁和消毒计划的回顾性评估，其中包括对清洁、消毒工艺和实践的相应整改措施以及完成时间表。提供设备清洁和消毒生命周期管理流程中漏洞的详细汇总。描述你公司对清洁和消毒计划的改进，包括提高清洁效果；改进对所有产品和设备的正确清洁和消毒执行的持续确认；以及所有其他需要的整改措施。

● Appropriate improvements to your cleaning validation program, with special emphasis on incorporating conditions identified as worst case in your drug manufacturing operation. This should include but not be limited to identification and evaluation of all worst-case：

● 适当地改进你公司的清洁验证计划，特别强调将确定为药品生产操作中最差情况的条件纳入其中。这应包括但不限于识别和评估所有最差情况：

○ drugs with higher toxicities

○ 具有较高毒性的药物

○ drugs with higher drug potencies

○ 具有较高药物活性的药物

○ drugs of lower solubility in their cleaning solvents

○ 在清洁溶剂中溶解度较低的药物

○ drugs with characteristics that make them difficult to clean

○ 具有难以清洁特性的药物

○ swabbing locations for areas that are most difficult to clean

○ 最难清洁区域的擦拭位置

○ maximum hold times before cleaning

○ 清洁前的最长存放时间

In addition, describe the steps that must be taken in your change management system before introduction of new manufacturing equipment or a new product.

此外，描述在引入新生产设备或新产品之前，在变更管理系统中必须采取的步骤。

● A summary of updated SOPs that ensure an appropriate program is in place for verification and validation of cleaning procedures for products, processes, and equipment.

● 更新的标准操作程序汇总，确保制定适当的计划来确认和验证产品、工艺和设备的清洁程序。

● A comprehensive, independent review of your personnel and environmental monitoring programs, including but not limited to, a plan to fully remediate these programs. For example, describe changes to equipment, procedures, and practices that will ensure meaningful ongoing data is collected to promptly detect and respond to emerging risks in your classified areas. Provide an updated timeline for implementation of your program, including a summary of the CAPA steps you will be undertaking to ensure effective remediation.

● 对你公司的人员和环境监测计划进行全面、独立的审查,包括但不限于全面整改这些程序的计划。例如,描述对设备、程序和实践的更改,以确保收集有意义的持续数据,以及时检测和回应洁净区新出现的风险。提供计划实施的最新时间表,包括你公司为确保有效整改而将采取的 CAPA 步骤的汇总。

检验方法

4. Your firm failed to establish the accuracy, sensitivity, specificity, and reproducibility of its test methods, and you also failed to conduct appropriate laboratory testing to determine whether each batch of drug product purporting to be sterile conforms to such requirements(21 CFR 211.165(e)and 211.167(a)).

4. 你公司未能建立其检验方法的精确度、灵敏度、专属性和重现性,并且也未能进行适当的实验室检验,来确定声称无菌的每批药品是否符合此类要求[21 CFR 211.165(e)和 211.167(a)]。

Your firm lacked adequate sterility testing, for example:

你公司缺乏充分的无菌性检验,例如:

A. You failed to show that your sterility test method was suitable to detect microorganisms in your ophthalmic drug products.

A. 你公司的无菌检验方法,未被证明适合检测你们的眼科药品中的微生物。

Method suitability testing ensures the method can reliably determine the presence of microbial growth in the product. Method validation and verification is necessary to support reliable determinations of identity, strength, quality, purity, and potency of drugs. Without evaluating the validity of methods, you lack the basic assurance that the data provided to customers was an accurate reflection of pharmaceutical product quality and safety.

方法适用性检验确保该方法能够可靠地确定产品中是否存在微生物生长。方法验证和确认对于支持药品的鉴别、规格、质量、纯度和效能的可靠测定是必要的。如果不评估方法的有效性,你公司就无法保证向客户提供的数据能够准确反映药品质量和安全性。

B. You lacked growth promotion tests of the media used for media fills and personnel monitoring.

B. 对于用于培养基模拟灌装和人员监控的培养基，你公司缺乏培养基的促生长检验。

The validity of your microbiological testing cannot be ensured without appropriate testing of media.

如果不对培养基进行适当的检验，就无法确保微生物检验的有效性。

In your response, you make commitments to review your sterility testing and other analytical method validations, initiate sterility method verification, and revise your media preparation procedures. Your response is inadequate because you fail to provide revised procedures and you do not address your failure to perform adequate sterility testing on your distributed finished drug products.

在回复中，你公司承诺审查你们的无菌检验和其他分析方法验证，启动无菌方法确认，并修订培养基制备程序。你公司的回复是不充分的，因为未能提供修订的程序，并且就已流通的成品，未能解决对其无充分无菌性检验的问题。

In response to this letter, provide the following:

在回复本函时，请提供以下信息：

● A comprehensive, independent assessment of your laboratory practices, procedures, methods, equipment, documentation, and analyst competencies. Based on this review, provide a detailed plan to remediate and evaluate the effectiveness of your laboratory system.

● 对你公司的实验室实践、程序、方法、设备、文件和分析员能力进行完整、全面、独立的评估。在此审查的基础上，提供详细的计划来整改和评估你公司实验室系统的有效性。

● A detailed risk assessment addressing the hazards posed by distributing contaminated drug products.

● 针对流通受污染药品造成的危害，进行详细的风险评估。

● Complete investigations into all batches with confirmed and potential microbial contamination. The investigations should detail your findings regarding the root causes of the contamination.

● 对所有已确认和潜在微生物污染的批次进行全面调查。调查应详细说明有关污染根本原因的调查结果。

- All chemical and microbial test methods used to analyze each of your drug products.

- 用于分析每种药品的所有化学和微生物检验方法。

质量部门

5. Your firm's quality control unit failed to exercise its responsibility to ensure drug products manufactured are in compliance with cGMP, and meet established specifications for identity, strength, quality, and purity(21 CFR 211.22).

5. 你公司的质量控制部门未能履行职责，以确保所生产的药品符合 cGMP 要求，并符合有关鉴别、规格、质量和纯度的既定质量标准（21 CFR 211.22）。

Your firm failed to establish an adequate quality unit(QU)with the responsibilities and authority to oversee the manufacture of your drug products. For example：

你公司未能建立一个合格的质量部门（QU）来负责监督药品的生产。例如：

A. You failed to perform adequate batch release to ensure the acceptability of all batches of Artificial Tears, prior to release for the U.S. market.

A. 在向美国市场放行之前，你公司未能进行充分的批放行，以确保所有批次的人工泪液是合格的。

B. Your quality system does not adequately ensure the accuracy and integrity of data to support the quality of the drugs you manufacture. For example, your firm permitted the unacceptable practice of using pre-filled batch release documents.

B. 你公司的质量体系不能充分确保数据的准确性和可靠性，以支持你公司生产的药品的质量。例如，你公司允许使用预先填写的批放行文件，这是一种不可接受的做法。

C. You failed to follow your change management procedure. The impact of the change to the specification for the inner cap(plug)used as part of your Artificial Tears container-closure system to a plug "with prehole" was not evaluated.

C. 你公司未能遵循变更管理程序。未评估将用作人工泪液容器封闭系统一部分的内盖（塞子）规格更改为"带预加工孔"塞子的影响。

In your response, you state you will perform an impact assessment for all change controls initiated. Your response is inadequate for reasons that include, but are not limited to, the following：

在回复中，你公司声称将对启动的所有变更控制进行影响评估。你公司的回复不充分，原因包括但不限于以下内容：

- You do not assess all records potentially affected by lapses in data integrity. You also do not assess how poor documentation practices affected distributed drug product nor how you could strengthen QU oversight. You also do not provide copies of the missing batch release documents you indicated that you have now recovered.

- 你公司未评估可能受数据可靠性缺陷影响的所有记录。也没有评估不良的记录实践如何影响已流通的药品，也没有评估如何加强 QU 监督。更没有提供你公司表示现已恢复的丢失批放行文档的副本。

- You do not perform a review and impact assessment for changes made outside of your change management system and not previously evaluated.

- 对于变更管理系统之外进行的且之前未评估过的变更，你公司未进行审查并评估影响。

In response to this letter, provide the following：

在回复本函时，请提供以下信息：

（略）

此处与 FDA 发给 Cosmobeauti Laboratories & Manufacturing Inc. 的警告信（编号：MARCS–CMS 657682，即"12 批生产记录存在倒记问题"）中有关 QU 的回应要求部分的内容类似，故略去。

- A comprehensive, independent assessment of your change management system. This assessment should include, but not be limited to, your procedure（s）to ensure changes are justified, reviewed, and approved by your quality unit. Your change management program should also include provisions for determining change effectiveness.

- 对你公司的变更管理系统进行全面、独立的评估。该评估应包括但不限于确保变更合理、经过质量部门审查和批准的程序。你公司的变更管理计划还应包括确定变更有效性的规定。

- A complete assessment of documentation systems used throughout your manufacturing and laboratory operations to determine where documentation practices are insufficient. Include a detailed CAPA plan that comprehensively remediates your firm's documentation practices to ensure you retain attributable, legible, complete, original, accurate, contemporaneous records throughout your operation.

- 对整个生产操作中使用的文档系统进行全面评估，以确定记录规范的不足之处。包括详细的 CAPA 计划，以全面整改公司的记录规范，确保你公司在整个运营过程中保存可追溯的、清晰的、完整的、原始的、准确的和同步的记录。

Drug Recalls | 药品召回

On January 30, 2023, FDA held a teleconference with you. We recommended you consider removing all batches of EzriCare Artificial Tears and Delsam Pharma's Artificial Tears in distribution from the U.S. market. On February 2, 2023, you initiated a voluntary recall of EzriCare Artificial Tears and Delsam Pharma's Artificial Tears based on bacterial contamination and cGMP concerns discussed with your firm. The company announcement was posted to the FDA website：https://www.fda.gov/safety/recalls-market-withdrawals-safety-alerts/global-pharma-healthcare-issues-voluntary-nationwide-recall-artificial-tears-lubricant-eye-drops-due.

2023 年 1 月 30 日，FDA 与你公司召开电话会议。我们建议你公司考虑下架美国市场上经销的所有批次的 EzriCare 人工泪液和 Delsam Pharma 人工泪液。2023 年 2 月 2 日，基于与你公司讨论的细菌污染和 cGMP 问题，你公司主动召回了 EzriCare 人工泪液和 Delsam Pharma 人工泪液。该公司公告发布在 FDA 网站上：网址（略，见上）。

On February 22, 2023, FDA held another teleconference with you. We recommended you remove batch H29 of Delsam Pharma's Artificial Eye Ointment in U.S. distribution. On February 24, 2023, you initiated a voluntary recall of Delsam Pharma's Artificial Eye Ointment due to non-sterility. The company announcement was posted to the FDA website：https://www.fda.gov/safety/recalls-market-withdrawals-safety-alerts/global-pharma-healthcare-issues-voluntary-nationwide-recall-delsam-pharma-artificial-eye-ointment.

2023 年 2 月 22 日，FDA 再次与你公司召开电话会议。我们建议你公司下架在美国上市的 H29 批次 Delsam Pharma 人工眼膏。2023 年 2 月 24 日，你公司因非无菌而主动召回 Delsam Pharma 人工眼膏。该公司公告发布在 FDA 网站上：网址（略，见上）。

Drug Production Suspended | 药品生产暂停

We acknowledge your commitment to suspend production of drugs for the U.S. market.

我们知晓，你公司承诺暂停为美国市场生产药品。

Given the egregious violations of cGMP at your facility, if you plan to resume drug manufacturing operations for the U.S. market, decide to transfer your ownership, contract out any processes, or move to a new location, notify this office.

鉴于你公司的设施严重违反 cGMP，如果你们计划恢复美国市场的药品生产业务或决定转让你公司的所有权、外包任何工艺或搬到新场所，请通知本办公室。

Based upon the nature of the violations we identified at your firm, you should engage a consultant qualified as set forth in 21 CFR 211.34, to assist your firm in meeting drug cGMP requirements, if your firm intends to resume manufacturing drugs for the U.S. market. The qualified consultant should also perform a comprehensive six-system audit of your entire operation for cGMP compliance and evaluate the completion and efficacy of all corrective actions and preventive actions before you pursue resolution of your firm's compliance status with FDA.

根据我们在你公司发现的违规情况的性质，如果你公司打算恢复为美国市场生产药品，应该聘请符合 21 CFR 211.34 规定的有资质的顾问，以协助你公司满足药品 cGMP 要求。有资质的顾问还应对你公司的整个运营进行全面的六大体系审核，以确保 cGMP 合规性，并在寻求解决你公司与 FDA 的合规状态之前，评估所有纠正和预防措施的完成情况和有效性。

Your use of a consultant does not relieve your firm's obligation to comply with cGMP. Your firm's executive management remains responsible for resolving all deficiencies and systemic flaws to ensure ongoing cGMP compliance.

你公司使用顾问并不能免除遵守 cGMP 的义务。你公司的高级管理层仍然负责解决所有缺陷和系统性问题，以确保持续遵守 cGMP。

投诉比例，不是产品质量指标

警告信编号： MARCS-CMS 660904

签发时间： 2023-11-17；**公示时间：** 2023-11-21

签发机构： 药物审评与研究中心 | CDER（Center for Drug Evaluation and Research | CDER）

公　　司： Cipla Limited

所在国家 / 地区： 印度

主　　题： cGMP/ 成品制剂 / 掺假（cGMP/Finished Pharmaceuticals/ Adulterated）

简　　介： 西普拉（Cipla）是印度的一家跨国制药和生物科技公司，总部位于孟买。其主要研发药物用于治疗心血管疾病、关节炎、糖尿病、肥胖症和抑郁等疾病。2023 年 2 月，FDA 对该公司位于印度的药品生产设施进行了检查。FDA 指出，他们对某吸入气雾剂质量缺陷的投诉调查不充分，缺乏适当和及时的纠正和预防措施，也未能将调查范围扩大到其他可能受影响的批次。该公司解释称，已经采取了充分的控制措施，其收到的产品质量问题投诉数量仅占销售量的 0.011%，并预期市场上不会出现更多有缺陷的产品，因此未按要求向 FDA 报告，并未考虑采取任何市场行动。FDA 对此表示不认可，认为该公司未采取市场行动的理由不充分。使用收到的顾客自发投诉数量与已流通产品总数的比率，这并不是可接受的产品质量指标，也不能保护消费者。随后，2023 年 6 月，该公司对六批吸入气雾剂发起了 I 级召回。然而，FDA 并不充分认可，认为该公司未能将调查范围扩大到可能受影响的其他批次，未能进行全面的风险评估以充分确定召回范围。

本警告信以下部分与本书此前其他警告信内容类似，故略去：前言、cGMP 顾 问 推 荐（cGMP Consultant Recommended）、 结 论（Conclusion）。

偏差调查

1. Your firm failed to thoroughly investigate any unexplained discrepancy or failure of a batch or any of its components to meet any of its specifications, whether or not the batch has already been distributed（21 CFR 211.192）.

1. 无论批次是否已经流通，对于该批次或其原辅料不满足其质量标准或存在无法解释的偏差或不合格，你公司未能进行彻底调查（21 CFR 211.192）。

Your investigations into quality defect complaints of Albuterol Sulfate Inhalation Aerosol were inadequate because they lacked appropriate and timely corrective actions and preventive actions（CAPAs）. You also failed to extend your investigations to other potentially affected batches.

你公司对硫酸沙丁胺醇吸入气雾剂质量缺陷投诉的调查不充分，因为缺乏适当和及时的纠正和预防措施（CAPA）。你公司也未能将调查范围扩大到其他可能受影响的批次。

Your firm received a very high number of complaints（approximately 3,000）from the start of commercial manufacturing in April 2020 to December 2022. In January 2021, you concluded that there was no risk to product quality and patient safety based on a risk assessment. Approximately 91% of these complaints were categorized as "no spray" or "empty/less weight." Furthermore, many of these complaints remained open for extended periods of time（up to 314 days）.

从 2020 年 4 月开始商业生产到 2022 年 12 月，你公司收到了大量投诉（约 3000 起）。2021 年 1 月，你们根据风险评估得出结论，产品质量和患者安全不存在风险。这些投诉中大约 91% 被归类为"无喷雾"或"空 / 重量轻"。此外，其中很多投诉持续很长一段时间（长达 314 天）未关闭。

You concluded that（b）（4）particles from the metered dose inhaler（MDI）valves became lodged in the actuators, blocking drug delivery. The MDI valve manufacturer,（b）（4）, identified four valve lots that were potentially affected by this issue. These four valve lots were used to manufacture over（b）（4）batches of Albuterol Sulfate Inhalation Aerosol. In addition, in at least two cases, your investigation into complaints received in 2021 confirmed inhalers were not able to deliver medication due to the defective valve lots.

你公司得出的结论是，来自计量吸入器（MDI）阀门的（b）（4）颗粒滞留在执行器中，阻碍了药品递送。MDI 阀门生产商（b）（4）确定了四个可能受此问题影响的阀门批次。这四个阀门批次用于生产超过（b）（4）批次的硫酸沙丁胺醇吸入气雾剂。此外，在至少两起案例中，你公司对 2021 年收到的投诉进行的调查证实，由于阀门批次存在缺陷，吸入器无法递送药品。

While your investigation identified a critical issue with the container-closure system in which particles were blocking the path of the drug delivery, you classified the "Final Severity of Complaint" as "Non-Critical," determined that no FAR was required, and concluded that no market action was warranted. The impacted Albuterol Sulfate Inhalation Aerosol batches remained on the market through expiry.

虽然你公司的调查发现了容器封闭系统的一个严重问题，其中颗粒阻塞了药品递送路径，但你公司将"投诉的最终严重程度"分类为"非严重"，确定不需要现场警戒报告（FAR），并得出结论没有必要采取任何市场行动。受影响的硫酸沙丁胺醇吸入气雾剂批次在效期内仍在市场上。

Inadequate container-closure parts or assembly processes can directly lead to production of poor-quality inhaler medicines with severe functionality or integrity defects, including but not limited to failure to dispense, inadequate dosing, or leaking units. It is essential that your manufacturing processes remain in a continued state of control to ensure that your rescue inhaler products reproducibly deliver the required dose for consumers who rely on your medicines.

不适当的容器封闭部件或组装工艺可直接导致生产劣质吸入器药品，这些药品具有严重的功能性或完整性缺陷，包括但不限于：分配失效、剂量不足或产品泄漏。你公司的生产工艺必须保持持续的受控状态，以确保救援性吸入器产品能够重复地为依赖你公司药品的消费者提供所需的剂量。

In your response, you state there are adequate controls in place and the number of complaints received through December 2022, for product quality issues represent 0.011% of total units distributed. You also state your belief that the two complaints with defective valve components verified in your laboratory investigation were "isolated events." Furthermore, you indicate that because you anticipate no additional defective units will be present in the market, you did not submit a FAR and no market action was being contemplated.

在回复中，你公司表示已经采取了充分的控制措施，截至 2022 年 12 月收到的产品质量问题投诉数量占已流通总单位的 0.011%。你公司还表示，你们相信，实验室调查中证实的两起有关有缺陷的阀门物料的投诉是"孤立事件"。此外，你公司指出，由于你们预测市场上不会出现更多有缺陷的产品，因此没有提交 FAR，并且没有考虑采取任何市场行动。

Your response is inadequate as the issue with defective valves appears to be unresolved. According to your response, you received numerous additional complaints (about 2, 000) between January 2023 and August 2023, with similar issues such as "no spray," "empty/less weight," and leaky containers. The batches associated with these complaints used valve lots beyond the four vendor lots previously identified as potentially affected. Many complaints are still under investigation.

你公司的回复不充分，因为阀门缺陷问题似乎尚未解决。根据你公司的回复，在 2023 年 1 月至 2023 年 8 月期间收到了大量额外投诉（约 2000 起），涉及类似问题，例如 "无喷雾""空 / 重量轻"和容器泄漏。与这些投诉相关的批次使用的阀门批次超出了先前确定为可能受影响的四个供应商批次。很多投诉仍在调查中。

Your justification for not taking market action is inadequate. The ratio of the number of spontaneous complaints received from customers to the total number of units distributed is not an acceptable indicator of product quality and does not safeguard consumers. You failed to demonstrate that your production design, controls, and input materials are capable of robustly producing units with reliable functionality.

你公司未采取市场行动，其理由不充分。使用收到的顾客自发投诉数量与已流通产品总数的比率，这并不是可接受的产品质量指标，也不能保护消费者。你公司未能证明你们的生产设计、控制和输入物料能够稳健地生产具有可靠功能性的产品。

The number of complaints you received showed a marked and adverse trend of critical drug delivery failures which fundamentally impacted the ability of patients to use your Albuterol Sulfate Inhalation Aerosol. Your complaint system was ineffective. For example, you emphasized the number of complaints verified in your laboratory investigation without appropriately evaluating the severity of the complaints. Also, passing results of retain sample testing cannot be used as a reason to disregard the validity of complaints that are of high severity and occur at a low frequency. For guidance on the principles and application of quality risk management, see FDA's guidance *Q9 Quality Risk Management* at https://www.fda.gov/media/167721/download.

你公司收到的投诉数量显示出关键性药品递送失效的明显不利趋势，这从根本上影响了患者使用硫酸沙丁胺醇吸入气雾剂的能力。你公司的投诉系统无效。例如，你公司强调了实验室调查中核实的投诉数量，但没有适当评估投诉的严重性。此外，留样检验的通过结果不能作为忽视严重程度高且发生频率低的投诉有效性的理由。有关质量风险管理原则和应用的指南，请参阅 FDA 指南，Q9 质量风险管理，网址（略，见上）。

We acknowledge your firm initiated a Class I recall on June 27, 2023, for six batches of Albuterol Sulfate Inhalation Aerosol due to a defective valve lot that had a partially missing bottom seat（gasket）. However, your firm failed to perform a comprehensive risk assessment by extending the investigations to other batches potentially impacted by defective container-closure components and to adequately determine the scope of the recall.

我们知晓，于 2023 年 6 月 27 日，你公司对六批硫酸沙丁胺醇吸入气雾剂发起了 I 级召回，原因是一批有缺陷的阀门批次，其底部底座（垫圈）部分缺失。然而，你公司未能将调查范围扩大到可能受有缺陷的容器封闭部件影响的其他批次，并充分确定召回范围，从而进行全面的风险评估。

In response to this letter, provide the following:

在回复本函时，请提供以下信息：

● A comprehensive, independent assessment of your overall system for investigating deviations, discrepancies, complaints, out-of-specification (OOS) results, and failures. Provide a detailed action plan to remediate this system. Your action plan should include, but not be limited to, significant improvements in investigation competencies, scope determination, root cause evaluation, CAPA effectiveness, quality unit (QU) oversight, and written procedures. Address how your firm will ensure all phases of investigations are appropriately conducted.

● 对整个系统进行全面、独立的评估，以调查偏差、差异、投诉、OOS 结果和不合格。提供详细的行动计划，以整改此系统。你公司的行动计划应包括但不限于：调查能力、范围确定、根本原因评估、CAPA 有效性、质量部门监督和书面程序方面的显著提高。说明你公司将如何确保：调查的所有阶段都得到适当实施。

● An independent assessment of your CAPA program. Based on this assessment, provide a plan that evaluates and remediates the program, including but not limited to ensuring robust:

● 对你公司的 CAPA 计划进行独立评估。根据此评估，提供评估和整改程序的计划，包括但不限于确保：

○ Triggers for fulfilling both corrective and preventive objectives

○ 实现纠正和预防目标的触发因素

○ Root cause analysis

○ 根本原因分析

○ CAPA effectiveness

○ CAPA 有效性

○ Analysis of investigations trends on a routine basis

    ○ 定期分析调查趋势

    ○ CAPA program improvements, whenever needed

    ○ 需要时改进 CAPA 计划

    ○ Implementation of final QU decisions

    ○ 实施最终 QU 决策

    ○ Support of the program by executive management

    ○ 高级管理层对计划的支持

● An independent, retrospective review of all complaints and associated investigations for Albuterol Sulfate Inhalation Aerosol batches manufactured since April 2020. Provide the consultant's recommendations based on a review that includes but is not limited to an evaluation of:

● 针对 2020 年 4 月以来生产的硫酸沙丁胺醇吸入气雾剂批次的所有投诉和相关调查，进行独立的回顾性审查。根据审查顾问的建议，包括但不限于评估：

    ○ All investigations related to "confirmed" and "unconfirmed" container-closure defects, the level of criticality for each defect, all potentially impacted batches (i.e., distributed, undistributed and rejected batches; approved and pending application drug products), and any associated issues identified during both product/process development and via commercial batch experience.

    ○ 与"已确认"和"未确认"容器封闭缺陷相关的所有调查、每个缺陷的严重程度、所有可能受影响的批次（即已流通、未流通和拒放的批次；已批准和待申请的药品），以及任何相关的在产品 / 工艺开发期间和商业批发现的问题。

    ○ The sufficiency (i.e., scope, trend analysis, root cause, CAPA) of the investigations, whether the complaint sample was obtained, all results of analysis of complaint and reserve samples.

    ○ 调查的充分性（即范围、趋势分析、根本原因、CAPA）；是否获取投诉样品；投诉和留样的所有分析结果。

● An independent, comprehensive review of your company's complaint handling program that identifies deficiencies and a corresponding CAPA.

● 对于你公司的投诉处理计划，进行独立、全面的审查，找出缺陷和相应的 CAPA。

● A management strategy including the interim measures describing the actions you have taken or will take to protect patients and to ensure the quality of your drugs, such as notifying your customers, recalling product, conducting additional testing, supplier changes, adding batches to your stability program to assure stability, drug application actions, and steps to enhance vigilance in response to serious quality complaints.

● 管理策略，包括描述你公司已采取或将采取的保护患者和确保药品质量的行动的临时措施，例如通知客户、召回产品、进行额外检验、供应商变更、在稳定性计划中添加批次确保稳定性、用药行动以及针对严重质量投诉提高警戒的步骤。

无菌和灭菌工艺验证

2. Your firm failed to establish and follow appropriate written procedures that are designed to prevent microbiological contamination of drug products purporting to be sterile, and that include validation of all aseptic and sterilization processes (21 CFR 211.113 (b)).

2. 你公司未能建立并遵循适当的书面程序，包括验证所有无菌和灭菌工艺的程序，以防止声称无菌的药品受到微生物污染 ［ 21 CFR 211.113 (b)］。

■ Media Fill Contamination Incidents ｜培养基模拟灌装污染事件

You failed to appropriately evaluate a pattern of media fill failures in your facility and afford sufficient attention to potential correlations among these contamination events. Between February 2021 and March 2022, there were multiple aborted and contaminated media fills on (b) (4) filling lines (b) (4) and (b) (4) (solution and suspension lines). For example,

你公司未能正确评估设施中的培养基模拟灌装不合格模式，也未能充分关注这些污染事件之间的潜在相关性。2021 年 2 月至 2022 年 3 月期间，(b) (4) 灌装线 (b) (4) 和 (b) (4)（溶液和混悬液生产线）上发生多次中止和污染的培养基模拟灌装。例如，

● In September 2021, you isolated a gram-negative microbe, Ralstonia picketii, from multiple media fill (b) (4) of Batch # (b) (4) manufactured on the (b) (4) suspension line. You identified multiple deviations such as damaged filter housing, choked (b) (4), dislocation of the filter, and ineffective (b) (4) processes.

● 2021 年 9 月，从 (b) (4) 混悬液生产线生产的批次 #(b) (4) 的多项培养基模拟灌装 (b) (4) 中，你公司分离出了一种革兰阴性微生物，皮氏罗尔斯顿氏菌。你公司发现了多个偏差，例如过滤器机壳受损、堵塞 (b) (4)、过滤器错位，以及 (b) (4) 工艺无效。

● In November 2021, you isolated *Pseudomonas stutzeri* from one (b) (4) of media fill Batch # (b)(4) manufactured on the (b)(4) suspension line. This media fill (Batch # (b)(4)) was performed as part of the initial qualification of the suspension line and as a corrective action for a previously failed media fill on the same line (Batch # (b)(4)). You identified *Pseudomonas stutzeri* to be a gram-negative opportunistic pathogen. Your investigation, reviewed during the inspection and further described in your response, indicated this contamination was due to a puncture in the body of the (b)(4) by a (b)(4) during handling or movement of the filled samples, storage, or visual inspection, prior to incubation. However, you lacked adequate evidence that described mishandling of (b)(4). Further, your investigation also does not include comprehensive steps to prevent future mishandling of incubated units, and indicates use of (b)(4) will still be permitted. Your QU approved the investigation and the media fill run for Batch # (b)(4), and you used this media fill as one of three successful runs required to qualify filling line (b)(4) for suspension products.

● 2021 年 11 月，你公司从（b）(4) 混悬液生产线上生产的培养基模拟灌装批中分离出了施氏假单胞菌。该培养基模拟灌装 [批次 #（b）(4)] 是作为混悬液生产线初始确认的一部分进行的，也是对同一生产线之前不合格的培养基模拟灌装 [批次 #（b）(4)] 的纠正措施。你公司确定施氏假单胞菌是一种革兰阴性机会致病菌。你公司在检查期间接受审查的，并在回复中进一步描述的调查，表明这种污染是由于在处理、移动、储存或目检灌装样品期间，培养前（b）(4) 在（b）(4) 主体上被刺穿而导致的。然而，你公司缺乏充分的证据，来描述（b）(4) 的不当处理。此外，你公司的调查也不包括防止未来对已培养产品进行不当处理的全面措施，并表明仍可以使用（b）(4)。你公司的 QU 批准了批次 #（b）(4) 的调查和培养基模拟灌装批，并且使用此培养基模拟灌装作为混悬液产品灌装线（b）(4) 确认所需的三个成功批之一。

● In March 2022, you isolated Stenotrophomonas maltophilia in multiple media fill (b)(4) of Batch # (b)(4). You identified Stenotrophomonas maltophilia to be a drug-resistant gram-negative emerging global opportunistic pathogen with a known propensity for biofilm formation. You determined the root cause to be a leakage caused by a damaged valve gasket and deformed filter.

● 2022 年 3 月，你公司在批次 #（b）(4) 的多种培养基灌装（b）(4) 中分离出了嗜麦芽寡养单胞菌。你公司确定嗜麦芽寡养单胞菌是一种耐药革兰阴性新兴机会性病原体，具有已知的生物膜形成倾向。你公司确定根本原因是由损坏的阀门垫圈和变形的过滤器引起的泄漏。

You failed to appropriately investigate root causes and implement effective CAPAs to prevent recurrence of contamination events. For example, you failed to substantively evaluate the personnel and environmental monitoring (EM) data obtained during the production of these media fill batches, and to comprehensively assess additional historical data from the manufacturing area.

你公司未能适当调查根本原因，并实施有效的 CAPA 来防止污染事件再次发生。例如，你公司未能对这些培养基模拟灌装批次的生产过程中获得的人员和环境监测（EM）数据进行实质性评估，也未能全面评估来自生产区域的其他历史数据。

Your response is inadequate because there is no overall assessment of these atypical invalidations of media fills, explanation of the adverse pattern of gram-negative microbe findings in your aseptic processing operational environment, or major improvements to ensure more reliable aseptic operational design and equipment maintenance.

你公司的回复是不充分的，因为没有对这些非典型的培养基模拟灌装不合格进行全面评估，没有对无菌工艺操作环境中革兰阴性微生物发现的不良模式进行解释，也没有进行重大改进以确保更可靠的无菌操作设计和设备维护。

The presence of any highly pathogenic microorganism in your aseptic processing environment presents a heightened risk to patients who are, for example, immunocompromised, have cystic fibrosis, or have chronic obstructive airway disease. Presence of such microbes should receive urgent investigation and effective remediation. Further, it is critical to ensure appropriate equipment design and maintenance, as equipment failures may not be easily observable and contamination events during commercial manufacturing may go undetected for substantial periods of time.

无菌工艺操作环境中任何高致病性微生物的存在都会给免疫功能低下、囊性纤维化或慢性阻塞性气道疾病等患者带来更高的风险。此类微生物的存在应接受紧急调查和有效的整改。此外，确保适当的设备设计和维护至关重要，因为设备故障可能不容易被观察到，并且商业生产期间的污染事件可能在很长一段时间内未被发现。

It is essential to address potential contamination hazards in your manufacturing environment in a timely manner. Any adverse microbiological trends and potential routes of contamination should be identified promptly, allowing for implementation of appropriate follow-up measures to prevent contamination. It should also be noted that finished product testing alone cannot establish sterility of all units because contamination is typically episodic and not uniformly distributed.

及时解决生产环境中潜在的污染危害至关重要。应立即确定任何不利的微生物趋势和潜在的污染途径，以便采取适当的后续措施来防止污染。还应该指出的是，仅靠成品检验并不能确定所有单元的无菌性，因为污染通常是偶发的且分布不均匀。

■ Environmental Monitoring ｜环境监测

You failed to provide adequate justification for the discontinuation of filling (b)(4) surface monitoring on your（b）（4）lines. For example, prior to January 2020, your EM plan required collection of surface samples from（b）（4）filling（b）（4）at the（b）（4）of filling of（b）（4）batch. However, from January 2020 to August 2022, you did not collect surface samples from the（b）（4）filling（b）（4）at the（b）（4）of filling of（b）（4）batch.

你公司未能提供充分的论证，来停止在（b）（4）线上就灌装（b）（4）进行表面监测。例如，在 2020 年 1 月之前，你公司的 EM 计划要求从（b）（4）批次灌装（b）（4）的（b）（4）灌装中收集表面样品。然而，从 2020 年 1 月至 2022 年 8 月，你公司没有在（b）（4）批次灌装（b）（4）时采集（b）（4）灌装（b）（4）的表面样品。

You revised your EM plan in August 2022 to perform surface monitoring of（b）（4）filling（b）（4）, the（b）（4）, at the（b）（4）of filling of（b）（4）batch. You lack a justification for sufficiency of your sampling plan, including its failure to rotate sampling among each of the（b）（4）.

你公司于 2022 年 8 月修订了 EM 计划，对（b）（4）灌装（b）（4），以及（b）（4）灌装（b）（4）、（b）（4）进行表面监测。你公司缺乏充分的论证，来证明取样计划的充分性，包括未能在每个（b）（4）之间轮换取样。

In your response, you state you have adequate controls in place to assure sterility of products manufactured on your（b）（4）lines and there is no impact on the sterility of batches manufactured on these lines.

在回复中，你公司声称采取了充分的控制措施，来确保（b）（4）生产线生产的产品的无菌性，并且对这些生产线生产的批次的无菌性没有影响。

Your response is inadequate in that it lacks a scientifically sound EM plan.

你公司的回应是不充分的，因为它缺乏科学合理的 EM 计划。

Vigilant and responsive EM programs should be designed to provide meaningful information on the state of control of your aseptic processing environment and ancillary classified areas.

应设计具有警戒性且反应灵敏的 EM 程序，以提供有关无菌工艺操作环境和辅助洁净级别区域的控制状态的有意义的信息。

In response to this letter, provide the following：

在回复本函时，请提供以下信息：

● A comprehensive, independent third-party review of your media fill program.

● 对你公司的培养基模拟灌装计划进行全面、独立的第三方审查。

● An independent review of the source of recurring gram negatives isolated from your aseptic processing equipment train.

● 就从你公司的无菌工艺操作设备系列中分离出的反复出现的革兰阴性菌的来源，进行独立审查。

● Your CAPA plan to implement routine, operations management oversight of facilities and equipment. This plan should include, at a minimum:

● 你公司的 CAPA 计划，对设施和设备实施日常运营管理监督。该计划至少应包括：

○ Improved production management oversight that ensures prompt detection of equipment, facility, and process performance issues

○ 改进生产管理监督，确保及时发现设备、设施和工艺性能问题

○ Timely upgrades to equipment and facilities

○ 及时升级设备和设施

○ Adherence to appropriate preventive maintenance schedules

○ 遵守适当的预防性维护计划

○ Effective execution of repairs

○ 有效执行维修

○ Allocation of appropriate resources, staffing, and competencies

○ 分配适当的资源、人员和能力

○ Appropriately qualified production supervisors and managers

○ 具有适当资质的生产主管和经理

○ Improved systems for ongoing management review

○ 改进的持续管理评审系统

○ A provision(s) that appropriate actions are taken throughout the company network

○ 在整个公司网络中采取适当措施的规定

○ A thorough evaluation and risk assessment that addresses the suitability of your equipment for its intended use. Include an evaluation whether equipment is of appropriate design and your ongoing control and maintenance program is effective.

○ 彻底的评估和风险评估，以解决设备对其预期用途的适用性。包括评估设备的设计是否合适以及你公司的持续控制和维护计划是否有效。

● A retrospective evaluation by a qualified consult of the sufficiency of investigations and the failure modes related to the capability of your aseptic processing operation to robustly produce sterile drugs including, but not limited, to:

● 由有资质的顾问对与你公司的无菌工艺操作稳健生产无菌药品的能力相关的调查的充分性和失效模式进行回顾性评估，包括但不限于：

○ All media fill contamination events, invalidated media fills, and sterility positive test results for the past four years, regardless of whether the batch was shipped to the U.S.

○ 过去四年的所有培养基模拟灌装污染事件、不合格的培养基模拟灌装和无菌阳性检验结果，无论该批次是否运往美国。

○ Identification of all potential failure modes associated with these media fill and sterility positives.

○ 识别与这些培养基模拟灌装和无菌阳性相关的所有潜在失效模式。

○ A detailed evaluation and description of each aseptic connection and manipulation made starting with, and downstream of, the（b）（4）filter including but not limited to any manipulations at sampling ports in the product flow pathway prior to filling.

○ 对从（b）（4）过滤器开始及其下游进行的每个无菌连接和操作进行详细评估和描述，包括但不限于在灌装之前在产品流路中的取样口处进行的任何操作。

○ A comparison of your aseptic manufacturing process to the process simulation protocol to identify areas in which media fills may be improved to simulate actual operations more accurately.

○ 将无菌生产工艺与工艺模拟方案进行比较，以确定可以改进培养基模拟灌装的区域，从而更准确地模拟实际操作。

○ Detailed media fill criteria used by your firm, and adequacy of provisions to ensure thorough investigation of any contamination.

○ 你公司使用的详细培养基模拟灌装标准以及充分的规定，以确保对任何污染进行彻底调查。

○ All changes implemented to your aseptic operations in response to any aseptic process simulation incidents and sterility failures for the past four years, including an evaluation of their adequacy and sufficiency, and a risk assessment of any distributed product affected by deficient aseptic processing operations that occurred during this period.

○ 为应对过去四年中的任何无菌工艺模拟事件和无菌不合格而对无菌操作实施的所有变更，包括对其充分性的评估，以及就此期间受无菌工艺操作缺陷影响的任何流通产品，进行风险评估。

○ Your plan to ensure appropriate aseptic practices and cleanroom behavior during production. Include steps to ensure routine and effective supervisory oversight for all production batches. Also, describe the frequency of QU oversight(e.g., audit)during aseptic processing and its support operations.

○ 确保生产过程中采取适当的无菌操作和洁净室行为的计划。包括确保对所有生产批次进行常规和有效监督的步骤。另外，描述无菌工艺操作过程中 QU 监督（例如审核）的频率及其支持操作。

● A comprehensive risk assessment of all contamination hazards with respect to your aseptic processes, equipment, and facilities, including an independent assessment that includes, but is not limited to:

● 就你公司的无菌工艺、设备和设施的所有污染危害，进行全面的风险评估，包含独立评估，这包括但不限于：

○ All human interactions within the ISO 5 area

○ ISO 5 区域内的所有人员交互

○ Equipment placement and ergonomics

○ 设备放置和人体工程学

○ Air quality in the ISO 5 area and surrounding room

○ ISO 5 区域和周围房间的空气质量

○ Facility layout

○ 设施布局

○ Personnel Flows and Material Flows (throughout all rooms used to conduct and support sterile operations)

○ 人流和物流（用于执行和支持无菌操作的所有房间）

● A detailed remediation plan with timelines to address the findings of the contamination hazards risk assessment. Describe specific tangible improvements to be made to aseptic processing operation design and control.

● 详细的整改计划和时间表，以解决污染危害风险评估所发现的问题。描述要对无菌工艺操作设计和控制进行的具体切实改进。

● A comprehensive assessment and CAPA plan for your EM program to ensure it supports robust environmental control in your aseptic processing facility. Your assessment should include justification of sampling locations, frequency of sampling, alert and action limits, the adequacy of your sampling techniques, and trending program.

● 针对你公司的 EM 计划的全面评估和 CAPA 计划，以确保其支持无菌工艺操作设施中稳健的环境控制。你公司的评估应包括取样位置的合理性、取样频率、警戒和行动限、取样技术的充分性以及趋势分析计划。

质量部门

3. Your firm failed to establish adequate written responsibilities and procedures applicable to the quality control unit and to follow such written procedures (21 CFR 211.22 (d)).

3. 你公司未能建立适用于质量控制部门的充分的书面职责和程序，也未能遵循此类书面程序 [21 CFR 211.22 (d)]。

Your QU failed to provide adequate oversight for the retention of original cGMP records. For example, our investigator observed a truck loaded with bags of scrap from Unit (b) (4), as well as bags stored at a central scrapyard intended for shredding. The bags of scrap included, but were not limited to, numerous torn pieces of printer weigh slips pertaining to drug product packaging, and a microbiology laboratory sample label with Quality Assurance wet signatures.

你公司的 QU 未能对原始 cGMP 记录的保存提供充分的监督。例如，我们的调查员观察到一辆卡车装载着来自（b）（4）单元的废品袋，以及存放在中央废品堆放场供粉碎的袋子。这些废品袋包括但不限于大量与药品包装有关的打印的称重单碎片，以及带有质量保证手写签名的微生物实验室样品标签。

Your QU is responsible for the oversight of your drug manufacturing operations, including the review and approval of documents and other document controls, to ensure a complete contemporaneous record of each batch of drug product manufactured. These and all cGMP record are retained for cGMP purposes, such as ongoing control, quality oversight, and periodic reviews. In addition to the critical responsibilities of individual departments to assure integrity of documents, your QU is also responsible for assuring production areas are adequately monitored and employees demonstrate understanding and adherence to your firm's procedures and assigned tasks.

你公司的 QU 负责监督药品生产操作，包括文件的审查和批准以及其他文件控制，以确保生产的每批药品都有完整的同步记录。这些和所有 cGMP 记录均出于 cGMP 目的而保存，例如持续控制、质量监督和定期审查。除了各个部门确保文件可靠性的关键职责外，你公司的 QU 还负责确保生产区域得到充分监控，并确保员工理解并遵守公司的程序和分配的任务。

The uncontrolled destruction of cGMP records, and your lack of adequate documentation practices, raise questions about the effectiveness of your operations management and QU in assuring the integrity and accuracy of your cGMP records.

cGMP 记录的不受控制的破坏以及缺乏充分的文件记录实践，引发了关于你公司的运营管理和 QU 在确保 cGMP 记录的可靠性和准确性方面有效性的问题。

In your response, you indicate you have created new procedures for document disposal, revised existing procedures to provide clarity for retaining intact or torn weigh slips with the batch packaging records, and trained your employees on new and revised procedures.

在回复中，你公司表示你们已经创建了新的文件处理程序，修订了现有程序，以清晰地保存完整或破损的称重单与批次包装记录，并对你公司的员工进行了有关新程序和修订程序的培训。

Your response is inadequate. It is unclear if you assessed other documents found in the scrap yard. Additionally, your response does not assess how poor documentation practices affected distributed drug product.

你公司的回应不够充分。目前尚不清楚你公司是否评估了在废品场发现的其他文件。此外，你公司的回复并未评估不良记录实践如何影响已流通的药品。

Your firm's quality systems are inadequate. See FDA's guidance document, *Quality Systems Approach to Pharmaceutical cGMP Regulations* for help implementing quality systems and risk management approaches to meet requirements of CGMP regulations 21 CFR, parts 210 and 211 at https://www.fda.gov/media/71023/download.

你公司的质量体系不够完善。请参阅 FDA 指南，药品 cGMP 法规的质量系统方法，以帮助实施质量系统和风险管理方法，以满足 cGMP 法规 21 CFR 第 210 和 211 部分的要求：网址（略，见上）。

Your quality system also does not adequately ensure the accuracy and integrity of data to support the safety, effectiveness, and quality of the drugs you manufacture. We strongly recommend that you retain a qualified consultant to assist in your remediation. See FDA's guidance document Data Integrity and Compliance With Drug CGMP for guidance on establishing and following CGMP compliant data integrity practices at https://www.fda.gov/

media/97005/download.

你公司的质量体系无法充分确保数据的准确性和可靠性，以支持你们所生产的药品的安全性、有效性和质量。我们强烈建议你公司聘请有资质的顾问来协助你们进行整改。有关建立和遵循 cGMP 合规数据可靠性实践的指南，请参阅 FDA 指南，数据可靠性和药品 cGMP 合规性，网址（略，见上）。

In response to this letter, provide the following:

在回复本函时，请提供以下信息：

● An assessment of the extent of data integrity deficiencies at your facility. Identify omissions, alterations, deletions, record destruction, non-contemporaneous record completion, and other deficiencies. Describe all parts of your facility's operations in which you discovered data integrity lapses.

● 对你公司设施的数据可靠性缺陷程度进行评估。识别遗漏、更改、删除、记录销毁、非同步记录完成和其他缺陷。描述你公司发现数据可靠性缺陷所涉及的设施运营的所有部分。

● A management strategy for your firm that includes the details of your global corrective action and preventive action plan. The detailed corrective action plan should describe how you intend to ensure the reliability and completeness of all the data you generate including analytical data, manufacturing records, and all data submitted to FDA.

● 你公司的管理策略，包括整体纠正和预防措施计划的详细信息。详细的纠正措施计划应描述你公司打算如何确保生成的所有数据（包括分析数据、生产记录和提交给 FDA 的所有数据）的可靠性和完整性。

● A complete assessment of documentation systems used throughout your manufacturing and laboratory operations to determine where documentation practices are insufficient. Include a detailed CAPA plan that comprehensively remediates your firm's documentation practices to ensure you retain contemporaneous, attributable, legible, complete, original, accurate, contemporaneous records throughout your operation.

● 对整个生产和实验室操作中使用的文档系统进行完整评估，以确定记录实践的不足之处。包括一份详细的 CAPA 计划，全面整改你公司的文件记录实践，以确保在整个运营过程中保存可追溯的、清晰的、完整的、原始的、准确的和同步的记录。

● A current risk assessment of the potential effects of the observed failures on the quality of your drugs. Your assessment should include analyses of the risks to patients caused by the release of drugs affected by a lapse of data integrity and analyses of the risks posed by ongoing operations.

● 当前观察到的不合格对药品质量的潜在影响的风险评估。你公司的评估应包括分析因数据可靠性缺失影响的药品放行对患者造成的风险，以及对正在进行的操作带来的风险的分析。

Repeat Observations at Multiple Sites
在多个场所中重复出现的违规行为

FDA has cited similar cGMP observations at other facilities in your company's network. On February 25, 2020, a Warning Letter was issued to Cipla Limited, Goa FEI 3004081307, citing deficiencies related to inadequate equipment cleaning procedures, inadequate investigations of high efficiency particulate air (HEPA) filter integrity test failures, and inadequate smoke studies to evaluate whether unidirectional air flow exists in your aseptic operations. Furthermore, during our August 26, 2022, inspection at your Goa site, the inspection team identified deficiencies for equipment cleaning procedures and (b)(4) surface sampling during EM of the (b)(4) aseptic filling lines from January 2019 to August 2022. These repeated failures at multiple sites demonstrate that your management's oversight and control over the manufacture of drugs is inadequate.

FDA 在你公司网络的其他设施中引用了类似的 cGMP 观察项。2020 年 2 月 25 日，向 Cipla Limited, Goa（FEI 3004081307）发出警告信，指出存在以下相关缺陷：设备清洁程序不充分，对高效颗粒空气（HEPA）过滤器完整性检验不合格，调查不充分，以及不充分的烟雾实验（用来评估无菌操作中是否存在单向气流）。此外，在 2022 年 8 月 26 日对 Goa 进行检查期间，就 2019 年 1 月至 2022 年 8 月对（b）(4) 无菌灌装线 EM 期间，检查小组发现了表面取样和设备清洁程序方面的缺陷。这些在多个场所中重复出现的不合格表明，你公司的管理层对药品生产的监督和控制是不够的。

Your executive management remains responsible for fully resolving all deficiencies and ensuring ongoing cGMP compliance. Executive management should immediately and comprehensively assess your company's global manufacturing operations to ensure that your systems, processes, and products conform to FDA requirements.

你公司的高级管理层仍然负责完全解决所有缺陷并确保持续符合 cGMP。高级管理层应立即全面评估你公司的整体生产操作，以确保你公司的系统、工艺和产品符合 FDA 的要求。

Field Alert Reporting Violations | 现场警戒报告违规情况

The NDA/ANDA Field Alert reporting requirements in 21 CFR 314.81 (b)(1)(ii), effective since May 23, 1985, require holders of NDAs and ANDAs to submit information concerning any bacteriological contamination, or any significant chemical, physical, or other change or deterioration in the distributed drug product to the appropriate FDA district office within three working days of receipt by the applicant. The intent of the 21 CFR 314.81（b）（1） regulation is to establish an early warning system so that significant problems are brought to the FDA's attention by applicant holders in order to prevent potential safety hazards from drug products already in distribution and also to prevent potential safety hazards with drug products manufactured in the future. FARs must be submitted for confirmed and unconfirmed problems meeting the definition of the regulation within three working days of becoming aware of the problem.

根据自 1985 年 5 月 23 日生效的 21 CFR 314.81（b）（1）（ii）中的 NDA/ANDA 现场警戒报告要求，NDA 和 ANDA 持有人必须在收到有关任何细菌污染或流通的药品出现任何重大化学、物理或其他变化或恶化的信息后的三个工作日内，将信息提交给相应的 FDA 地区办事处。21 CFR 314.81（b）（1）规定的目的是建立一个早期警戒系统，以便申请人持有者及时引起 FDA 对重大问题的关注，防止已经流通的药品可能存在的安全隐患，同时也防止未来生产的药品可能存在的安全隐患。对于符合规定定义的已确认和未确认问题，必须在发现问题后的三个工作日内提交 FAR 报告。

From this inspection, in addition to the aforementioned cGMP violations, your firm is in violation of the Field Alert reporting requirements set forth in 21 CFR 314.81（b）（1）（ii）. FARs related to Albuterol Sulfate Inhalation Aerosol were not provided to FDA within three working days. Specifically, you received thousands of complaints related to the failure of Albuterol Sulfate Inhalation Aerosol to appropriately deliver medication. No FAR was submitted until after the close of this inspection.

根据这次检查，除了上述的 cGMP 违规情况外，你公司还违反了 21 CFR 314.81（b）（1）（ii）规定的现场警戒报告要求。与沙丁胺醇硫酸盐吸入气雾剂相关的 FAR 未在三个工作日内提供给 FDA。具体来说，你公司收到了数千起与硫酸沙丁胺醇吸入气雾剂未能正确递送药品相关的投诉。直到本次检查结束后才提交 FAR。

第六部分

其他成品制剂

1 质量部门未能履行职责

警告信编号： MARCS-CMS 636200

签发时间： 2023-1-23；**公示时间：** 2023-2-28

签发机构： 药品质量业务二处（Division of Pharmaceutical Quality Operations Ⅱ）

公　　司： Skyless，LLC

所在国家 / 地区： 波多黎各

主　　题： cGMP/ 成品制剂 / 掺假（cGMP/Finished Pharmaceuticals/ Adulterated）

简　　介： 2022 年 5 月，FDA 检查了位于波多黎各的药品生产设施。结果显示，该公司未能在放行前对每批药品进行相应的实验室测定，以确保符合药品的最终质量标准。同时，该公司也未能在相应的时间间隔内验证和确定其物料供应商检验分析的可靠性。基于这些发现，FDA 认为质量部门未能履行职责，未能确保所生产的药品符合 cGMP 要求，因此该公司的质量体系存在不足。例如，该公司未能为质量部门的角色和职责制定并编写相应的程序，使其有责任和权力审查、批准影响产品质量的相关职能。

本警告信以下部分与本书此前其他警告信内容类似，故略去：前言、未经批准的新药和标识错误违规情况（Unapproved New Drug and Misbranding Violations）、cGMP 顾 问 推 荐（cGMP Consultant Recommended）、结论（Conclusion）。

产品检验

1. Your firm failed to have, for each batch of drug product, appropriate laboratory determination of satisfactory conformance to final specifications for the drug product, including the

identity and strength of each active ingredient, prior to release（21 CFR 211.165（a））.

1. 你公司未能在放行前对每批药品进行适当的实验室测定，以确保其符合药品的最终质量标准，包括每种原料药的鉴别和规格［21 CFR 211.165（a）］。

You failed to perform analytical and microbiological release testing for each batch of your over-the-counter（OTC）topical drug products prior to distribution, including Xpasmo Manteca de Ubre（Cow's Udder grease）and Xpasmo Arthritis Formula.

你公司未能在流通前对每批非处方（OTC）外用药品进行分析和微生物放行检验，包括 Xpasmo Manteca de Ubre（牛乳房油脂）和 Xpasmo 关节炎处方。

Drug product batches must be tested for identity, strength, quality, and purity prior to release. Testing is an essential part of ensuring that the drug products you manufacture conform to all predetermined quality attributes and are appropriate for their intended use. Without adequate testing, you lack basic data to support that each drug product batch conforms to appropriate specifications before release.

药品批次在放行前，必须进行鉴别、规格、质量和纯度检验。对于确保所生产的药品符合所有预定质量属性并适合其预期用途，检验是重要的组成部分。如果没有充分的检验，就缺乏基本数据，来支持每个药品批次在放行前符合相应的质量标准。

Your response is inadequate because your firm did not provide a procedure describing how your firm will ensure your finished products meet the appropriate quality standards prior to release.

你公司的回复不充分，因为没有提供描述你公司如何确保成品在放行前符合相应的质量标准的程序。

In response to this letter, provide：

在回复本函时，请提供：

● A comprehensive, independent assessment of your laboratory practices, procedures, methods, equipment, documentation, and analyst competencies. Based on this review, provide a detailed plan to remediate and evaluate the effectiveness of your laboratory system.

● 对你公司的实验室实践、程序、方法、设备、文件和分析人员能力进行全面、独立的评估。在此审查的基础上，提供一个详细的计划来整改和评估你公司实验室系统的有效性。

● A list of chemical and microbial specifications, including test methods, used to analyze each lot of your drug product before making a batch disposition decision, and the associated written procedures.

● 化学和微生物质量标准清单，包括检验方法，用于在做出批次处置决定之前分析每批药品，以及相关的书面程序。

物料检验

2. Your firm failed to conduct at least one test to verify the identity of each component of a drug product. Your firm also failed to validate and establish the reliability of your component supplier's test analyses at appropriate intervals（21 CFR 211.84（d）（1）and 211.84（d）（2））.

2. 你公司未进行至少一项检验来确认药品中每种原辅料都被鉴别。你公司也未能在适当的时间间隔内，验证和确定你公司物料供应商的检验分析的可靠性［21 CFR 211.84（d）（1）和（2）］。

You failed to test all your incoming raw materials including active pharmaceutical ingredients（API）and other components. You relied on your supplier's certificate of analysis（COA）in lieu of testing each component lot for purity, strength, identity, and quality. You also did not establish a supplier qualification program to assess（i.e., initially and periodically）the reliability of your suppliers' test results for these attributes.

你公司未能检验所有进场原料，包括原料药（API）和其他原辅料。你公司依靠供应商的分析证书（COA）来代替检验每个原辅料批次的纯度、规格、鉴别和质量。此外，你公司也没有建立供应商确认计划（即初始和定期确认），来评估供应商这些属性检验结果的可靠性。

Your response is inadequate. You intend to establish necessary procedures to evaluate all raw materials to determine if they are acceptable for further manufacturing. However, you did not provide any procedures or testing methods for review. In addition, you did not provide a plan for your supplier qualification program. Furthermore, you did not commit to testing reserve samples of your raw materials to verify the identity of components used in your distributed OTC drug products.

你公司的回应不充分。你公司打算建立必要的程序来评估所有原料，以确定它们是否适合进一步生产。然而，却没有提供任何程序或检验方法供审查。此外，你公司没有提供供应商确认程序的计划。此外，你公司没有承诺检验原料的留样，来确认你公司流通的非处方药产品中使用的原辅料的鉴别。

In response to this letter, provide:

在回复本函时，请提供：

● A comprehensive, independent review of your material system to determine whether all suppliers of components, containers, and closures, are each qualified and the materials are assigned appropriate expiration or retest dates. The review should also determine whether incoming material controls are adequate to prevent use of unsuitable components, containers, and closures.

● 对你公司的物料系统进行全面、独立的审查，以确定所有物料、容器和密封件的供应商是否均有资质，并为物料指定了适当的有效期或复验期。审查还应确定进场物料控制是否足以防止使用不适当的物料、容器和密封件。

● The chemical and microbiological quality control specifications you use to test and release each incoming lot of components for use in manufacturing.

● 针对每批用于生产目的的进场物料，用于检验和放行的化学和微生物质控标准。

● A description of how you will test each component lot for conformity with all appropriate specifications for identity, strength, quality, and purity. If you intend to accept any results from your supplier's COA instead of testing each component lot for strength, quality, and purity, specify how you will robustly establish the reliability of your supplier's results through initial validation as well as periodic re-validation. In addition, include a commitment to always conduct at least one specific identity test for each incoming component lot.

● 说明如何检验每个批次，确定其是否符合有关鉴别、规格、质量和纯度的质量标准。如果你公司打算接受供应商的COA结果，而不是检验每个物料批次的规格、质量和纯度，请说明如何进行初始验证和定期再验证，从而稳健地确保供应商结果的可靠性。此外，还应承诺：对于每个进场原辅料批次，至少进行一个专属鉴别检验。

● A summary of results obtained from testing all components to evaluate the reliability of the COA from each component manufacturer. Include your SOP that describes this COA validation program.

● 一份所有物料检验的结果汇总，以评估每个物料生产商的COA的可靠性。包括描述此COA验证计划的程序。

质量部门

3. Your firm's quality control unit failed to exercise its responsibility to ensure drug products manufactured are in compliance with cGMP, and meet established specifications for identity, strength, quality, and purity(21 CFR 211.22)

3. 你公司的质量控制部门未能履行职责，以确保所生产的药品符合cGMP要求，并符合有关鉴别、规格、质量和纯度的既定质量标准（21 CFR 211.22）。

Your firm failed to establish an adequate Quality Unit（QU）to ensure that：

你公司未能建立合格的质量部门（QU），来确保：

● Adequate procedures were established and written for roles and responsibilities of the QU to have the responsibility and authority to review and approve quality related functions that impact product quality（21 CFR 211.22（d））.

● 为 QU 的角色和职责制定并编写了适当的程序，使其有责任和权力审查、批准影响产品质量的相关职能［21 CFR 211.22（d）］。

● An ongoing written program for monitoring process control was established to ensure stable manufacturing operations and consistent drug quality（21 CFR 211.100（a））.

● 制定持续的工艺控制监测书面计划，以确保稳定的生产操作和一致的药品质量［21 CFR 211.100（a）］。

● Cleaning processes were written, validated, reviewed, and approved for cleaning nondedicated manufacturing equipment to ensure that residues are adequately removed from the product contact surfaces of manufacturing equipment during cleaning（21 CFR 211.67（b））.

● 已编写、验证、审查和批准用于清洁非专用生产设备的清洁工艺，以确保在清洁过程中充分清除生产设备的产品接触表面上的残留物［21 CFR 211.67（b）］。

● Equipment maintenance procedures were established, written, reviewed, and approved for your drug manufacturing equipment to ensure robust equipment operations（21 CFR 211.67（b））.

● 为你公司的药品生产设备制定、编写、审查和批准设备维护程序，以确保设备稳健运行［21 CFR 211.67（b）］。

Your response is inadequate. You intend to establish and implement procedures to comply with cGMPs. However, you did not provide detailed corrective action and preventive actions（CAPA）plan to systematically address the deficiency.

你公司的回应不充分。你公司本打算建立并实施符合 cGMP 的程序。但是，没有提供详细的纠正和预防措施（CAPA）计划来系统地解决缺陷。

Your firm's quality systems are inadequate. See FDA's guidance document *Quality Systems Approach to Pharmaceutical cGMP Regulations* for help implementing quality systems and risk management approaches to meet the requirements of cGMP regulations 21

CFR, parts 210 and 211 at https://www.fda.gov/media/71023/download.

你公司的质量体系不够完善。请参阅 FDA 指南，药品 cGMP 法规的质量系统方法，以帮助实施质量系统和风险管理方法，以满足 cGMP 法规 21 CFR 第 210 和 211 部分的要求：网址（略，见上）。

In response to this letter, provide the following:

在回复本函时，请提供以下信息：

（略）

此处与 FDA 发给 Cosmobeauti Laboratories & Manufacturing Inc. 的警告信（编号：MARCS-CMS 657682，即 "12 批生产记录存在倒记问题"）中有关 QU 的回应要求部分的内容类似，故略去。

● A detailed summary of your validation program for ensuring a state of control throughout the product lifecycle, along with associated procedures. Describe your program for process performance qualification, and ongoing monitoring of both intra-batch and inter-batch variation to ensure a continuing state of control.

● 用于确保整个产品生命周期控制状态的验证计划的详细摘要以及相关程序。描述你公司的工艺性能确认计划，以及对批次内和批次间变化的持续监控，以确保持续的控制状态。

● A timeline for performing appropriate process performance qualification (PPQ) for each of your marketed drug products.

● 为每种上市药品执行适当的工艺性能确认（PPQ）的时间表。

● An assessment of each drug product process to ensure that there is a data-driven and scientifically sound program that identifies and controls all sources of variability, such that your production processes will consistently meet appropriate specifications and manufacturing standards. This includes, but is not limited to, evaluating suitability of equipment for its intended use, sufficiency of detectability in your monitoring and testing systems, quality of input materials, and reliability of each manufacturing process step and control.

● 每个药品工艺的评估，以确保有一个以数据为依据的、科学合理的程序，该程序可以识别和控制所有波动来源，并始终符合相应的质量标准和生产标准。这包括但不限于评估设备的预期用途适用性，监测和检验系统中检测能力是否充分，输入物料的质量，以及每个生产工艺步骤和控制的可靠性。

○ See FDA's guidance document *Process Validation: General Principles and Practices* for general principles and approaches that FDA considers appropriate elements of process validation at https://www.fda.gov/regulatory–information/search–fda–guidancedocuments/process–validation–general–principles–and–practices.

○ 有关 FDA 认为适当的工艺验证要素的一般原则和方法，请参阅 FDA 指南，工艺验证：一般原则和实践，网址（略，见上）。

● Appropriate improvements to your cleaning validation program, with special emphasis on incorporating conditions identified as worst case in your drug manufacturing operation. This should include but not be limited to identification and evaluation of all worst–case：

● 适当改进你公司的清洁验证计划，特别强调将确定为药品生产操作中最差情况的条件纳入其中。这应包括但不限于识别和评估所有最差情况：

○ drugs with higher toxicities

○ 具有较高毒性的药物

○ drugs with higher drug potencies

○ 具有较高药物活性的药物

○ drugs of lower solubility in their cleaning solvents

○ 在清洁溶剂中溶解度较低的药物

○ drugs with characteristics that make them difficult tclean

○ 具有难以清洁特性的药物

○ swabbing locations for areas that are most difficult tclean

○ 最难清洁区域的擦拭位置

○ maximum hold times before cleaning

○ 清洁前的最长存放时间

In addition，describe the steps that must be taken in your change management system before introduction of new manufacturing equipment or a new product.

此外，描述在引入新生产设备或新产品之前，在变更管理系统中必须采取的步骤。

● A summary of updated SOPs that ensure an appropriate program is in place for verification and validation of cleaning procedures for products，processes，and equipment.

● 更新的标准操作程序的汇总，确保制定适当的计划来确认和验证产品、工艺和设备的清洁程序。

● Your CAPA plan to implement routine, vigilant operations management oversight of facilities and equipment. This plan should ensure, among other things, prompt detection of equipment/facilities performance issues, effective execution of repairs, adherence to appropriate preventive maintenance schedules, timely technological upgrades to the equipment/facility infrastructure, and improved systems for ongoing management review.

● 你公司的 CAPA 计划，对设施和设备实施日常、警戒性的运营管理监督。至少，该计划应确保及时发现设备 / 设施性能问题，有效执行维修，遵守适当的预防性维护计划，及时对设备 / 设施进行技术升级，并对持续管理评审的系统进行改进。

2 OOS 调查不充分

警告信编号： MARCS-CMS 647232

签发时间： 2023-4-6；**公示时间：** 2023-4-18

签发机构： 药物审评与研究中心 | CDER（Center for Drug Evaluation and Research | CDER）

公　　司： Zermat International S.A. de C.V.

所在国家 / 地区： 美国

主　　题： cGMP/ 成品制剂 / 掺假（cGMP/Finished Pharmaceuticals/ Adulterated）

简　　介： 2022 年 10 月，FDA 对位于美国本土的药品生产设施进行了检查。检查中发现，该公司没有充分调查不合格（OOS）结果。举例来说，在出现了 OOS 黏度结果的情况下，该公司未经调查就放行并流通了一批非处方药品。FDA 的审查还指出，某个批次的比重也出现了 OOS，但该公司未能进行进一步的调查。公司辩称，药品的质量标准不正确，导致结果与错误的可接受标准进行了比较。而 FDA 强调指出，公司没有提供全面的回顾性审查资料，无法确保已经完全识别并彻底调查了所有 OOS 结果和差异。FDA 建议，如需了解更多处理 OOS、超常或其他非预期结果的相关信息，可以参阅 FDA 指南，调查药品生产的不合格（OOS）检验结果。

本警告信以下部分与本书此前其他警告信内容类似，故略去：前言、结论（Conclusion）。

偏差调查

1. Your firm failed to thoroughly investigate any unexplained discrepancy or failure of a batch or any of its components to meet any of its specifications，whether or not the batch has

already been distributed（21 CFR 211.192）.

1. 无论批次是否已经流通，对于该批次或其原辅料不满足质量标准、存在无法解释的偏差或不合格，你公司未能进行彻底调查（21 CFR 211.192）。

Your firm did not adequately investigate out-of-specification（OOS）results. Specifically, you released and distributed batches of over-the-counter（OTC）（b）（4）drug product lots#（b）（4）and（b）（4）with OOS results for viscosity without an investigation. Our review also noted that lot#（b）（4）was OOS for specific gravity and no further investigation occurred.

你公司没有充分调查不合格（OOS）结果。具体来说，在出现 OOS 黏度结果且未经调查的情况下，你公司放行并分销了一批非处方药（OTC）（b）（4）药品，批号#（b）（4）和（b）（4）。我们的审查还注意到，批号（b）（4）的比重为 OOS，却未能进行进一步调查。

In your response, you acknowledge that you do not have a procedure to handle OOS results. You state that the specification of the drug product was incorrect, and the results were compared against the wrong acceptance criteria. However, the certificates of analysis of these lots included a note stating that the product was approved with high viscosity. You also acknowledge a low specific gravity result for lot#（b）（4）.

在回复中，你公司承认你们没有处理 OOS 结果的程序。你公司声称药品的质量标准不正确，导致根据错误的合格标准来对各项结果进行比较。然而，这些批次的分析证书包含一条注释，表明该产品的高黏度得到批准。你公司还确认批次#（b）（4）的比重较低。

Your response is inadequate. You do not provide a retrospective review to ensure that you have fully identified and thoroughly investigated all OOS results and discrepancies. In addition, you do not provide your OOS procedure or an implementation date. You also do not include supporting evidence and a scientific rationale for the modified specification included in your response.

你公司的回应不充分。没有提供回顾性审查，来确保你公司已完全识别并彻底调查所有 OOS 结果和偏差。此外，你公司没有提供 OOS 程序或实施日期。也没有在回复中提供支持证据以及修订后的质量标准的科学论证。

For more information about handling failing, out-of-specification, out-of-trend, or other unexpected results and documentation of your investigations, see FDA's guidance document Investigating Out-of-Specification（OOS）Test Results for Pharmaceutical Production at https://www.fda.gov/media/158416/download.

有关处理不合格、OOS、超常或其他非预期结果以及调查记录的更多信息，请参阅 FDA 指南，调查药品生产的不合格（OOS）检验结果，网址（略，见上）。

In response to this letter, provide the following：

在回复本函时，请提供以下信息：

（略）

此处与 FDA 发给 Dunagin Pharmaceuticals Inc. dba Massco Dental 的警告信（编号：MARCS–CMS 644335，即"3 与非药用产品的共线生产问题"）中的 OOS 调查要求类似，故略去。

稳定性研究

2. Your firm failed to establish and follow an adequate written testing program designed to assess the stability characteristics of drug products and to use results of stability testing to determine appropriate storage conditions and expiration dates（21 CFR 211.166（a））.

2. 你公司未能遵循适当的书面检验程序，以评估药品的稳定性特征；未能使用稳定性检验结果，来确定适当的储存条件和有效期［21 CFR 211.166（a）］。

You did not have stability data that adequately demonstrates your drug products met established chemical and microbial specifications throughout their assigned shelf life.

你公司没有充分的稳定性数据，来证明药品在指定的有效期内符合既定的化学和微生物质量标准。

For example, your stability procedure requires an organoleptic assessment（odor, color, appearance）of your OTC drug products only at four–weeks. Although, your procedure references long–term stability at ambient temperature, your firm did not provide evidence of long–term stability. In addition, the temperature storage condition is not monitored throughout the study and there are no protocols for humidity.

例如，你公司的稳定性程序要求仅在四周内对 OTC 药品进行感官评估（气味、颜色、外观）。尽管你公司的程序提到了环境温度下的长期稳定性，但没有提供长期稳定性的证据。此外，在整个研究过程中没有监测温度储存条件，也没有湿度方案。

In your response, you state that you will test existing lots of drug product to confirm the expiration date. You commit to identifying a third party for the storage of stability samples. Additionally, you claim to have created a testing program to assess the stability characteristics of drug products.

在回复中，你公司声称将检验现有批次的药品以确认有效期。并承诺指定第三方来存储稳定性样品。此外，你公司还声称已经创建了一个检验程序，来评估药品的稳定性特征。

Your response is inadequate. You have not provided your stability protocols, any updates regarding the new testing results, and interim actions with specified implementation dates.

你公司的回应不够充分。尚未提供：稳定性方案，有关新检验结果的任何更新，以及指定实施日期的临时行动。

In response to this letter, provide the following:

在回复本函时，请提供以下信息：

（略）

此处与 FDA 发给 Cosmobeauti Laboratories & Manufacturing Inc. 的警告信（编号：MARCS-CMS 657682，即"12 批生产记录存在倒记问题"）中有关稳定性研究的回应要求部分的内容类似，故略去。

工艺验证

3. Your firm failed to establish adequate written procedures for production and process control designed to assure that the drug products you manufacture have the identity, strength, quality, and purity they purport or are represented to possess(21 CFR 211.100(a)).

3. 你公司未能建立充分的书面生产和过程控制程序，来确保生产的药品具有其声称或陈述的鉴别、规格、质量和纯度［21 CFR 211.100(a)］。

You failed to adequately validate your manufacturing processes for(b)(4)produced in the(b)(4)filling line. You are responsible for assuring your manufacturing processes will consistently result in drug products meeting predefined quality attributes.

你公司未能充分验证（b）(4）灌装线生产的（b）(4）的生产工艺。你公司有责任确保生产工艺始终能够生产出符合预定质量属性的药品。

In your response, you include process qualification protocols for your OTC drug products.

在你公司的回复中，应包含 OTC 药品的工艺确认方案。

Your response is inadequate. You have not demonstrated that your manufacturing process is designed, controlled and reproducible to yield a product of uniform character and quality.

Failure to perform adequate process validation can result in product quality attribute failure. In addition, your response does not include timeframes and interim actions.

你公司的回应不够充分。没有证明你们的生产工艺是经过设计的、可控制和可重现的，并能够生产出具有统一特性和质量的产品。未能进行充分的工艺验证可能会导致产品质量属性不合格。此外，你公司的回复不包括时间表和临时行动。

Your firm lacks an ongoing program for monitoring process control to ensure stable manufacturing operations and consistent drug quality.

你公司缺乏用于监控过程控制的持续计划，以确保稳定的生产操作和一致的药品质量。

（略）

<u>此处与 FDA 发给 Profounda, Inc. 的警告信（编号：MARCS-CMS 642595，即"2 未能提供生产工艺的验证数据"）中有关工艺验证的重要性部分的内容类似，故略去。</u>

In response to this letter, provide the following：

在回复本函时，请提供以下信息：

● A detailed summary of your validation program for ensuring a state of control throughout the product lifecycle, along with associated procedures. Describe your program for process performance qualification, and ongoing monitoring of both intra-batch and inter-batch variation to ensure a continuing state of control.

● 有关确保整个产品生命周期中控制状态的验证项目的详细汇总，以及相关程序。描述你公司的程序，以进行工艺性能确认，并持续监控批内和批间变化，以确保持续的控制状态。此外，还需包括你公司的设备和设施确认计划。

● A timeline for performing appropriate process performance qualification（PPQ）for each of your marketed drug products.

● 为每种上市药品执行适当的工艺性能确认（PPQ）的时间表。

● Include your updated process performance protocol（s）, and written procedures for qualification of equipment and facilities.

● 包括更新的工艺性能方案以及设备和设施确认的书面程序。

● Provide a detailed program for designing, validating, maintaining, controlling and monitoring each of your manufacturing processes that includes vigilant monitoring of intra-batch and inter-batch variation to ensure an ongoing state of control. Also, include your program for qualification of your equipment and facility.

● 提供用于设计、验证、维护、控制和监测每个生产工艺的详细计划，包括对批内和批间变化进行警戒性的监测，以确保持续的控制状态。另外，需包括设备和设施确认计划。

质量部门

4. Your firm's quality control unit failed to exercise its responsibility to ensure drug products manufactured are in compliance with cGMP, and meet established specifications for identity, strength, quality, and purity (21 CFR 211.22).

4. 你公司的质量控制部门未能履行职责，以确保所生产的药品符合 cGMP 要求，并符合有关鉴别、规格、质量和纯度的既定质量标准（21 CFR 211.22）。

Your quality unit (QU) did not provide adequate oversight for the manufacture of your OTC drug products. For example, your QU failed to ensure an adequate written procedure for annual product review and an adequate written procedure for complaint handling. In addition, discrepancies related to OOS values were noted during the inspection but not identified by your quality unit at the time of release.

你公司的质量部门（QU）没有对 OTC 药品的生产提供充分的监督。例如，你公司的 QU 未能确保制定适当的年度产品回顾书面程序和适当的投诉处理书面程序。此外，在检查过程中注意到了与 OOS 值相关的偏差，但在放行时你公司的质量部门未能识别出。

In your response, you state that a written procedure has been established for annual product review. You also commit to updating the complaint procedure to include your QU's involvement, root cause analysis, and corrective actions and preventive actions.

在回复中，你公司声称已制定了年度产品回顾的书面程序。还承诺更新投诉程序，包括你公司 QU 的参与、根本原因分析以及纠正和预防措施。

Your response is inadequate. You do not provide evidence of the procedures and timeframes of implementation. You also do not indicate how your QU will provide oversight of your operations to ensure that errors are identified prior to the release of batches.

你公司的回应不够充分。没有提供实施程序和时间表的证据。也没有说明你公司的 QU 将如何监督你们的操作，以确保在批放行之前发现错误。

Significant findings in this letter demonstrate that your firm does not operate an effective quality system in accordance with cGMP. In addition to the lack of effective production operations oversight to ensure reliable facilities and equipment, we found your quality unit is not enabled to exercise proper authority and/or has insufficiently implemented its responsibilities. You should immediately and comprehensively assess your company's global manufacturing operations to ensure that systems, processes, and the products manufactured conform to FDA requirements.

本函中的重要调查结果表明，你公司没有按照 cGMP 运行有效的质量体系。除了缺乏有效的生产操作监督，来确保设施和设备可靠之外，我们还发现你公司的质量部门无法行使适当的权力和（或）没有充分履行其职责。你公司应立即全面评估你们的整体生产操作，以确保系统、工艺和所生产的产品符合 FDA 的要求。

■ Quality Systems ｜质量体系

Your firm's quality systems are inadequate. See FDA's guidance document *Quality Systems Approach to Pharmaceutical cGMP Regulations* for help implementing quality systems and risk management approaches to meet the requirements of cGMP regulations 21 CFR, parts 210 and 211 at https://www.fda.gov/media/71023/download.

你公司的质量体系不够完善。请参阅 FDA 指南，药品 cGMP 法规的质量系统方法，以帮助实施质量系统和风险管理方法，以满足 cGMP 法规 21 CFR 第 210 和 211 部分的要求：网址（略，见上）。

In response to this letter, provide the following:

在回复本函时，请提供以下信息：

（略）

此处与 FDA 发给 Cosmobeauti Laboratories & Manufacturing Inc. 的警告信（编号：MARCS-CMS 657682，即 "12 批生产记录存在倒记问题"）中有关 QU 的回应要求部分的内容类似，故略去。

Our review also found you manufacture OTC drug products with the active ingredient（b）（4）without determining the levels of "arsenic" and a "limit of（b）（4）", as required by the United States Pharmacopeia（USP）.

我们的审查还发现，你公司生产的含有原料药（b）（4）的非处方药品，未按照 USP 的要求确定"砷"含量和"（b）（4）限量"。

In response to this letter, provide a copy of the certificate of analysis for all（b）（4）lots received by your firm during the last 3 years and your firm's procedure for testing incoming raw materials.

作为对本函的回复，请提供你公司在过去 3 年中收到的所有（b）（4）批货物的分析证书副本，以及你公司检验进场原料的程序。

FDA cited similar cGMP violations at your site in a previous inspection that covered another type of OTC drug product. At that time, your firm discontinued the distribution and manufacturing of that drug product. However, the current inspection found repeated violations related to process validation and stability. These repeated failures demonstrate that management oversight and control over the manufacture of drug products are inadequate.

FDA 在之前的一次检查中指出，你公司的设施存在类似的 cGMP 违规情况，该检查涵盖了另一种类型的 OTC 药品。当时，你公司停止了该药品的流通和生产。然而，目前的检查发现，工艺验证和稳定性方面依旧屡屡违规。这些重复的不合格表明你公司对药品生产的管理监督和控制不充分。

cGMP Consultant Recommended | cGMP 顾问推荐

Because you failed to correct repeat violations, we strongly recommend engaging a consultant qualified as set forth in 21 CFR 211.34 to assist your firm in meeting cGMP requirements. Your use of a consultant does not relieve your firm's obligation to comply with cGMP. Your firm's executive management remains responsible for resolving all deficiencies and systemic flaws to ensure ongoing cGMP compliance.

由于你公司未能纠正重复违规情况，我们强烈建议你公司聘请符合 21 CFR 211.34 规定的有资质的顾问，来协助你公司满足 cGMP 要求。使用顾问并不能免除你公司遵守 cGMP 的义务。你公司的高级管理层仍然负责解决所有缺陷和系统性问题，以确保持续符合 cGMP。

Your quality system does not adequately ensure the accuracy and integrity of data to support the safety, effectiveness, and quality of the drugs you manufacture. See FDA's guidance document *Data Integrity and Compliance With Drug cGMP* for guidance on establishing and following cGMP compliant data integrity practices at https://www.fda.gov/media/119267/download.

你公司的质量体系也无法充分确保数据的准确性和可靠性，以支持你们所生产的药品的安全性、有效性和质量。有关建立和遵循 cGMP 合规数据可靠性实践的指南，请参阅 FDA 指南，数据可靠性和药品 cGMP 合规性，网址（略，见上）。

We strongly recommend that you retain a qualified consultant to assist in your remediation. In response to this letter, provide:

我们强烈建议你公司聘请有资质的顾问来协助你们进行整改。在回复本函时，请提供：

A. A comprehensive investigation into the extent of the inaccuracies in data records and reporting including results of the data review for drugs distributed to the United States. Include a detailed description of the scope and root causes of your data integrity lapses.

A. 对数据记录和报告的不准确程度进行全面调查，包括对销往美国的药品的数据审查结果。包括数据可靠性缺陷的范围和根本原因的详细描述。

B. A current risk assessment of the potential effects of the observed failures on the quality of your drugs. Your assessment should include analyses of the risks to patients caused by the release of drugs affected by a lapse of data integrity and analyses of the risks posed by ongoing operations.

B. 对观察到的不合格对药品质量的潜在影响进行风险评估。你公司的评估应包括分析因数据可靠性失效影响的药品放行对患者造成的风险，以及对正在进行的操作带来的风险的分析。

C. A management strategy for your firm that includes the details of your global corrective action and preventive action plan. The detailed corrective action plan should describe how you intend to ensure the reliability and completeness of all data generated by your firm including microbiological and analytical data, manufacturing records, and all data submitted to FDA.

C. 你公司的管理策略，包括整体纠正行动和预防行动计划的详细信息。详细的纠正措施计划应描述你公司打算如何确保所生成的所有数据的可靠性和完整性，包括微生物和分析数据、生产记录以及提交给 FDA 的所有数据。

3 清洁验证未考虑转运容器

警告信编号： MARCS-CMS 648883

签发时间： 2023-4-13；**公示时间：** 2023-4-25

签发机构： 药物审评与研究中心 | CDER（Center for Drug Evaluation and Research | CDER）

公　　司： Pharmaplast S.A.E.

所在国家 / 地区： 埃及

主　　题： cGMP/ 成品制剂 / 掺假（cGMP/Finished Pharmaceuticals/ Adulterated）

简　　介： 2022 年 11 月，FDA 检查了位于埃及的药品生产设施。FDA 指出，该公司未对每个物料批次进行充分的鉴别检验，其中包括药品中的原料药乙醇。此外，原料药乙醇未检验甲醇含量，也未能确保检测甘油中是否存在二甘醇或乙二醇。这些污染物已经在全球范围内导致了多起人类致命中毒事件。此外，该公司还未将用于生产药品和器械产品的所有产品接触设备纳入清洁验证方案和程序中。其清洁验证方案和程序没有包括用于生产过程中移动药品和物料的转运容器，这增加了交叉污染的风险。

本警告信以下部分与本书此前其他警告信内容类似，故略去：前言、结论（Conclusion）。

物料检验

1. Your firm failed to test samples of each component for identity and conformity with all appropriate written specifications for purity，strength，and quality. Your firm also failed to validate and establish the reliability of your component supplier's test analyses at appropriate intervals（21 CFR 211.84（d）（1）and（2））.

1. 你公司未进行至少一项检验来确认药品中每种原辅料都被鉴别，并使其符合所有适当的纯度、规格和质量的书面标准。你公司也未能在适当的时间间隔内，验证和确定你们的物料供应商的检验分析的可靠性 [21 CFR 211.84（d）（1）和（2）]。

You failed to perform adequate identity testing for each component lot used in the production of your（b）（4）drug products，including ethanol，your active pharmaceutical ingredient（API）. Additionally，your API，ethanol，is not tested for methanol content，and your procedures did not ensure that you test glycerin for presence of diethylene glycol（DEG）or ethylene glycol（EG）. For example，you failed to test your incoming components for identity prior to manufacturing（b）（4）Gel，batch（b）（4）.

你公司未能对（b）（4）药品生产中使用的每个原辅料批次进行充分的鉴别检验，包括乙醇，即药品中的原料药（API）。此外，你公司的 API（乙醇）未检验甲醇含量，并且你们的程序无法确保甘油中是否存在二甘醇（DEG）或乙二醇（EG）。例如，在生产（b）（4）凝胶，批次（b）（4）之前，你公司未能进行进场原辅料的鉴别。

Component testing is fundamental to quality. Without adequate testing，you do not have scientific evidence that your incoming components conform to appropriate specifications before use in the manufacture of drug products.

物料检验是质量的基础。如果没有充分的检验，就没有科学证据证明你公司的进场原辅料在用于药品生产之前符合相应的质量标准。

In your response，you provide a corrective action and preventive action（CAPA）that states samples of your raw materials in your warehouse will be tested for conformance to the supplier's certificate of analysis（COA）. You also state that glycerin will be tested for DEG and EG.

在回复中，你公司提供了纠正和预防措施（CAPA），其中声明将对你公司仓库中的原料样品进行检验，以确保其符合供应商的分析证书（COA）。你公司还指出将对甘油进行 DEG 和 EG 检测。

Your response is inadequate because it fails to include a detailed plan for how raw materials will be tested such as test method and review of compendial requirements. Your proposed action plan does not include a strategy to implement corrective actions. Also，you do not provide a detailed plan to ensure that previously distributed drug products were manufactured with incoming components that meet the identity and impurity testing requirements.

你公司的回复不充分，因为它没有包括如何检验原料的详细计划，例如检验方法和药典要求审查。你公司提出的行动计划不包括实施纠正措施的策略。此外，没有提供详细的计划，来确保以前流通的药品是用符合鉴别和杂质检验要求的进场物料生产的。

■ Products Contain Glycerin ｜产品含有甘油

You manufacture drugs that contain glycerin. The use of glycerin contaminated with diethylene glycol（DEG）has resulted in various lethal poisoning incidents in humans worldwide.

你公司生产含有甘油的药品。在全球范围内，使用受二甘醇（DEG）污染的甘油已导致多起人类致命中毒事件。

See FDA's guidance document *Testing of Glycerin for Diethylene Glycol* to help you meet the cGMP requirements when manufacturing drugs containing glycerin at https://www.fda.gov/regulatory-information/search-fda-guidance-documents/testing-glycerin-diethylene-glycol.

请参阅 FDA 指南，甘油中二甘醇检验，以帮助你公司在生产含有甘油的药品时满足 cGMP 要求：网址（略，见上）。

■ Products Contain Ethanol ｜产品含有乙醇

You manufacture drugs that contain ethanol. The use of ethanol contaminated with methanol has resulted in various lethal poisoning incidents in humans worldwide.

你公司生产含有乙醇的药品。在全球范围内，使用被甲醇污染的乙醇已导致多起人类致命中毒事件。

See FDA's guidance document *Policy for Testing of Alcohol（Ethanol）and Isopropyl Alcohol for Methanol, Including During the Public Health Emergency（COVID-19）* at：https://www.fda.gov/media/145262/download.

请参阅 FDA 指南，酒精（乙醇）和异丙醇检验政策——包括在公共卫生紧急事件（COVID-19）期间的要求，网址（略，见上）。

In response to this letter, provide：

在回复本函时，请提供：

● A comprehensive review of your material system to determine whether all suppliers of components, containers, and closures, are each qualified and the materials are assigned appropriate expiration or retest dates. The review should also determine whether incoming material controls are adequate to prevent use of unsuitable components, containers, and closures.

● 对你公司的物料系统进行全面审查，以确定所有物料、容器和密封件的供应商是否均合格，并为物料指定适当的有效期或复验日期。审查还应确定进场物料控制是否足以防止使用不合适的物料、容器和密封件。

● A description of how you will test each component lot for conformity with all appropriate specifications for identity, strength, quality, and purity. If you intend to accept any results from your supplier's COA instead of testing each component lot for strength, quality, and purity, specify how you will robustly establish the reliability of your supplier's results through initial validation as well as periodic revalidation. In addition, include a commitment to always conduct at least one specific identity test for each incoming component lot.

● 说明如何检验每个批次，确定其是否符合有关鉴别、规格、质量和纯度的质量标准。如果你公司打算接受供应商 COA 的结果，而不是检验每个物料批次的规格、质量和纯度，请说明如何进行初始验证和定期再验证，从而稳健地确保供应商结果的可靠性。此外，还应承诺：对于每个进场原辅料批次，至少进行一个专属鉴别检验。

● Results of tests for DEG and EG in retain samples of all glycerin lots used to manufacture your drug products.

● 用于生产药品的所有甘油批次的留样中 DEG 和 EG 的检验结果。

● A full risk assessment for drug products that contain glycerin and are within expiry in the U.S. market. Take prompt corrective actions and preventive actions and detail your future actions to ensure appropriate selection of your suppliers, ongoing scrutiny of their supply chain, and appropriate incoming lot controls.

● 对美国市场上含有甘油且在有效期内的药品进行全面的风险评估。立即采取纠正和预防措施，并详细说明将来的措施，以确保正确选择供应商、持续审查其供应链以及适当的进场批次控制措施。

● Limit test of methanol and test results for all（b）（4）batches released and distributed.

● 甲醇的限度检测，以及所有放行和流通（b）（4）批的检验结果。

清洁验证

2. Your firm failed to establish and follow adequate written procedures for cleaning and maintenance of equipment（21 CFR 211.67（b））.

2. 你公司未建立并遵循适当的书面程序，来清洁和维护设备［21 CFR 211.67（b）］。

You failed to include all pieces of product-contact equipment used for manufacturing your drug and device products in your cleaning validation protocols and procedures. Your cleaning validation protocols and procedures did not include the transfer carriage vessels that are used for moving drug and chemical device component during manufacturing, creating a risk of cross contamination.

你公司未能将用于生产药品和器械产品的所有产品接触设备纳入清洁验证方案和程序中。你公司的清洁验证方案和程序不包括在生产过程中用于移动药品和器械产品化学原辅料的转运容器，从而产生交叉污染的风险。

In your response, you provide a CAPA and cleaning validation for the transfer carriage vessel. Your CAPA contains a list of products evaluated for use of the transfer carriage vessel.

在回复中，你公司提供了转运容器的 CAPA 和清洁验证。你公司的 CAPA 包含评估转运容器涉及的产品清单。

Your response is inadequate because the list of products provided in the CAPA contained products without "orders" and therefore lacks a complete evaluation of all possible uses of the transfer carriage vessel. You state that (b)(4) and (b)(4) finished products are the worst-case product to clean. Your response, however, does not provide information on products listed in your CAPA without "orders," whether those products use the transfer carriage vessel, and what impact those products had on your worst-case product selection.

你公司的回复不充分，因为 CAPA 中提供的产品清单包含没有"订单"的产品，因此缺乏对转运容器所有可能用途的完整评估。你公司指出（b）(4) 和（b）(4) 成品是最难清洁的产品。然而，你公司的回复中并未提供：有关 CAPA 中列出的没有"订单"的产品的信息，这些产品是否使用转运容器，以及这些产品对最差情况下的产品选择有何影响。

In response to this letter, provide:

在回复本函时，请提供：

（略）

此处与 FDA 发给 Cosmetic Science Laboratories LLC 的警告信（编号：MARCS-CMS 645558，即"5 水系统未经充分设计与监控"）中有关清洁验证的回应要求部分的内容类似，故略去。

4 标识为"已清洁"的设备不洁净

警告信编号： MARCS-CMS 650263

签发时间： 2023-5-26；**公示时间：** 2023-7-11

签发机构： 药品质量业务四处（Division of Pharmaceutical Quality Operations IV）

公　　司： NeilMed Pharmaceuticals Inc.

所在国家 / 地区： 美国

主　　题： cGMP/ 成品制剂 / 掺假（cGMP/Finished Pharmaceuticals/ Adulterated）

简　　介： 据称 NeilMed 是全球最大的 LVLP（大容量低压）盐水鼻腔冲洗系统制造商和供应商。FDA 在 2022 年 11 月至 12 月检查了该公司位于加利福尼亚州的药品生产设施。检查发现，该公司未能充分检验用于生产非处方药品的进场物料。特别是甘油和其他高风险原辅料应根据 USP 进行鉴别检验，以确保符合污染物二甘醇或乙二醇的安全限度。FDA 提醒指出，甘油和丙二醇都是药品中常用的原辅料，全球范围内甘油和丙二醇中的污染已导致多起人类致命中毒事件。作为药品生产商，其有责任在放行物料用于生产之前，对所有进场原辅料批次进行专属鉴别检验。此外，在设备清洁方面，该公司未能充分清洁和维护用于生产药品的设备。例如，FDA 的调查员在被标识为"已清洁"的非专用混合罐的直接产品接触表面上发现了不明的可见残留物。此外，该公司也未能按时清洁这些非专用混合罐并维护使用台账。

本警告信以下部分与本书此前其他警告信内容类似，故略去：前言、cGMP 顾问推荐（cGMP Consultant Recommended）、结论（Conclusion）。

物料检验

1. Your firm failed to conduct at least one test to verify the identity of each component of

a drug product. Your firm also failed to validate and establish the reliability of your component supplier's test analyses at appropriate intervals (21 CFR 211.84 (d) (1) and 211.84 (d) (2)).

1. 你公司未进行至少一项检验来确认药品中每种原辅料都被鉴别。也未能在适当的时间间隔内，验证和确定你公司的物料供应商检验分析的可靠性［21 CFR 211.84（d）（1）和（2）］。

Your firm failed to adequately test incoming components used to manufacture over-the-counter (OTC) drug products. Glycerin, along with other high-risk components, requires identification testing per the United States Pharmacopeia (USP) to ensure that it meets safety limits for diethylene (DEG) or ethylene glycol (EG). Because you did not perform the identity testing on each shipment of each glycerin lot using the USP identification test method that detects these hazardous impurities, you failed to assure the acceptability of glycerin used to manufacture your drug products. Furthermore, your firm relied on the manufacturer's certificate of analysis (COA) and released one lot of glycerin from an unqualified supplier to manufacture (b) (4) batches of Clear Canal.

你公司未能充分检验用于生产非处方（OTC）药品的进场原辅料。甘油以及其他高风险原辅料需要根据 USP 进行鉴别检验，以确保其符合二甘醇（DEG）或乙二醇（EG）的安全限度。你公司没有使用检测这些有害杂质的 USP 鉴别检验方法，对每批甘油的每批货物进行鉴别检验，因此无法确保用于生产药品的甘油是否合格。此外，你公司依赖生产商的分析证书（COA），从未经确认的供应商处放行了一批甘油，用于生产（b）（4）批次的 Clear Canal。

Both glycerin and propylene glycol are ingredients used in your drug products. DEG contamination in glycerin and propylene glycol has resulted in various lethal poisoning incidents in humans worldwide. As a drug manufacturer, you are responsible for performing specific identity tests for all incoming shipments of component lots prior to release for use in manufacturing.

甘油和丙二醇都是药品中使用的原辅料。在全球范围内，甘油和丙二醇中的 DEG 污染已导致多起人类致命中毒事件。作为药品生产商，你公司有责任在放行物料用于生产之前，对所有进场原辅料批次进行专属鉴别检验。

In your response, you commit to revise the material specifications for glycerin to include identity testing prior to release for drug product manufacturing. Your response is inadequate. You failed to perform identity testing on glycerin lots currently in your inventory. With respect to your glycerin-containing products, you have not addressed whether your evaluation will include all lots of glycerin for each drug product already released for distribution and within expiry. Without appropriate testing of components and ingredients, you cannot ensure the quality and safety of your drug products.

在回复中，你公司承诺修订甘油的物料质量标准，从而在药品生产放行之前对其进行鉴别检验。你公司的回应不够充分。未能对库存中当前的甘油批次执行鉴别检验。就含甘油的产品而言，尚未说明的问题是，你公司的评估是否将包括已放行流通且在效期内药品所涉及的所有甘油批次。如果不对原辅料进行适当的检验，就无法确保药品的质量和安全性。

See the FDA's guidance document *Testing of Glycerin*, *Propylene Glycol*, *Maltitol Solution*, *Hydrogenated Starch Hydrolysate*, *Sorbitol Solution*, *and Other High-Risk Drug Components for Diethylene Glycol and Ethylene Glycol*, to help you meet the cGMP requirements when manufacturing drugs containing ingredients at risk for DEG or EG contamination, at https://www.fda.gov/regulatory-information/search-fda-guidance-documents/testing-glycerin-propylene-glycol-maltitol-solution-hydrogenated-starch-hydrolysate-sorbitol.

请参阅 FDA 指南，甘油、丙二醇、麦芽糖醇溶液、氢化淀粉水解物、山梨醇溶液和其他高风险药品原辅料中二甘醇和乙二醇的检验，以帮助你公司在生产含有 DEG 或 EG 污染风险原辅料的药品时，满足 cGMP 要求，网址（略，见上）。

In response to this letter, provide:

在回复本函时，请提供：

（略）

此处与 FDA 发给 Profounda，Inc. 的警告信（编号：MARCS-CMS 642595，即"2 未能提供生产工艺的验证数据"）中有关物料检验回应要求内容类似，故略去。

设备清洁

2. Your firm failed to clean, maintain, and, as appropriate for the nature of the drug, sanitize and/or sterilize equipment and utensils at appropriate intervals to prevent malfunctions or contamination that would alter the safety, identity, strength, quality, or purity of the drug product beyond the official or other established requirements(21 CFR 211.67(a)).

2. 你公司未能根据药品的性质，按照适当的时间间隔对设备和器具进行消毒和（或）灭菌，以防止出现改变药品安全性、鉴别、规格、质量或纯度使其超过 USP 或其他既定要求的故障或污染［21 CFR 211.67(a)］。

You failed to adequately clean and maintain equipment used for manufacturing your drug products. For example, our investigator observed unidentified visible residues on direct product contact surfaces in (b)(4) non-dedicated mixing tanks labeled as "Cleaned" in (b)(4).

Furthermore, you failed to maintain cleaning and usage logs for these non-dedicated mixing tanks.

你公司未能充分清洁和维护用于生产药品的设备。例如，在（b）（4）中标识为"已清洁"的非专用混合罐的直接产品接触表面上，我们的调查员观察到不明的可见残留物。此外，你公司未能维护及时清洁这些非专用混合罐和并维护使用台账。

In addition, we note that you have reported multiple findings of objectionable microbial contamination in several of your finished drug products that were manufactured using non-dedicated mixing tanks in（b）（4）. Your corrective actions and preventive action（CAPA）indicated that the probable root causes were inadequate cleaning of mixing tank closures and valves, as well as a lack of Quality Assurance（QA）oversight of these activities. However, it did not mention the failure of operations management to oversee daily cleaning activities are performed satisfactorily.

此外，我们注意到，你公司报告了多个发现项，涉及在（b）（4）中使用非专用混合罐生产的几种成品中存在有害微生物污染。你公司的纠正和预防措施（CAPA）表明，可能的根本原因是混合罐密封件和阀门清洁不充分，以及缺乏对这些活动的质量保证（QA）监督。然而，并未提及运营管理部门未能监督日常清洁活动的执行的失败。

In your response, you commit to revise cleaning procedures and mandate utilization of logbooks. Your response is inadequate. You do not provide a comprehensive assessment of your cleaning effectiveness in determining the identity of the residues, assess whether other manufacturing equipment had been improperly cleaned, and evaluate if any cross-contaminated products were released for distribution. Additionally, you do not commit to holistically review the scope and effectiveness of daily operations management and QA oversight activities.

在回复中，你公司承诺修订清洁程序并强制使用台账。你公司的回应不够充分。没有对清洁效果进行全面评估，以确定残留物的鉴别，评估其他生产设备是否清洁不当，以及评估是否放行了任何交叉污染的产品进行流通。此外，你公司未承诺全面审查日常运营管理和质量保证监督活动的范围和有效性。

In response to this letter, provide the following:

在回复本函时，请提供以下信息：

● A comprehensive, independent retrospective assessment of your cleaning effectiveness to evaluate the scope of cross-contamination hazards. Include the identity of residues, other manufacturing equipment that may have been improperly cleaned, and an assessment whether cross-contaminated products may have been released for distribution. The assessment should identify any inadequacies of cleaning procedures and practices, and encompass each piece of manufacturing equipment used to manufacture more than one product.

● 对清洁效果进行全面、独立的回顾性评估，以评估交叉污染危害的范围。包括残留物的鉴别、其他可能未正确清洁的生产设备，以及对交叉污染的药品是否可能已被放行以供流通的评估。评估应确定清洁程序和实践的任何不足之处，并涵盖用于生产多个产品的每台生产设备。

● A CAPA plan, based on the comprehensive assessment of your cleaning program, that includes appropriate remediations to your cleaning processes and practices, timelines for completion, as well as a plan to implement routine, vigilant operations management, and QA oversight. Provide a detailed summary of vulnerabilities in your process for lifecycle management of equipment cleaning. Describe improvements to your cleaning program, including enhancements to cleaning effectiveness; improvements to ensure ongoing verification of proper cleaning and execution for all products and equipment; and all other needed remediations. Also describe how your cleaning validation studies will be updated based on your comprehensive assessment of the cleaning program.

● CAPA 计划，基于对清洁计划的全面评估，包括对清洁工艺和实践的相应整改措施、完成时间表，以及实施例行、警戒性的运营管理和 QA 监督的计划。提供设备清洁生命周期管理流程中漏洞的详细汇总。描述对清洁计划的改进，包括清洁效果的增强；改进以确保对所有产品和设备的正确清洁和执行进行持续确认；以及所有其他需要的整改措施。并说明如何根据对清洁计划的综合评估，来更新你公司的清洁验证研究。

● A CAPA plan to implement routine oversight of facilities and equipment. This plan should ensure, among other things, prompt detection of equipment/facilities performance issues, effective execution of repairs, adherence to appropriate preventive maintenance schedules, timely technological upgrades to the equipment/facility infrastructure, and improved systems for ongoing management review.

● 对设施和设备实施日常、警戒性的运营管理监督的 CAPA 计划。至少，该计划应确保及时发现设备 / 设施性能问题，有效执行维修，遵守适当的预防性维护计划，及时对设备 / 设施进行技术升级，并对持续管理评审的系统进行改进。

● A retrospective, independent review of water system failures, batch failures, rejected batches, returned drug products, complaints, and deviations that may have been related to microbiological contamination over the last three years.

● 对过去三年中可能与微生物污染相关的水系统不合格、批次不合格、拒收批次、退回药品、投诉和偏差，进行回顾性的独立审查。

Additional Concerns Related to Investigation of OOS Bioburden Test Results | 与 OOS 微生物负荷检验结果调查相关的其他问题

During our review, we noticed deficiencies in your investigation for out-of-specification (OOS) bioburden results involving *Burkholderia cepacia complex* (BCC), or yeast and mold in your finished drug products.

在审核过程中，我们注意到，对成品中涉及洋葱伯克霍尔德菌复合体（BCC）或酵母和霉菌的不合格（OOS）微生物负荷结果，你公司的调查存在缺陷。

For example, from February 2020 to September 2020, your firm recovered OOS results for BCC or, yeast and mold in multiple finished drug product batches that were manufactured using non-dedicated equipment in (b)(4). Per your investigation, CAPA 20-005 was deemed effective and was subsequently closed on April 2, 2021, approximately eight months later. However, you did not extend the investigation to other potentially impacted drug product batches manufactured around the timeframe when objectionable microorganisms were recovered. You did not implement an effective and timely CAPA to prevent the recurrence of bioburden excursions.

例如，从 2020 年 2 月到 2020 年 9 月，在（b）(4) 中使用非专用设备生产的多个成品制剂批次中，你公司回收到了 BCC 或酵母和霉菌的 OOS 结果。根据你公司的调查，CAPA 20-005 被视为有效，并随后于 2021 年 4 月 2 日（大约八个月后）关闭。然而，你公司没有将调查范围扩大，以涵盖在回收有害微生物的时间范围内生产的其他可能受影响的药品批次。你公司没有实施有效且及时的 CAPA，来防止微生物负荷偏差情况再次发生。

Although CAPA 20-005 identified a probable root cause, the scope of the investigation did not include all potentially affected drug product batches.

尽管 CAPA 20-005 确定了可能的根本原因，但调查范围并未包括所有可能受影响的药品批次。

For further information regarding the significance of BCC and other objectionable contamination of non-sterile, water-based drug products, see the FDA's advisory notice posted on April 21, 2023, at https://www.fda.gov/drugs/drug-safety-and-availability/fda-advises-drug-manufacturers-burkholderia-cepacia-complex-poses-contamination-risk-non-sterile.

有关 BCC 和非无菌水基药品其他不良污染重要性的更多信息，请参阅 FDA 于 2023 年 4 月 21 日发布的咨询通知，网址（略，见上）。

5 不良卫生条件下生产

警告信编号： MARCS-CMS 654464

签发时间： 2023-7-13；**公示时间：** 2023-8-1

签发机构： 药品质量业务一处（Division of Pharmaceutical Quality Operations I）

公　　司： Jamol Laboratories，Inc.

所在国家/地区： 美国

主　　题： cGMP/成品制剂/掺假（cGMP/Finished Pharmaceuticals/ Adulterated）

简　　介： 在 2022 年 12 月至 2023 年 1 月期间，FDA 对位于新泽西州的药品生产设施进行了检查。他们发现，药品生产发生在一个未经控制的空间里，这个空间用于各种多功能活动。调查员指出，这个空间年久失修，清洁和维护情况糟糕，有死虫、暴露的天花板和不足的通风等问题。由于缺乏足够的控制措施，这导致无法维持清洁的生产环境，也未能有效防止药品污染。在警告信中，第一个缺陷项针对质量部门。FDA 指出，质量部门没有对药品生产提供充分的监督。例如，他们没有规范描述质量部门的角色和职责的程序，也未能对不合格品进行调查或处理其他存在偏离的结果和偏差。

本警告信以下部分与本书此前其他警告信内容类似，故略去：前言、结论（Conclusion）。

Insanitary Conditions │ 不良卫生条件

Your firm manufactures an over-the-counter（OTC）drug product, Ponaris® NASAL EMOLLIENT（Ponaris）. Your Ponaris drug product is adulterated under section 501（a）（2）（A）of the FD&C Act because it was prepared, packed, or held under insanitary conditions.

你公司生产非处方（OTC）药品 Ponaris® NASAL EMOLLIENT（Ponaris）。根据 FD&C 法案第 501（a）（2）（A）条，Ponaris 因在不良卫生条件下制备、包装和保存而被视为掺假。

Your drug manufacturing occurs in a multipurpose uncontrolled space used for a variety of activities. FDA investigators observed this space to be in a state of disrepair, poorly cleaned and maintained, as evidenced by a dead insect, exposed ceiling, and inadequate ventilation. For example, you conduct a portion of your manufacturing in a corridor using a stained and debris covered fan surrounded by cardboard. You lack adequate controls in place to maintain a clean production environment and prevent contamination of drug products.

你公司的药品生产发生在不受控制的空间中，该空间用于各种多功能的活动。FDA 调查员发现，这个空间年久失修，清洁和维护不善，死虫、暴露的天花板和通风不足就证明了这一点。例如，你公司使用被纸板包围的污迹斑斑且覆盖碎片的风扇，并在使用这些风扇的走廊中进行部分生产。你公司缺乏充分的控制措施，来维持清洁的生产环境，并防止药品被污染。

cGMP Violations ｜ cGMP 违规

During our inspection, our investigators observed specific violations including, but not limited to, the following.

在检查过程中，我们的调查员发现了具体的违规情况，包括但不限于以下内容。

质量部门

1. Your firm lacks an adequate quality control unit with adequate facilities and procedures to ensure that drugs are manufactured in compliance with cGMP regulations and meet established specifications for identity, strength, quality, and purity（21 CFR 211.22）.

1. 你公司缺乏合格的质量控制部门，以及充分的设施和程序，以确保药品的生产符合 cGMP 法规，并符合既定的鉴别、规格、质量和纯度标准（21 CFR 211.22）。

Your quality unit（QU）did not provide adequate oversight for the manufacture of your drug product. For example, you lacked procedures describing the roles and responsibilities of the QU, investigations of out-of-specification（OOS）and other discrepant results and deviations. Additionally, your QU failed to ensure that all batch records are complete.

你公司的质量部门（QU）没有对药品的生产提供充分的监督。例如，缺乏描述 QU 角色和职责的程序、对不合格（OOS）以及其他存在偏离的结果和偏差的调查。此外，你公司的 QU 未能确保所有批记录完整。

Your response is inadequate because you failed to perform a review of your standard operating procedures（SOPs）and other governing documents to identify and address deficiencies in a holistic manner.

你公司的回复不充分，因为未能对标准操作程序（SOP）和其他管理文件进行审查，以全面识别和解决缺陷。

In response to this letter, provide：

在回复本函时，请提供：

● A comprehensive assessment and remediation plan to ensure your QU is given the authority and resources to effectively function. The assessment should also include, but not be limited to：

● 全面的评估和整改计划，以确保你公司的 QU 获得有效运作的权限和资源。评估还应包括但不限于以下内容：

○ A determination of whether procedures used by your firm are robust and appropriate.

○ 确定你公司使用的程序是否可靠和适当。

○ Provisions for QU oversight throughout your operations to evaluate adherence to appropriate practices.

○ 在整个运营过程中 QU 进行监督的规定，以评估对相应规范的遵守情况。

○ A complete and final review of each batch and its related information before the QU disposition decision.

○ 在 QU 决定处置之前，对每批产品及其相关信息进行完整和最终审查。

○ Oversight and approval of investigations and discharging of all other QU duties to ensure identity, strength, quality, and purity of all products

○ 监督和批准调查以及履行所有其他 QU 职责，以确保所有产品的鉴别、规格、质量和纯度。

○ A complete assessment of documentation systems used throughout your manufacturing operations to determine where documentation practices are inadequate. Include a detailed CAPA plan that remedies documentation practices and ensures that you retain complete and accurate records.

○ 对整个生产操作中使用的文档系统进行全面评估，以确定记录实践的不足之处。

包括详细的 CAPA 计划，以纠正记录实践并确保你公司保存完整且准确的记录。

● A retrospective evaluation of your drug product in the U.S. market and within expiry to identify and take appropriate action on any product quality or patient safety risks.

● 对你公司在美国市场上和有效期内的药品进行回顾性评估，以识别任何产品质量或患者安全风险，并采取适当的措施。

● A comprehensive assessment of your overall system for investigating deviations, discrepancies, complaints, OOS results, and failures. Provide a detailed action plan to remediate this system. Your action plan should include, but not be limited to, significant improvements in investigation competencies, scope determination, root cause evaluation, CAPA effectiveness, QU oversight, and written procedures. Address how your firm will ensure all phases of investigations are appropriately conducted.

● 对整个系统进行全面评估，以调查偏差、差异、投诉、OOS 结果和不合格。提供详细的行动计划来整改该系统。你公司的行动计划应包括但不限于调查能力、范围确定、根本原因评估、CAPA 有效性、QU 监督和书面程序方面的显著提高。说明你公司将如何确保适当进行所有阶段的调查。

See FDA's guidance document *Quality Systems Approach to Pharmaceutical cGMP Regulations* for help in implementing quality systems and risk management approaches to meet the requirements of cGMP regulations 21 CFR parts 210 and 211, at https://www.fda.gov/media/71023/download.

你公司的质量体系不够完善。请参阅 FDA 指南，药品 cGMP 法规的质量系统方法，以帮助实施质量系统和风险管理方法，以满足 cGMP 法规 21 CFR 第 210 和 211 部分的要求：网址（略，见上）。

物料检验

2. Your firm failed to establish laboratory controls that include scientifically sound and appropriate specifications, standards, sampling plans, and test procedures designed to assure that components conform to appropriate standards of identity, strength, quality, and purity, and conduct for each batch of drug product, appropriate laboratory testing, as necessary, required to be free of objectionable microorganisms (21 CFR 211.160(b) and 211.165(b)).

2. 你公司未能建立实验室控制措施，其中包括科学合理且相应的规范、标准、取样计划和检验程序，旨在确保原辅料符合适当的鉴别、规格、质量和纯度标准，并为每批产品进行检验。必要时进行适当的实验室检验，要求不含有害微生物 [21 CFR 211.160(b) 和 211.165(b)]。

You failed to establish an identification test with adequate specificity to appropriately test incoming lots of Eucalyptus Oil to meet the United States Pharmacopoeia（USP）monograph. Specifically, your test procedure fails to include an appropriate test using infrared spectroscopy for identification.

你公司未能建立具有足够专属性的鉴别方法，来适当检验进场的桉树油批次，使其满足 USP 专论的要求。具体来说，你公司的检验程序未包括使用红外光谱进行识别的检验。

Your firm also failed to conduct appropriate laboratory testing for each batch of drug product that is required to be free of objectionable microorganisms. Your practice of conducting microbiological testing on（b）（4）of Ponaris selected（b）（4）is inadequate. Additionally, as your drug product contains ingredients of botanical origin, an assessment for the absence of aflatoxins or other mycotoxins should be conducted.

你公司也未能对每批药品进行适当的实验室检验，以确保不含有害微生物。你们进行微生物检验的实践是不充分的。此外，由于你公司的药品含有植物来源的原辅料，因此应评估是否含有黄曲霉毒素或其他霉菌毒素。

In your response you state that you will continue to test（b）（4）of Ponaris for "microcontaminants" and heavy metals（b）（4）, in addition to the rancidity test you already perform. Your response is inadequate because you did not provide scientific justification for conducting microbiological testing only（b）（4）, nor recognize the need for conducting analysis showing your products are free of aflatoxins and other mycotoxins.

在回复中，你公司声称除了已经执行的酸败度检验之外，你们还将继续检验 Ponaris 的（b）（4）中的"微污染物"和重金属（b）（4）。你公司的回复不充分，因为没有提供仅进行微生物检验的科学论证（b）（4），也没有认识到需要进行分析以表明你公司的产品不含黄曲霉毒素和其他霉菌毒素。

In your response to this letter：

在你公司对本函的回复中：

● Provide a timeline to complete retroactive identification tests using an appropriate identification method for all potentially compromised batches. Respond promptly with all results. If your data indicates that defective products are in the U.S. marketplace, commit to recall the products.

● 应提供一个时间表，使用适当的鉴别方法对所有可能受影响的批次完成追溯鉴别检验。及时回复所有结果。如果你公司的数据表明美国市场上存在有缺陷产品，请承诺召回这些产品。

● Determine if all methods used to test your raw and in-process materials and finished drug products use USP-NF, or if not, employ an equivalent or better method. Provide a CAPA to address any inadequate methods that are identified.

● 确定用于检验原料、中间物料和成品的所有方法是否都使用 USP-NF，如果没有，则应采用等效或更好的方法。提供 CAPA，来解决已发现的任何不适当的方法。

● A list of chemical and microbial specifications, including test methods, used to analyze each lot of your drug products before a lot disposition decision.

● 在做出批处置决定之前，用于分析每批药品的化学和微生物质量标准（包括检验方法）的清单。

○ An action plan and timelines for conducting full chemical and microbiological testing of retain samples to determine the quality of all batches of drug product distributed to the United States that are within expiry as of the date of this letter.

○ 行动计划和时间表：对留样进行全面的化学和微生物检验，对于流通给美国的所有效期内（本函发出之日计）药品批次，确定其质量。

○ A summary of all results obtained from testing retain samples from each batch. If such testing reveals substandard quality drug products, take rapid corrective actions, such as notifying customers and product recalls.

○ 所有批次的留样检验汇总。如果此类检验表明药品质量不合格，请迅速采取整改措施，例如通知客户和产品召回。

工艺验证

3. Your firm failed to establish written procedures for production and process control designed to assure that the drug products you manufacture have the identity, strength, quality, and purity they purport or are represented to possess(21 CFR 211.100(a)).

3. 你公司未能建立充分的书面生产和过程控制程序，旨在确保所生产的药品具有其声称或表示具备的鉴别、规格、质量和纯度［21 CFR 211.100(a)］。

You failed to adequately validate the processes used to manufacture Ponaris, and do not have an ongoing program for monitoring process control, to ensure stable manufacturing operations and consistent drug quality.

你公司未能充分验证用于生产 Ponaris 的工艺，并且没有持续的工艺控制监控计划，以确保稳定的生产操作和一致的药品质量。

For example, you have not identified the component attributes (e.g., solubility, viscosity, and density) and the process parameters (e.g., speed, temperature, and (b)(4)) that are important to produce this product with a consistent quality.

例如，对于生产具有一致质量的产品而言重要的原辅料属性（例如溶解度、黏度和密度）和工艺参数［例如速度、温度和（b）(4)］，你公司尚未明确。

（略）

此处与 FDA 发给 Profounda, Inc. 的警告信（编号：MARCS-CMS 642595，即"2 未能提供生产工艺的验证数据"）中有关工艺验证的重要性部分的内容类似，故略去。

In your response you state that you will begin recording mixing times for each lot that is manufactured to ensure consistency and quality of the product. Your response is inadequate because recording mixing times or performing a single "Uniformity in Drum" test does not itself provide adequate evidence of process control at each step of the manufacturing process and show lot-to-lot consistency.

在回复中，你公司声明将开始记录每批生产的混合时间，以确保产品的一致性和质量。你公司的回复是不充分的，因为记录混合时间或执行单个"滚筒均匀性"检验本身，并不能提供生产工艺每个步骤的过程被控制的充分证据，也不能显示批次之间的一致性。

In response to this letter, provide the following:

在回复本函时，请提供以下信息：

（略）

此处与 FDA 发给 Dunagin Pharmaceuticals Inc. dba Massco Dental 的警告信（编号：MARCS-CMS 644335，即"3 与非药用产品的共线生产问题"）中的工艺验证回应要求类似，故略去。

6 判定 OOS 结果无效，依据不充分

警告信编号： MARCS-CMS 654085

签发时间： 2023-7-20；**公示时间：** 2023-8-1

签发机构： 药物审评与研究中心 | CDER（Center for Drug Evaluation and Research | CDER）

公　司： Medgel Private Limited

所在国家 / 地区： 印度

主　题： cGMP/ 成品制剂 / 掺假（cGMP/Finished Pharmaceuticals/ Adulterated）

简　介： FDA 在 2023 年 1 月对位于印度的药品生产设施进行了检查。FDA 指出该公司将不合格结果判定为无效，缺乏充分的科学论证。对于多个 OOS 结果，公司假设可能的根本原因是样品制备中的错误，但缺乏充分的科学论证。随后，他们进行了复验，并在获得合格结果后放行了相关批次。在其回复中，该公司承认对 OOS 无效缺乏充分的科学论证，并提出了 CAPA。然而，这些 CAPA 被认为不够充分，因为虽然 CAPA 狭隘地阐述了 FDA 调查员注意到的 OOS 事件和该公司独特的假设，但在整体范围和深度上仍然存在不足。

本警告信以下部分与本书此前其他警告信内容类似，故略去：前言、质量体系（Quality Systems）、cGMP 顾问推荐（cGMP Consultant Recommended）、结论（Conclusion）。

偏差调查

1. Your firm failed to thoroughly investigate any unexplained discrepancy or failure of a batch or any of its components to meet any of its specifications, whether or not the batch has already been distributed（21 CFR 211.192）.

1. 无论批次是否已经流通，对于该批次或其原辅料不满足质量标准、存在无法解释的偏差或不合格，你公司未能进行彻底调查（21 CFR 211.192）。

Invalidated out-of-specification results lacked adequate scientific justification ｜ 无效的不合格结果，缺乏充分的科学论证

Your firm manufactures numerous over-the-counter (OTC) drug products in (b)(4) capsule form. Your investigations into bulk drug product assay out-of-specification (OOS) test results for batches (b)(4) were inadequate, as they lacked adequate hypothesis testing and evidence to support the root cause. Specifically, you hypothesized that the probable root cause was an error in sample preparation, but you did not have an adequate scientific basis. You subsequently retested and released the batch in question after obtaining passing results.

你公司生产多种（b)(4）胶囊形式的非处方（OTC）药品。你公司对批次（b)(4）的原料药检测不合格（OOS）检验结果的调查不充分，因为它们缺乏充分的假设检验和证据，来支持根本原因。具体来说，你公司假设可能的根本原因是样品制备中的错误，但没有充分的科学论证。你公司随后进行复验，并在获得合格结果后，放行了相关批次。

Additionally, in several assay OOS investigations from 2019, to 2022, you attributed the root cause to sample preparation error without identifying the appropriate corrective action and preventive action (CAPA) from these investigations to prevent recurrence of such events.

此外，在 2019 年至 2022 年的多项分析 OOS 调查中，你公司将根本原因归因于样品制备错误，但没有从这些调查中确定适当的纠正和预防措施（CAPA），以防止此类事件再次发生。

In your response, you acknowledge that you lack adequate scientific justification for the OOS invalidations and proposed CAPA that narrowly addresses the OOS events noted by FDA investigators and your unique hypotheses. However, your CAPAs were inadequate because they were specific to your inadequate investigations and lacked a comprehensive scope.

在回复中，你公司承认对 OOS 无效的判定缺乏充分的科学论证，并提出了 CAPA，该 CAPA 仅仅解决了 FDA 调查员注意到的 OOS 事件和你公司唯一的假设。但是，你公司的 CAPA 是不够的，因为它们是针对你们不充分的调查而制定的，并缺乏全面的范围。

Inadequate investigation of humidity excursions ｜ 对湿度偏移的调查不充分

You did not adequately investigate several humidity excursions beyond your specification limits during the production of your drug products as well as in your stability chambers. Furthermore, our investigators could not review portions of humidity data between December 2022, and January 2023, because the raw data is not backed up and deleted every month. High levels of humidity can impact the properties of (b)(4) capsules and make them vulnerable to undesirable microbiological contamination.

对于在药品生产过程中以及稳定性考察箱中几次超出规格限度的湿度偏差，你公司没有充分调查。此外，我们的调查员无法审查 2022 年 12 月至 2023 年 1 月期间的部分湿度数据，因为原始数据每月删除，并未备份。高湿度会影响（b）(4) 胶囊的特性，并使它们容易受到有害微生物污染。

In your response, you attribute the humidity excursions to a defective dehumidifier but do not provide information on the steps taken to ensure that your dehumidifier and the overall conditions at your facility are maintained optimally. You also state that you reviewed your humidity monitoring data from January to December 2022, and concluded that there was no impact to the product because the (b)(4) and assay results for the affected batches were within specifications. Your response was inadequate because (b)(4) and does not measure (b)(4) content.

在回复中，你公司将湿度异常归因于除湿机有缺陷，但没有提供有关信息，来确保你公司为除湿机和设施的整体条件保持最佳状态而采取的步骤。你公司还指出，你们审查了 2022 年 1 月至 12 月的湿度监测数据，并得出结论认为对产品没有影响，因为受影响批次的（b）(4) 和检验结果符合质量标准。你公司的回应不充分，因为（b）(4) 并没有衡量（b）(4) 内容。

In response to this letter, provide:

在回复本函时，请提供:

（略）

此处与 FDA 发给 Dunagin Pharmaceuticals Inc. dba Massco Dental 的警告信（编号: MARCS-CMS 644335，即 "3 与非药用产品的共线生产问题"）中的 OOS 调查要求类似，故略去。

质量部门

2. Your firm's quality control unit failed to exercise its responsibility to ensure drug products manufactured are in compliance with cGMP, and meet established specifications for identity, strength, quality, and purity (21 CFR 211.22).

2. 你公司的质量控制部门未能履行职责，以确保所生产的药品符合 cGMP 要求，并符合有关鉴别、规格、质量和纯度的既定质量标准（21 CFR 211.22）。

Your QU did not provide adequate oversight and control over your drug manufacturing operations. For example, your QU failed to ensure the following:

你公司的 QU 没有对药品生产业务提供充分的监督和控制。例如，你公司的 QU 未能确保以下事项：

- Controlled access to master batch records and issuance of batch records.

- 对工艺规程的受控访问和对批记录的受控发布。

- Controlled correction and disposal of cGMP documentation.

- cGMP 文件的受控纠正和处置。

- Contemporaneous documentation of laboratory data that would support batch release (e.g., you had destroyed microbiological plates before recording the data).

- 支持批放行的实验室数据的同步记录（例如，你公司在记录数据之前已销毁微生物培养皿）。

- Appropriate data integrity controls (e.g., your QU failed to adequately restrict access to analytical instruments; you used shared usernames and passwords).

- 适当的数据可靠性控制（例如，你公司的 QU 未能充分限制对分析仪器的访问；你公司使用了共享的用户名和密码）。

- Procedures for review of raw data and audit trails.

- 原始数据和审计追踪的审查程序。

In your response, you state that you revised your procedures with additional instructions for issuing and disposing cGMP documents. You attribute the root cause of the non-contemporaneous documentation to human error and instituted a second person check for microbiological testing and data recording. You also commit to reviewing audit trails and retraining your analysts.

在回复中，你公司声称你们修订了程序，并添加了有关发布和处置 cGMP 文件的附加说明。你公司将非同步记录的根本原因归因于人为错误，并针对微生物检验和数据记录进行了第二人复核。你公司还承诺审查审计追踪，并重新培训你们的分析人员。

Your response was inadequate because it lacked details on how your QU would oversee the implementation of the CAPAs and check their effectiveness. Furthermore, the CAPAs were specific to the examples FDA noted during the inspection and did not extend to a comprehensive review of your cGMP documentation systems, laboratory systems, and data integrity systems. This was a repeat observation from FDA's 2019 inspection where you also attributed the root cause of non-contemporaneous documentation of microbiological plates to human error and implemented CAPAs including cGMP documentation training, which were ultimately ineffective.

你公司的回复不充分，因为它缺乏关于 QU 将如何监督 CAPA 的实施并检查其有效性的详细信息。此外，CAPA 专门针对 FDA 在检查期间注意到的例子，并未扩展到对你公司的 cGMP 文件系统、实验室系统和数据可靠性系统的全面审查。这是 FDA 2019 年检查中已出现的违规行为，当时你公司将微生物培养皿非同步记录的根本原因归于人为错误，并实施了包括 cGMP 文件培训在内的 CAPA，但最终证明 CAPA 无效。

■ Data Integrity Remediation 数据可靠性整改

Your quality system does not adequately ensure the accuracy and integrity of data to support the safety, effectiveness, and quality of the drugs you manufacture. See FDA's guidance document *Data Integrity and Compliance With Drug cGMP* for guidance on establishing and following cGMP compliant data integrity practices at https://www.fda.gov/media/119267/download.

你公司的质量体系也无法充分确保数据的准确性和可靠性，以支持你们所生产的药品的安全性、有效性和质量。有关建立和遵循 cGMP 合规数据可靠性实践的指南，请参阅 FDA 指南，数据可靠性和药品 cGMP 合规性，网址（略，见上）。

In response to this letter, provide：

在回复本函时，请提供：

● A comprehensive investigation into the extent of the inaccuracies in data records and reporting including results of the data review for drugs distributed to the United States. Include a detailed description of the scope and root causes of your data integrity lapses.

● 对数据记录和报告的不准确程度进行全面调查，包括对销往美国的药品的数据审查结果。包括数据可靠性缺陷的范围和根本原因的详细描述。

● A current risk assessment of the potential effects of the observed failures on the quality of your drugs. Your assessment should include analyses of the risks to patients caused by the release of drugs affected by a lapse of data integrity and analyses of the risks posed by ongoing operations.

● 当前观察到的不合格对药品质量潜在影响的风险评估。你公司的评估应包括分析因数据可靠性失效影响的药品放行对患者造成的风险，以及对正在进行的操作带来的风险的分析。

● A management strategy for your firm that includes the details of your global CAPA plan. The detailed corrective action plan should describe how you intend to ensure the reliability and completeness of all data generated by your firm including microbiological and analytical data, manufacturing records, and all data submitted to FDA.

● 你公司的管理策略，其中包括整体 CAPA 计划的详细信息。详细的纠正措施计划应描述你公司打算如何确保生成的所有数据的可靠性和完整性，包括微生物和分析数据、生产记录以及提交给 FDA 的所有数据。

物料检验

3. Your firm failed to test samples of each component for identity and conformity with all appropriate written specifications for purity, strength, and quality. Your firm also failed to validate and establish the reliability of your component supplier's test analyses at appropriate intervals(21 CFR 211.84(d)(1)and 211.84(d)(2)).

3. 你公司未能对每种原辅料的样品进行鉴别，以及判断其是否符合所有适当的纯度、规格和质量的书面标准。你公司也未能以适当的时间间隔验证和建立物料供应商检验分析的可靠性［21 CFR 211.84(d)(1) 和 211.84(d)(2)］。

You failed to conduct adequate testing on each component lot used to manufacture your drug products. For example, your component identity testing did not include a limit test for diethylene glycol(DEG)and ethylene glycol(EG)on all lots of glycerin, propylene glycol, (b)(4), and sorbitol solution before use in the manufacture or preparation of your drug products. Similarly, your component impurity testing for polyethylene glycol did not include a limit test for diethylene glycol(DEG)and ethylene glycol(EG). In addition, except for(b) (4), you accepted the impurities listed on your API suppliers' certificate of analyses(COAs), without performing impurity testing on your active pharmaceutical ingredients(APIs).

你公司未能对用于生产药品的每个原辅料批次进行充分的检验。例如，在药品生产或制备之前，对所有批次的甘油、丙二醇、(b)(4)和山梨醇溶液进行二甘醇（DEG）和乙二醇（EG）的限度检验，你公司的原辅料鉴别检验未能将其纳入考虑。同样，对于聚乙二醇原辅料杂质检验，也没有包括二甘醇（DEG）和乙二醇（EG）的限度检验。此外，除（b）(4)之外，你公司仅仅依赖 API 供应商的分析证书（COA）上列出的杂质，而没有对你公司的原料药（API）进行杂质检验。

Without adequate testing, you do not have scientific evidence that your incoming components conform to appropriate specifications before use in the manufacture of drug products.

如果没有充分的检验，你公司就没有科学证据，来证明进场物料在用于药品生产之前符合相应的质量标准。

In your response to our request for additional information, you stated that you analyzed DEG/EG results on your suppliers' COAs from 2018 and 2019 and all were either not detected or within specifications. You stated that you sent all existing raw material retains from 2020 to 2022 for third-party testing and revised procedures to test for DEG/EG in your incoming component going forward. You committed to test for DEG/EG in all lots of finished drug products within expiry that were intended for the U.S. market. You stated that you revised your vendor qualification procedure to specify the requirement of impurity testing according to the monograph. You also stated that you would perform impurity testing for three recent batches of API for existing vendors and subsequently perform periodic impurity testing of each API for all vendors and that you would qualify your vendors by June 2023 to accept their impurity specifications.

在你公司对我们提供更多信息的要求的回复中，表示你们分析了 2018 年和 2019 年供应商 COA 的 DEG/EG 结果，所有结果或未检测到，或符合质量标准。你公司表示，已将 2020 年至 2022 年保留的所有现有原料发送给第三方检验，并修订了程序以检验未来进场物料中的 DEG/EG。还承诺在有效期内对销往美国市场的所有批次成品进行 DEG/EG 检测。你公司表示，你们修订了供应商资质确认审查程序，以根据专论规定杂质检验的要求。还表示，将为现有供应商最近三批 API 进行杂质检验，随后对所有供应商的每个 API 进行定期杂质检验，并且将在 2023 年 6 月之前确认你公司供应商的资质，从而接受其杂质质量标准。

Your response is inadequate because you did not provide a risk assessment for finished products on the market and within expiry manufactured with glycerin, polyethylene glycol, propylene glycol, (b)(4), and sorbitol solution. Additionally, your response lacked details regarding your plans in the interim regarding products already on the market and within expiry.

你公司的回复不充分，对市场上和在有效期内使用甘油、聚乙二醇、丙二醇、(b)(4) 和山梨糖醇溶液生产的成品，没有提供风险评估。此外，有关你公司已上市且在有效期内的产品的临时计划，你们的回复缺乏详细信息。

In response to this letter, provide:

在回复本函时，请提供:

- A comprehensive, independent review of your material system to determine whether all suppliers of components, containers, and closures, are each qualified and the materials are assigned appropriate expiration or retest dates. The review should also determine whether incoming material controls are adequate to prevent use of unsuitable components, containers, and closures.

● 对你公司的物料系统进行全面、独立的审查，以确定所有物料、容器和密封件的供应商是否均合格，并为物料指定适当的有效期或复验日期。审查还应确定进场物料控制是否足以防止使用不合适的物料、容器和密封件。

● A summary of test results for reserve samples of all finished product lots manufactured with glycerin, polyethylene glycol, propylene glycol, (b)(4), and sorbitol solution.

● 针对甘油、聚乙二醇、丙二醇、(b)(4) 和山梨糖醇溶液生产的所有成品批次，其留样的检验结果汇总。

● The chemical and microbiological quality control specifications you use to test and release each incoming lot of component for use in manufacturing.

● 针对每批用于生产目的的进场物料，用于检验和放行的化学和微生物质控标准。

● A description of how you will test each component lot for conformity with all appropriate specifications for identity, strength, quality, and purity. If you intend to accept any results from your supplier's COAs instead of testing each component lot for strength, quality, and purity, specify how you will robustly establish the reliability of your supplier's results through initial validation as well as periodic re-validation. In addition, include a commitment to always conduct at least one specific identity test for each incoming component lot.

● 说明如何检验每个批次，确定其是否符合有关鉴别、规格、质量和纯度的标准。如果你公司打算接受供应商 COA 的结果，而不是检验每个物料批次的规格、质量和纯度，请说明如何进行初始验证和定期再验证，从而稳健地确保供应商结果的可靠性。此外，还应承诺：对于每个进场原辅料批次，至少进行一个专属鉴别检验。

● A summary of results obtained from testing all components to evaluate the reliability of the COA from each component manufacturer. Include your procedures that describe this COA validation program.

● 从所有原辅料检验中获得的结果汇总，以评估每个物料生产商的 COA 的可靠性。包括描述此 COA 验证计划的程序。

● A summary of your program for qualifying and overseeing contract testing facilities.

● 你公司委托检验设施确认和监督计划的汇总。

The use of ingredients contaminated with DEG or EG has resulted in various lethal poisoning incidents in humans worldwide. See FDA's guidance document *Testing of Glycerin, Propylene Glycol, Maltitol Solution, Hydrogenated Starch Hydrolysate, Sorbitol Solution, and Other High-Risk Drug Components for Diethylene Glycol and Ethylene Glycol* to help you meet the cGMP requirements when manufacturing drugs containing ingredients at risk for DEG or EG contamination, at https://www.fda.gov/media/167974/download.

在全球范围内，使用受 DEG 或 EG 污染的原辅料已导致多起人类致命中毒事件。请参阅 FDA 指南，甘油、丙二醇、麦芽糖醇溶液、氢化淀粉水解物、山梨醇溶液和其他高风险药品原辅料中二甘醇和乙二醇的检验，以帮助你公司在生产含有 DEG 或 EG 污染风险原辅料的药品时，满足 cGMP 要求，请访问：网址（略，见上）。

7 药品存在交叉污染风险

警告信编号： MARCS-CMS 655231

签发时间： 2023-7-25；**公示时间：** 2023-8-1

签发机构： 药物审评与研究中心 | CDER（Center for Drug Evaluation and Research | CDER）

公　　司： Centaur Pharmaceuticals Private Ltd.

所在国家 / 地区： 印度

主　　题： cGMP/ 成品制剂 / 掺假（cGMP/Finished Pharmaceuticals/ Adulterated）

简　　介： FDA 在 2023 年 1 月至 2 月期间检查了位于印度的药品生产设施。在检查中，FDA 发现该公司对非专用设备的清洁和维护程序不充分，导致直接和间接产品接触表面上似乎存在不同产品的残留物。该公司在回复中声称已经生产了安慰剂批次，以评估药品交叉污染的可能性。根据他们的结论，没有对市售批次的产品产生质量影响，患者的健康和安全也不会面临风险，并且称"物料不存在污染的可能性"。然而，FDA 认为该公司的回应不够充分。他们指出，交叉污染并不均匀，对对照样品和安慰剂批次的检验不能科学地证明产品不含明显肮脏设备造成的污染。因此，FDA 要求该公司进行全面、独立的回顾性审查，来评估交叉污染危害的范围。这包括对残留物的鉴别、可能未正确清洁的其他生产设备的评估，以及对已放行用于流通的可能存在交叉污染的药品的评估。

本警告信以下部分与本书此前其他警告信内容类似，故略去：前言、结论（Conclusion）。

设备清洁

1. Your firm failed to clean, maintain, and, as appropriate for the nature of the drug, sanitize and/or sterilize equipment and utensils at appropriate intervals to prevent malfunctions or contamination that would alter the safety, identity, strength, quality, or purity of the drug product beyond the official or other established requirements (21 CFR 211.67 (a)).

1. 你公司未能根据药品的性质，按照适当的时间间隔对设备和器具进行消毒和（或）灭菌，以防止出现故障或污染，从而改变药品安全性、鉴别、规格、质量或纯度，超过 USP 或其他既定要求［21 CFR 211.67 (a)］。

Your cleaning and maintenance procedures for non-dedicated (b)(4) equipment (b)(4), including your (b)(4) and (b)(4), are inadequate. Our inspection identified residues of what appeared to be different products on direct and indirect product contact surfaces, including those located inside (b)(4) systems, (b)(4) units (b)(4), and (b)(4). Your firm acknowledged that sections of the (b)(4), (b)(4), and (b)(4) have not been cleaned or examined for cleanliness since they were installed over 14 years ago. During the inspection, your analytical testing confirmed these residues contained multiple active ingredients. Furthermore, during the inspection, you collected residue samples at the end of placebo batches and subsequent cleaning, which also demonstrated active ingredient cross-contamination on surfaces.

你公司对非专用（b）(4) 设备（b）(4)，包括（b）(4) 和（b）(4) 的清洁和维护程序不充分。我们的检查发现直接和间接产品接触表面上似乎存在不同产品的残留物，包括位于（b）(4) 系统、（b）(4) 单元（b）(4) 和（b）(4)。你公司承认，对于（b）(4)、（b）(4) 和（b）(4) 部分，自 14 年前安装以来，都未进行过清洁或清洁度检查。在检查过程中，你们的分析检验证实这些残留物含有多种原料药。此外，在检查过程中，你公司在安慰剂批次结束和随后的清洁时收集了残留样品，这也证明了表面上的原料药交叉污染。

(b)(4) over dirty surfaces can facilitate contamination of the drug being processed in an (b)(4). Robust design, cleaning, and maintenance of this and other equipment is critical to prevent cross-contamination.

在肮脏表面上的（b）(4)，可能会促进在（b）(4) 中处理的药品受到污染。对于防止交叉污染，该设备和其他设备的稳健设计、清洁和维护是至关重要的。

The inspection also noted missing or faulty (b)(4) in (b)(4), as well as material back flow, which resulted in equipment contamination. For example, you stated the manually operated (b)(4) inside (b)(4) number CP/PT/(b)(4)-01 in (b)(4) Area (b)(4) is always in the open position. You also indicated the buildup of powder inside the（b）（4）and（b）（4）of this equipment was caused by the back flow of materials during equipment（b）（4）.

检查还发现（b）（4）中的（b）（4）缺失或有缺陷，并存在物料回流的现象，导致设备污染。例如，你公司在（b）（4）区域（b）（4）中指定人工操作（b）（4）内的（b）（4）编号 CP/PT/（b）（4）–01 始终处于打开位置。你公司还指出，该设备（b）（4）和（b）（4）内的粉末堆积是由于设备（b）（4）期间物料回流造成的。

As a result of these inspectional findings, you communicated with your client, Breckenridge Pharmaceutical, Inc., who initiated a recall of numerous batches of alprazolam tablets and clobazam tablets manufactured in your（b）（4）. We also acknowledge the recall initiated by（b）（4）of（b）（4）tablets you manufactured.

根据这些检查结果，你公司与你们的客户 Breckenridge Pharmaceutical, Inc. 进行了沟通，后者发起了对你公司（b）（4）生产的多批阿普唑仑片剂和氯巴扎姆片剂的召回。我们还知晓，由（b）（4）发起的对你公司生产的（b）（4）片剂的召回。

In your response, you state all（b）（4）and（b）（4）used for multiple products have been taken out of service, and you have cleaned, replaced, and improved（b）（4）processing and cleaning equipment. You also indicate you have revised your cleaning procedures, and you explain that（b）（4）and（b）（4）are now appropriately inspected to verify cleanliness, which is recorded in your cleaning records. Further, you state you have manufactured placebo batches to assess the potential for cross-contamination of drug products. Through your testing of control and placebo batch samples, you conclude there is no product quality impact on commercially distributed batches of alprazolam tablets and clobazam tablets. You also state there is no risk to patients' health and safety, and "no probability of contamination of material."

在回复中，你公司声称用于多种产品的所有（b）（4）和（b）（4）均已停止使用，并且你们已清洁、更换和改进（b）（4）加工和清洁设备。你公司还表明你们已经修订了清洁程序，并解释说现在对（b）（4）和（b）（4）进行了适当检查，以确认清洁度，并将其记录在清洁记录中。此外，你公司声称已经生产了安慰剂批次，来评估药品交叉污染的可能性。通过对对照和安慰剂批次样品的检验，你公司得出结论，对于市售批次的阿普唑仑片剂和氯巴扎姆片剂，没有产品质量影响。你公司还表示，患者的健康和安全不会面临风险，并且"物料不存在污染的可能性"。

Your response is inadequate. Cross-contamination is not uniform, and your testing of control samples and placebo batches failed to scientifically prove your products are free of contaminants from your visibly dirty equipment. Additionally, you state the active ingredient recovered after placebo batch manufacturing was from "mostly indirect contact surfaces." You did not sufficiently address contamination recovered from product contact surfaces, and you failed to acknowledge that other locations and other sampling may reveal higher levels of contamination. FDA is aware of other instances where such lack of cleaning in（b）（4）handling has led to cross-contamination between drug products.

你公司的回应不够充分。交叉污染并不均匀，你公司对对照样品和安慰剂批次的检验，未能科学地证明产品不含明显滞脏设备造成的污染物。此外，你公司还指出，安慰剂批生产后回收的原料药来源"主要是间接接触表面"。你公司没有充分解决从产品接触表面回收的污染问题，也没有指出其他位置和取样可能会显示出更高水平的污染。FDA 意识到，（b）（4）处理中缺乏清洁，这会导致药品之间交叉污染的其他情况。

In response to this letter, provide：

在回复本函时，请提供：

● A comprehensive, independent retrospective assessment of your cleaning effectiveness to evaluate the scope of cross-contamination hazards. Include the identity of residues, other manufacturing equipment that may have been improperly cleaned, and an assessment whether cross-contaminated products may have been released for distribution. The assessment should identify any inadequacies of cleaning procedures and practices, and encompass each piece of manufacturing equipment used to manufacture more than one product.

● 对清洁效果进行全面、独立的回顾性评估，以评估交叉污染危害的范围。包括残留物的鉴别、其他可能未正确清洁的生产设备，以及对交叉污染的药品是否可能已被放行以供流通的评估。评估应确定清洁程序和实践的任何不足之处，并涵盖用于生产多个产品的每台生产设备。

● A corrective action and preventive action（CAPA）plan based on the retrospective assessment of your cleaning program, that includes appropriate remediations to your cleaning processes and practices, and timelines for completion. Provide a detailed summary of vulnerabilities in your process for lifecycle management of equipment cleaning. Describe improvements to your cleaning program, including enhancements to cleaning effectiveness；improved ongoing verification of proper cleaning execution for all products and equipment；and all other needed remediations.

● 一项 CAPA 计划，基于对你公司的清洁和预防性维护计划的回顾性评估，其中包括对工艺和实践的相应整改、频率评估和完成时间表。提供设备清洁和预防性维护生命周期管理流程中漏洞的详细总结。描述对清洁计划的改进，包括提高清洁效果；改进对所有药品和设备清洁正确执行的持续确认；以及所有其他需要的整改措施。

● Appropriate improvements to your cleaning validation program, with special emphasis on incorporating conditions identified as worst case in your drug manufacturing operation. This should include but not be limited to identification and evaluation of all worst-case：

● 适当改进你公司的清洁验证计划，特别强调将确定为药品生产操作中最差情况的条件纳入其中。这应包括但不限于识别和评估所有最差情况：

○ drugs with higher toxicities

○ 具有较高毒性的药物

○ drugs with higher drug potencies

○ 具有较高药物活性的药物

○ drugs of lower solubility in their cleaning solvents

○ 在清洁溶剂中溶解度较低的药物

○ drugs with characteristics that make them difficult to clean

○ 具有难以清洁特性的药物

○ swabbing locations for areas that are most difficult to clean

○ 最难清洁区域的擦拭位置

○ maximum hold times before cleaning

○ 清洁前的最长存放时间

In addition, ensure use of appropriate limits that take into account recovery study results and describe the steps that must be taken in your change management system before introduction of new manufacturing equipment or a new product.

此外，确保使用适当的限度，考虑回收研究结果，描述在引入新生产设备或新产品之前，于变更管理系统中必须采取的步骤。

● A summary of updated standard operating procedures（SOPs）that ensure an appropriate program is in place for verification and validation of cleaning procedures for products, processes, and equipment.

● 更新的标准操作程序（SOP）的汇总，确保制定适当的程序来验证和确认产品、工艺和设备的清洁程序。

● A holistic review of cleaning procedures and the associated cleaning validation strategy for all manufacturing equipment to determine whether similar deficiencies exist.

● 对所有生产设备的清洁程序和相关清洁验证策略，进行整体审查，以确定是否存在类似缺陷。

质量部门

2. Your firm failed to establish an adequate quality unit and the responsibilities and procedures applicable to the quality control unit are not in writing and fully followed（21 CFR 211.22（a）and（d））.

2. 你公司未能建立适当的质量部门，用于质量部门的责任和程序未以书面形式形成，且未得到完全遵守［21 CFR 211.22（a）和（d）］。

Your quality unit（QU）failed to adequately implement the facility's quality function and ensure quality oversight. For example：

你公司的质量部门（QU）未能充分履行设施的质量职能并确保质量监督。例如：

A. Inadequate cleaning procedures

A. 清洁程序不充分

Your procedure to clean（b）（4）lacked sufficient requirements to clean（b）（4）and（b）（4），which had not been cleaned since they were installed more than 14 years ago. Also，your procedure for visually ensuring cleanliness of equipment failed to identify visible contamination.

你公司的清洁（b）（4）程序缺乏清洁（b）（4）和（b）（4）的充分要求，因为它们自 14 年前安装以来一直没有被清洁过。此外，你公司的目视确保设备清洁度的程序未能识别出可见的污染。

In your response，you state that you have improved your standards for visual verification of（b）（4）equipment part cleanliness. The verification is then documented in the equipment cleaning record. You also indicate you have updated your cleaning procedures.

在回复中，你公司声称已经提高了（b）（4）设备零件清洁度的目视标准。然后将确认结果记录在设备清洁记录中。你公司还表明已经更新了清洁程序。

Your response is inadequate. You failed to provide evidence you have implemented CAPA measures to ensure written procedures are sufficiently written and reviewed for adequacy prior to implementing.

你公司的回应不够充分。未能提供证据，证明你公司已实施 CAPA 措施，确保在实施之前充分编写书面程序，并对其进行充分审查。

In response to this letter, provide：

在回复本函时，请提供：

● A comprehensive assessment and remediation plan to ensure your QU is given the authority and resources to effectively function. The assessment should also include, but not be limited to：

● 全面的评估和整改计划，以确保你公司的 QU 获得有效发挥职能的权限和资源。评估还应包括但不限于以下内容：

○ A determination of whether procedures used by your firm are robust and appropriate.

○ 确定你公司使用的程序是否可靠和适当。

○ Provisions for QU oversight throughout your operations to evaluate adherence to appropriate practices.

○ 在整个运营过程中 QU 进行监督的规定，以评估对相应规范的遵守情况。

○ A complete and final review of each batch and its related information before the QU disposition decision.

○ 在 QU 决定处置之前，对每批产品及其相关信息进行完整的、最终的审查。

○ Oversight and approval of investigations and discharging of all other QU duties to ensure identity, strength, quality, and purity of all products

○ 监督和批准调查以及履行所有其他 QU 职责，以确保所有产品的鉴别、规格、质量和纯度。

○ A complete assessment of documentation systems used throughout your manufacturing operations to determine where documentation practices are inadequate. Include a detailed CAPA plan that remedies documentation practices and ensures that you retain complete and accurate records.

○ 对整个生产操作中使用的文档系统进行全面评估，以确定记录实践的不足之处。包括详细的 CAPA 计划，以整改记录实践并确保你公司保存完整且准确的记录。

B. Inadequate Investigations

B. 调查不充分

Your QU failed to adequately investigate extraneous peaks observed in long-term stability samples tested for dissolution by high-performance liquid chromatography（HPLC）. Your investigation dated January 24, 2020, identified varying intensities in the peak response, and noted the peak eluted in some tablets, but not in others from the same batch. You determined the root cause to be interference from excipients used during manufacturing and concluded the peaks do not impact product quality. However, you provided no scientific explanation for this conclusion.

在通过高效液相色谱（HPLC）进行长期稳定性样品溶出度检验时，观察到了杂质峰，对此你公司的 QU 未能进行充分调查。你公司的调查日期为 2020 年 1 月 24 日，确定了峰回应的不同强度，并注意到峰在某些药片中洗脱，但在同批次的其他药片中未洗脱。你公司确定根本原因是生产过程中使用的辅料的干扰，并得出结论这些峰不会影响产品质量。但是，没有对这一结论提供科学解释。

In your response, you describe further investigations that you performed, and conclude the inconsistent peaks were due to insufficient saturation of the filter used to prepare samples.

在回复中，你公司描述了你们进行的进一步调查，并得出结论，峰不一致是由于用于制备样品的过滤器饱和度不足造成的。

Your response is inadequate. You lacked an appropriate assessment of your procedures for investigating discrepancies. Furthermore, you failed to provide evidence that you have implemented sufficient corrective actions or interim controls to ensure investigations contain adequate root cause determination, CAPA, and effectiveness checks.

你公司的回应不够充分。缺乏对调查差异的程序进行适当的评估。此外，你公司未能提供证据证明已实施充分的纠正措施或临时控制措施，以确保调查包含充分的根本原因确定、CAPA 和有效性检查。

In response to this letter, provide:

在回复本函时，请提供：

● A comprehensive assessment of your overall system for investigating deviations, discrepancies, complaints, out-of-specification（OOS）results, and failures. Provide a detailed action plan to remediate this system. Your action plan should include, but not be limited to, significant improvements in investigation competencies, scope determination, root cause evaluation, CAPA effectiveness, quality assurance oversight, and written procedures. Address how your firm will ensure all phases of investigations are appropriately conducted.

● 对整个系统进行全面评估，以调查偏差、差异、投诉、OOS 结果和不合格。提供详细的行动计划来整改该系统。你公司的行动计划应包括但不限于调查能力、范围确定、根本原因评估、CAPA 有效性、质量保证监督和书面程序方面的显著提高。说明你公司将如何确保适当进行所有阶段的调查。

● A detailed, independent assessment of all test methods to ensure they include specific instructions to ensure repeatability and system suitability, are supported by adequate validation（or verification, for United States Pharmacopeia（USP）compendial methods）studies and are appropriate for their intended use. The assessment should also determine whether test methods used in the stability program are stability-indicating. The scope of the assessment should encompass any tests conducted by your firm or its contract laboratories.

● 对所有检验方法进行详细、独立的评估，以确保它们包含具体说明，并确保重复性和系统适应性得到充分验证研究（或被确认，USP 方法），并适合其预期用途。评估还应确定稳定性计划中使用的检验方法是否表明稳定性。评估范围应涵盖你公司或其委托实验室进行的任何检验。

Drug Recall and Production Suspended | 药品召回和暂停生产

We acknowledge your commitment to temporarily suspend production and distribution of certain drugs intended for the U.S. market. In response to this letter, clarify which products you are continuing to manufacture and distribute to the U.S. market, and whether you intend to resume manufacturing drugs for the U.S. market at this facility in the future.

我们知晓，你公司承诺暂时停止生产和流通某些供美国市场上市的药品。在回复本函时，请澄清你公司将继续生产并向美国市场上市哪些产品，以及将来是否打算恢复在该设施为美国市场生产药品。

If you plan to resume manufacturing drugs for the U.S. market, notify this office before resuming your operations.

如果你公司计划恢复为美国市场生产药品，请在恢复运营之前通知本办公室。

We also acknowledge recalls of alprazolam tablets and clobazam tablets manufactured at this facility that remain within expiry.

我们还知晓，你公司设施生产的仍在有效期内的阿普唑仑片剂和氯巴扎姆片剂被召回。

对于脆弱患者存在重大安全风险

警告信编号： MARCS-CMS 655929

签发时间： 2023-8-15；**公示时间：** 2023-8-29

签发机构： 药品质量业务二处（Division of Pharmaceutical Quality Operations II）

公　　司： Gadal Laboratories Inc.

所在国家/地区： 美国

主　　题： cGMP/成品制剂/掺假（cGMP/Finished Pharmaceuticals/Adulterated）

简　　介： 2023年2月，FDA对位于佛罗里达州的药品生产设施进行了检查。在检查中，FDA指出该公司未能按适当的时间间隔，验证和确定物料供应商检验分析的可靠性。举例来说，该公司供应商资质确认文件中辅料的微生物检验仅包括一般性声明，即它应不含病原体，但缺乏有害微生物的任何进一步具体信息。在该公司的回复中提到，一批物料已经送去进行微生物检验，以完成供应商确认。该公司还表示，由于成品制剂中没有发现不合格微生物结果，因此他们并不担心风险。然而，FDA认为该公司的回应不够充分，尤其该物料是肉毒杆菌孢子的已知来源，并且与婴儿肉毒杆菌中毒病例有关。用于婴儿制剂产品的生产时，物料应符合USP和国家处方集（NF）中不含梭菌属的要求。而该公司的儿科产品标明适合用于两岁以下的儿童，因此存在对于脆弱患者的重大安全风险。

本警告信以下部分与本书此前其他警告信内容类似，故略去：前言、质量体系失效（Ineffective Quality Systems）、质量部门授权（Quality Unit Authority）、cGMP顾问推荐（cGMP Consultant Recommended）、结论（Conclusion）。

物料检验

1. Your firm failed to validate and establish the reliability of your component supplier's test analyses at appropriate intervals（21 CFR 211.84（d）（2））.

1. 你公司未能按适当的时间间隔，来验证和确定物料供应商检验分析的可靠性［21 CFR 211.84（d）（2）］。

Your firm failed to qualify your suppliers and adequately test the components used to manufacture your finished drug products, including pediatric over-the-counter（OTC）（b）（4）products. For example,

你公司未能对供应商进行确认，也未能充分检验用于生产成品的原辅料，包括儿科非处方药（OTC）（b）（4）产品。例如，

A.（b）（4）, one of your active ingredients is sourced from an unqualified supplier and was approved for use without establishing the reliability of your suppliers' certificate of analysis（COA）.

A.（b）（4），一种来自未经确认的供应商的原料药，在未建立供应商分析证书（COA）可靠性的情况下被批准使用。

In your response you state that assay testing for（b）（4）has been completed to address the observation, and you will "complete the qualification of this vendor" after receiving the microbiological results.

在回复中，你公司声明已完成（b）（4）的含量检验，以解决观察到的问题，并将在收到微生物结果后"完成该供应商的确认"。

Your response is inadequate. You do not provide a detailed plan demonstrating how you will appropriately validate and establish the reliability of your supplier's COA results. It is unclear if you will validate all tests on the supplier's COA. Additionally, you do not provide the completed assay results for（b）（4）with your response, nor address the other active pharmaceutical ingredient（API）and materials you use to manufacture drug products.

你公司的回应不够充分。没有提供详细的计划，来证明你公司将如何正确验证和建立供应商 COA 结果的可靠性。目前尚不清楚你公司是否会验证供应商 COA 的所有检验。此外，回复中没有提供（b）（4）的完整检测结果，也没有提及你公司用于生产药品的其他原料药（API）和物料。

B. The microbiological testing of（b）（4）excipient in your supplier qualification document only included a general statement that it should be free from pathogens but lacked any further specificity on microorganisms that your firm considers to be objectionable.

B. 你公司供应商资质确认文件中的（b）（4）辅料的微生物检验仅包括一般性声明，即它应不含病原体，但缺乏有害微生物的任何进一步具体信息。

You state in your response that the "last batches of（b）（4）" were sent for microbiological testing to complete vendor qualification, and you do not have concerns because you did not detect out-of-specification（OOS）microbiological results in your finished drug product.

你公司在回复中提到，"最后一批（b）（4）"已经送去进行微生物检验，以完成供应商确认。你公司还声称，由于成品制剂中没有发现不合格（OOS）微生物结果，因此你公司并不担心这一情况。

Your response is inadequate.（b）（4）is a known source of *Clostridium botulinum* spores and has been implicated in cases of infant botulism.（b）（4）used in preparations for infants should meet the requirements for absence of *Clostridium species* per United States Pharmacopeia（USP）, National Formulary（NF）. Your pediatric products（i.e., OTC（b）（4））are labeled for use in children younger than two years of age under a doctor's guidance. It is unclear what specification your firm uses, or microbial identification tests will be performed on each lot, or if any specific objectionable organisms are the focus of testing. You do not propose a revision to this specification or review of other specifications that may be similarly insufficient.

你公司的回应不够充分。（b）（4）是肉毒杆菌孢子的已知来源，并与婴儿肉毒杆菌中毒病例有关。（b）（4）用于婴儿制剂的产品，应符合 USP、国家处方集（NF）中不含梭菌属的要求。你公司的儿科产品［即 OTC（b）（4）］标明适合在医生指导下，用于两岁以下的儿童。目前尚不清楚你公司使用什么质量标准，或者是否对每批产品进行微生物鉴别检验，或者是否有特定的有害微生物作为检验的重点。你公司未建议修订本质量标准，或审查可能同样不充分的其他质量标准。

C. You lacked a specific identity test to detect（b）（4）and（b）（4）in all shipments, containers, and lots of（b）（4）and（b）（4）before use in the manufacturing of drug products. Some of your drug products containing these ingredients are intended for oral use in pediatric populations.

C. 在用于生产之前，你公司缺乏专属鉴别检验，来检测所有货物、容器和批次（b）（4）和（b）（4）中的（b）（4）和（b）（4）药品。你公司的一些药品含有这些原辅料，旨在供儿童口服使用。

Your response includes updated（b）（4）and（b）（4）specifications that incorporate（b）（4）and（b）（4）testing, and states that analysts must sample each lot for（b）（4）and（b）（4）contamination.

你公司的回复包括更新的（b）（4）和（b）（4）质量标准，其中包含（b）（4）和（b）（4）检验，并声称分析人员必须对每批样品进行取样，以检验（b）（4）（b）（4）污染。

Your response is inadequate, you fail to provide sufficient evidence demonstrating adequate identity testing on all containers of all lots of (b)(4) and (b)(4) prior to its use in the manufacture of drug products. Your specifications lack appropriate testing of representative samples of each lot of high-risk components.

你公司的回复不充分，未能提供充分的证据，来证明在用于药品生产之前，对所有批次的（b）（4）和（b）（4）的所有容器进行了充分的鉴别检验。对于每批高风险物料的代表性样品，你公司的质量标准对其缺乏适当的检验。

After the inspection and after a discussion with FDA on June 1, 2023, you stated you would test and provide your (b)(4) or (b)(4) results for your bulk retains of (b)(4) and (b)(4) lots used to manufacture finished drugs. You also provided finished products manufactured with high-risk components that are in distribution and within expiry for analysis of potential (b)(4) or (b)(4) contamination. Based on the provided results, it is unclear what tests were performed to detect (b)(4) or (b)(4). On August 8, 2023, we requested additional information and specified the testing required to ensure potential (b)(4) or (b)(4) contamination is detected.

此次检查后，你公司于 2023 年 6 月 1 日与 FDA 进行了讨论，之后，你们表示，将检验你公司的（b）（4）和（b）（4）半成品留样并提供（b）（4）或（b）（4）结果，这些半成品批次用于生产成品制剂。就使用高风险物料生产的成品（这些成品正在流通且在有效期内），你公司还提供了潜在（b）（4）或（b）（4）污染的分析。根据提供的结果，尚不清楚进行了哪些检验，来检测（b）（4）或（b）（4）。2023 年 8 月 8 日，我们要求提供更多信息，并指定了确保检测到潜在（b）（4）或（b）（4）污染所需的检验。

In the discussion with FDA, you also stated you would test appropriate representative samples of incoming high-risk component lots for potential (b)(4) or (b)(4) contamination prior to manufacturing drug products.

在与 FDA 的讨论中，你公司还表示，将在生产药品之前，针对进场高风险原辅料批次的适当代表性样品，检验其是否存在潜在的（b）（4）或（b）（4）污染。

The use of ingredients contaminated with (b)(4) or (b)(4) has resulted in various lethal poisoning incidents in humans worldwide. See FDA's guidance document *Testing of Glycerin, Propylene Glycol, Maltitol Solution, Hydrogenated Starch Hydrolysate, Sorbitol Solution, and Other High-Risk Drug Components for Diethylene Glycol and Ethylene Glycol* to help you meet the cGMP requirements when manufacturing drugs containing ingredients at risk for（b）（4）or（b）（4）contamination, at https://www.fda.gov/media/167974/download.

使用受（b）（4）或（b）（4）污染的原辅料已导致全世界范围内多起人类致命中毒事件。请参阅 FDA 指南，甘油、丙二醇、麦芽糖醇溶液、氢化淀粉水解物、山梨醇溶液和其他高风险药品原辅料中二甘醇和乙二醇的检验，以帮助你公司在生产含有 DEG 或 EG 污染风险原辅料的药品时，满足 cGMP 要求，请访问网址（略，见上）。

In response to this letter, provide：

在回复本函时，请提供：

● A comprehensive, independent review of your material system to determine whether all suppliers of components, containers, and closures, are each qualified and the materials are assigned appropriate expiration or retest dates. The review should also determine whether incoming material controls are adequate to prevent use of unsuitable components, containers, and closures.

● 对你公司的物料系统进行全面、独立的审查，以确定所有物料、容器和密封件的供应商是否均合格，并为物料指定适当的有效期或复验日期。审查还应确定进场物料控制是否足以防止使用不合适的物料、容器和密封件。

● The remaining（b）（4）and（b）（4）test results for finished products and for retains of high-risk components no later than 30 calendar days from the date of this letter.

● 在收到本函之日后 的 30 个日历日内，提供成品和高风险物料留样的剩余（b）（4）和（b）（4）检验结果。

● A full risk assessment for drug products that are within expiry which contain any ingredient at risk for（b）（4）or（b）（4）contamination（including but not limited to（b）（4））. Take prompt and appropriate actions to determine the safety of all lots of the component（s）and any related drug product that could contain（b）（4）or（b）（4）, including customer notifications and product recalls for any contaminated lots. Identify additional appropriate corrective actions and preventive actions that secure supply chains in the future, including but not limited to ensuring that all incoming raw material lots are from fully qualified manufacturers and free from unsafe impurities. Detail these actions in your response to this letter.

● 对在效期内、含有任何有（b）（4）或（b）（4）污染风险的原辅料〔包括但不限于（b）（4）〕的药品，进行全面风险评估。立即采取适当的措施，就所有批次原辅料，以及可能含有（b）（4）或（b）（4）的所有相关药品，确定其安全性，措施包括针对任何受污染批次的客户通知和产品召回。确定其他适当的纠正和预防措施，以确保未来的供应链安全，包括但不限于确保：所有进场原料批次均来自完全有资质的生产商，并且不含不安全的杂质。在你公司对本函的回复中详细说明这些行动。

● A risk assessment of components qualified and released for use in manufacturing without appropriate testing for purity, strength, and quality.

● 对用于生产的物料进行风险评估，这些物料被判为合格并放行但未对纯度、规格和质量进行适当的检验。

● A review of completion status and adequacy of microbial effectiveness testing studies for your multi-use non-sterile drug products. Based on this review, provide a detailed summary and corrective action and preventive action (CAPA), with timelines for completion for any gaps in your studies.

● 就多用途非无菌药品的微生物效能研究，对其完成状态和充分性进行审查。根据此审查，提供详细的总结以及纠正和预防措施（CAPA），并就研究中所有差距，提供完成的时间表。

● The chemical and microbiological quality control specifications you use to test and determine suitability of each incoming lot of components for use in manufacturing.

● 针对每批用于生产目的的进场物料，用于检验和放行的化学和微生物质控标准。

● A description of how you will test each component lot for conformity with all appropriate specifications for identity, strength, quality, and purity. If you intend to accept any results from your supplier's COA instead of testing each component lot for strength, quality, and purity, specify how you will robustly establish the reliability of your supplier's results through initial validation as well as periodic revalidation. In addition, include a commitment to always conduct at least one specific identity test for each incoming component lot. In the case of (b)(4), (b)(4), and certain additional high-risk components we note that this includes the performance of parts A, B, and C of the United States Pharmacopeia (USP)monograph. Include your standard operating procedure(SOP)that describes this COA validation program.

● 说明如何检验每个批次，确定是否符合有关鉴别、规格、质量和纯度的质量标准。如果你公司打算接受供应商 COA 的结果，而不是检验每个物料批次的规格、质量和纯度，请说明如何进行初始验证和定期再验证，从而稳健地确定供应商结果的可靠性。此外，还应承诺：对于每个进场原辅料批次，至少进行一个专属鉴别检验。对于（b）（4）、（b）（4）和某些其他高风险原辅料，我们注意到这包括 USP 专论 A、B 和 C 部分的性能表现。包括描述此 COA 验证计划的标准操作程序（SOP）。

● A summary of results obtained from testing all components to evaluate the reliability of the COA from each component manufacturer. Include your standard operating procedure（SOP）that describes this COA validation program.

● 一份从所有物料检验获得的结果汇总，以评估每个物料生产商 COA 的可靠性。包括描述此 COA 验证计划的程序。

生产和过程控制

2. Your firm's quality control unit did not review and approve written procedures for production and process control, including any changes to them, designed to ensure that the drug products you manufacture have the identity, strength, quality, and/or purity they purport or are represented to possess（21 CFR 211.100（a））.

2. 你公司的质量控制部门没有审查和批准生产和过程控制（包括对其进行的任何变更）的书面程序，以确保你公司生产的药品具有其声称或陈述的鉴别、规格、质量和（或）纯度［21 CFR 211.100（a）］。

A. You failed to adequately validate your production and process controls. You did not have assurance that you are capable of consistently manufacturing OTC drug products with defined quality attributes. During the inspection, you acknowledged that none of your initial process validation studies（i.e., process performance qualification（PPQ））were complete.

A. 你公司未能充分验证你们的生产和过程控制。无法保证自己有能力，来稳定地生产具有明确质量属性的非处方药产品。在检查过程中，你公司承认你们的初始工艺验证研究［即工艺性能确认（PPQ）］均未完成。

In your response you commit to review all studies in your process validation program. Your response is inadequate. You do not adequately specify how you will evaluate the information collected and compare it to appropriate predetermined protocol requirements. Your validation studies should document whether your process is reproducible, and your products perform as expected using your actual facility, utilities, equipment, personnel, controls, and other variables unique to your operation.

在回复中，你公司承诺审查工艺验证计划中的所有研究。你公司的回应不够充分。没有充分说明如何评估所收集的信息，并将其与适当的预定方案要求进行比较。你公司的验证研究应记录你们的工艺是否可重现，以及你们的产品是否通过使用实际设施、公用系统、设备、人员、控制装置和其他操作上所特有的变量按照预期来进行。

In addition, your response does not address or otherwise include a risk assessment for any marketed drug products manufactured and distributed with a lack of adequate validation.

此外，你公司的回复并未涉及或以其他方式包括对任何在缺乏充分验证的情况下生产和流通的市售药品的风险评估。

Successful process qualification studies are necessary before commercial distribution. Thereafter, ongoing vigilant oversight of process performance and product quality is necessary to ensure you maintain a stable manufacturing operation throughout the product lifecycle.

在商业流通之前，成功的工艺确认研究是必要的。此后，需要对工艺性能和产品质量进行持续的警戒性监督，以确保你公司在整个产品生命周期中保持稳定的生产操作。

We also note you did not define an assay specification range in your process validation report for your（b）（4）finished drug product. Additionally, you did not investigate multiple out-of-specification assay results in your process validation studies for（b）（4）finished drug product.

我们还注意到，你公司没有在（b）（4）成品的工艺验证报告中定义含量质量标准范围。此外，在（b）（4）成品的工艺验证研究中，没有调查多个不符合质量标准的测定结果。

See FDA's guidance document Process Validation: General Principles and Practices for general principles and approaches that FDA considers appropriate elements of process validation at https://www.fda.gov/media/71021/download.

有关 FDA 认为适当的工艺验证要素的一般原则和方法，请参阅 FDA 指南，工艺验证：一般原则和实践，网址（略，见上）。

B. You also failed to adequately qualify and test your（b）（4）system to assure the（b）（4）produced from the system consistently meets chemical and microbiological standards and is suitable for use as a raw material in drug manufacturing or for cleaning.

B. 你公司也未能充分验证和检验（b）（4）系统，以确保该系统生产的（b）（4）始终符合化学和微生物标准，并且适合用作药品生产的原料或用于清洁。

In your response you provide the performance qualification protocol for your（b）（4）system. You state that you will begin performance qualification with an intermittent sampling frequency described in the protocol.

在回复中，你公司提供了（b）（4）系统的性能确认方案。你们声称将以方案中描述的间歇取样频率开始性能确认。

Your response is inadequate. You fail to describe how your（b）（4）system maintenance, cleaning process, seasonal variations, and other actual conditions of use are being considered during your "validation" efforts. You do not provide an adequate justification for the performance qualification sampling frequency, the sampling plan in the protocol, (b)(4) sampling from only one of the (b)(4), and your proposed sampling frequency is not justified for the qualification period.

你公司的回应不够充分。未能描述在"验证"期间，如何考虑你公司的 (b)(4) 系统维护、清洁工艺、季节变化和其他实际使用条件。就性能确认取样频率、方案中的取样计划、(b)(4) 仅从 (b)(4) 之一进行取样，你公司没有提供充分的论证，并且你公司建议的取样频率不适合确认的时期。

You are responsible for ensuring the (b)(4) for equipment cleaning and manufacturing is of suitable quality, reproducibly conforms to (b)(4) standards, and does not potentially contribute microbial contamination to manufacturing processes.

你公司有责任确保设备清洁和生产的 (b)(4) 具有适当的质量，可重现地符合 (b)(4) 标准，并且不会对生产工艺造成潜在的微生物污染。

C. You have not thoroughly validated your cleaning processes and your cleaning verification program does not adequately detect potential cross-contamination between products or microbiological contamination.

C. 你公司没有彻底验证清洁工艺，并且你公司的清洁验证程序没有充分检测产品之间潜在的交叉污染或微生物污染。

In your response, you commit to finalizing your cleaning validation reports and continuing cleaning verification.

在回复中，你公司承诺完成清洁验证报告并继续清洁确认。

Your response is inadequate. Your cleaning validation and verification program does not adequately evaluate the effectiveness of your cleaning procedures. You lack a scientific justification for the sole use of pH testing to verify the effectiveness of your cleaning operations. Your cleaning verification lacks the ability to detect cross-contamination from carryover, microbiological contamination, or traces of cleaning solution.

你公司的回应不够充分。你们的清洁验证和验证计划没有充分评估清洁程序的有效性。就单独使用 pH 检验来确认清洁操作的有效性，你公司缺乏科学论证。你们的清洁确认无法检测残留物、微生物污染或微量清洁溶液造成的交叉污染。

In response to this letter, provide:

在回复本函时，请提供:

- A detailed summary of your validation program for ensuring a state of control throughout the product lifecycle, along with associated procedures. Describe your program for PPQ, and ongoing monitoring of both intra-batch and inter-batch variation to ensure a continuing state of control.

● 用于确保整个产品生命周期控制状态的验证计划的详细汇总以及相关程序。描述你公司的 PPQ 计划，并持续监控批内和批间变化，以确保持续的控制状态。

● A timeline for performing appropriate PPQ for each of your marketed drug products.

● 为你公司的每种上市药品执行适当的 PPQ 的时间表。

● Include your process performance protocol（s）, and written procedures for qualification of equipment and facilities.

● 包括你公司的工艺性能方案以及设备和设施确认的书面程序。

● Provide a detailed program for designing, validating, maintaining, controlling and monitoring each of your manufacturing processes that includes vigilant monitoring of intra-batch and inter-batch variation to ensure an ongoing state of control. Also, include your program for qualification of your equipment and facility.

● 提供用于设计、验证、维护、控制和监测每个生产工艺的详细计划，包括对批内和批间变化进行警戒性的监测，以确保持续的控制状态。另外，请包括设备和设施确认计划。

● A comprehensive remediation plan for the design, control, and maintenance of the（b）（4）system.

● 针对（b）（4）系统的设计、控制和维护的全面整改计划。

● A（b）（4）system validation report. Also include the summary of any improvements made to system design and to the program for ongoing control and maintenance.

●（b）（4）系统验证报告。还包括对系统设计以及持续控制和维护程序所做的任何改进的汇总。

● A comprehensive, independent retrospective assessment of your cleaning effectiveness to evaluate the scope of cross-contamination hazards. Include the identity of residues, other manufacturing equipment that may have been improperly cleaned, and an assessment whether cross-contaminated products may have been released for distribution. The assessment should identify any inadequacies of cleaning procedures and practices and encompass each piece of manufacturing equipment used to manufacture more than one product.

● 对清洁效果进行全面、独立的回顾性评估，以评估交叉污染危害的范围。包括残留物的鉴别、其他可能未正确清洁的生产设备，以及对交叉污染的药品是否可能已被放行以供流通的评估。评估应确定清洁程序和实践的任何不足之处，并涵盖用于生产多个产品的每台生产设备。

● Appropriate improvements to your cleaning validation program, with special emphasis on incorporating conditions identified as worst case in your drug manufacturing operation. This should include but not be limited to identification and evaluation of all worst-case:

● 适当改进你们的清洁验证计划，特别强调将确定为药品生产操作中最差情况的条件纳入其中。这应包括但不限于识别和评估所有最差情况：

○ drugs with higher toxicities

○ 具有较高毒性的药物

○ drugs with higher drug potencies

○ 具有较高药物活性的药物

○ drugs of lower solubility in their cleaning solvents

○ 在清洁溶剂中溶解度较低的药物

○ drugs with characteristics that make them difficult to clean

○ 具有难以清洁特性的药物

○ swabbing locations for areas that are most difficult to clean

○ 最难清洁区域的擦拭位置

○ maximum hold times before cleaning

○ 清洁前的最长存放时间

● A summary of updated SOPs that ensure an appropriate program is in place for verification and validation of cleaning procedures for products, processes, and equipment.

● 更新的标准操作程序汇总，确保制定适当的计划来确认和验证产品、工艺和设备的清洁程序。

质量部门

3. Your firm failed to establish adequate written responsibilities and procedures applicable to the quality control unit and to follow such written procedure（21 CFR 211.22（d））.

3. 你公司未能建立足够的适用于质量控制部门的书面职责和程序，也未能遵循此类书面程序［21 CFR 211.22（d）］。

Your quality unit（QU）did not provide adequate oversight for the manufacture of your OTC drug products. For example，

你公司的质量部门（QU）没有对 OTC 药品的生产提供充分的监督。例如，

A. You replaced the inactive ingredient with another inactive ingredient，without documented scientific rationale and justification，in multiple batches of your OTC drug products. For example，while manufacturing（b）（4）batch（b）（4），you replaced（b）（4）with（b）（4），without appropriate documentation or a product risk assessment. Your firm failed to perform adequate change management. You failed to perform stability studies to show equivalency between the original and substituted ingredient. Additionally，you failed to update the product label to list the actual inactive ingredient used.

A. 你公司在多个批次的 OTC 药品中用另一种辅料替换了原来的辅料，但没有记录科学原理和论证。例如，在生产（b）（4）批次（b）（4）时，你公司将（b）（4）替换为（b）（4），而没有适当的记录支持或进行产品风险评估。你公司未能执行适当的变更管理。未能进行稳定性研究，来证明原始原辅料和替代原辅料之间的等效性。此外，你公司未更新产品标签以列出实际使用的辅料。

You also used multiple specification ranges for the same quality attribute in the same OTC drug product.

你公司还在同一非处方药品中对同一质量属性使用了多个质量标准范围。

In your response you state that you will no longer permit ingredient substitution. You note that your previous substitution with（b）（4）was expected to provide the same emulsifier function. Your response is inadequate. You fail to address if appropriate studies were performed to show equivalency with the substituted ingredient. In addition，your response does not include a risk assessment for any marketed drug products manufactured and distributed with substituted ingredients that lack supportive validation studies.

在回复中，你公司声称将不再允许原辅料替代。你们解释到，之前用（b）（4）进行的替换预期会提供相同的乳化剂功能。你公司的回应不够充分。未能说明是否进行

了适当的研究，以证明其与替代原辅料的等效性。此外，就使用缺乏支持性验证研究的替代原辅料生产和流通的市售药品，你公司的回复未包括相应的风险评估。

Your response also commits to perform a detailed investigation and to scientifically determine the correct specification for your OTC（b）（4）drug product. Your response is inadequate. Your response does not address or otherwise include a risk assessment for the distributed drug products manufactured and tested using different specification ranges. Additionally, your response does not commit to investigate the specification ranges in other drug products.

你公司在回复中还承诺进行详细调查，并科学地确定 OTC（b）（4）药品的正确质量标准。你公司的回应不够充分。对使用不同质量标准范围生产和检验的流通药品，你公司的回复未涉及或以其他方式包括相应的风险评估。此外，你公司的回复未承诺调查其他药品的质量标准范围。

B. Analysts documented original laboratory data on uncontrolled sheets of paper. Analysts also recorded raw data in pencil and changed written data using correction fluid to obscure the original result.

B. 分析人员将原始实验室数据记录在不受控制的纸张上。此外，分析人员还用铅笔记录原始数据，并使用修正液更改书面数据，以掩盖原始结果。

Your response to the use of uncontrolled sheets, correction fluid, and pencil in the Quality Control（QC）laboratory is inadequate. You do not specify the changes in your procedures you intend to implement to address these deficiencies. Additionally, there is no commitment to perform a retrospective review and risk assessment for potentially impacted data obtained for finished drug products manufactured, tested, and distributed.

就对质量控制（QC）实验室使用不受控制的纸张、涂改液和铅笔，你公司的回应是不充分的。没有具体说明你公司打算对程序进行哪些更改来解决这些缺陷。此外，对可能影响已生产、检验和流通的成品制剂的数据，你公司没有承诺进行回顾性审查和风险评估。

An adequate QU overseeing all elements of CGMP is necessary to consistently ensure drug quality. Your firm's quality systems are inadequate. See FDA's guidance document *Quality Systems Approach to Pharmaceutical cGMP Regulations* for help in implementing quality systems and risk management approaches to meet the requirements of cGMP regulations 21 CFR parts 210 and 211, at https://www.fda.gov/media/71023/download.

需要有充分的 QU 来监督所有生产操作，以始终如一地确保药品质量。你公司的质量体系不完善。请参阅 FDA 指南，药品 cGMP 法规的质量体系方法，帮助你公司实施质量体系和风险管理方法，以满足 cGMP 法规 21 CFR 第 210 和 211 部分的要求，网址

（略，见上）。

In response to this letter, provide：

在回复本函时，请提供：

● A comprehensive, independent assessment and remediation plan to ensure your QU is given the authority and resources to effectively function. The assessment should also include, but not be limited to：

● 全面的评估和整改计划，以确保你公司的 QU 获得有效发挥职能的权限和资源。评估还应包括但不限于以下内容：

○ A determination of whether procedures used by your firm are robust and appropriate.

○ 确定你公司使用的程序是否可靠和适当。

○ Provisions for QU oversight throughout your operations to evaluate adherence to appropriate practices.

○ 在整个运营过程中 QU 进行监督的规定，以评估对相应规范的遵守情况。

○ A complete and final review of each batch and its related information before the QU disposition decision.

○ 在 QU 决定处置之前，对每批产品及其相关信息进行完整和最终审查。

○ Oversight and approval of investigations and discharging of all other QU duties to ensure identity, strength, quality, and purity of all products

○ 监督和批准调查以及履行所有其他 QU 职责，以确保所有产品的鉴别、规格、质量和纯度。

Also describe how top management supports quality assurance and reliable operations, including but not limited to timely provision of resources to proactively address emerging manufacturing/quality issues and to assure a continuing state of control.

并说明高层管理人员如何支持质量保证和可靠运营，包括但不限于及时提供资源以主动解决新出现的生产 / 质量问题，并确保持续的控制状态。

● A comprehensive, independent assessment of your overall system for investigating deviations, discrepancies, complaints, OOS results, and failures. Provide a detailed action plan to remediate this system. Your action plan should include, but not be limited to, significant improvements in investigation competencies, scope determination, root cause evaluation, CAPA effectiveness, quality assurance unit oversight, and written procedures.

Address how your firm will ensure all phases of investigations are appropriately conducted.

● 对整个系统进行全面、独立的评估，以调查偏差、差异、投诉、OOS 结果和不合格。提供详细的行动计划，以整改此系统。你公司的行动计划应包括但不限于：调查能力、范围确定、根本原因评估、CAPA 有效性、质量部门监督和书面程序方面的显著提高。说明你公司将如何确保：调查的所有阶段都得到适当实施。

● A comprehensive, independent assessment of your change management system. This assessment should include, but not be limited to, your procedure（s）to ensure changes are justified, reviewed, and approved by your quality assurance unit. Your change management program should also include provisions for determining change effectiveness.

● 对你公司的变更管理系统进行全面、独立的评估。该评估应包括但不限于确保变更经过合理论证、经过质量部门审查和批准的程序。你公司的变更管理计划还应包括确定变更有效性的规定。

● A complete assessment of documentation systems used throughout your manufacturing and laboratory operations to determine where documentation practices are insufficient. Include a detailed CAPA plan that comprehensively remediates your firm's documentation practices to ensure you retain attributable, legible, complete, original, accurate, contemporaneous records throughout your operation.

● 对整个生产和实验室操作中使用的文档系统进行完整评估，以确定记录实践的不足之处。包括一份详细的 CAPA 计划，全面整改你公司的文件记录实践，以确保在整个运营过程中你公司保存可追溯的、清晰的、完整的、原始的、准确的和同步的记录。

● A complete assessment of all drug product batch records that included substituted ingredients without appropriate validation（including stability）studies to support the change. Provide a risk assessment for impacted distributed drug products that are within expiry, and your action plan to address any product quality or patient safety risks for your drug product in U.S. distribution, including potential customer notifications and recalls.

● 对所有药品批记录进行完整评估，其中包括替代原辅料，但没有适当的验证（包括稳定性）研究来支持变更。提供对在有效期内受影响的流通药品的风险评估，以及你公司的行动计划，以解决你公司在美国流通的药品的任何产品质量或患者安全风险，包括潜在的客户通知和召回。

● A comprehensive comparison of all drug product specifications defined in your batch records, process validation studies, annual product reviews, and certificates of analysis. This comparison should record any differences in specification ranges for the quality attribute for the same product. Perform a thorough investigation for any inconsistent drug product specifications and include a detailed CAPA plan to remediate the specifications.

● 对批记录、工艺验证研究、年度产品回顾和分析证书中定义的所有药品质量标准进行全面比较。这种比较应记录同一产品质量属性标准范围内的任何差异。对任何不一致的药品质量标准进行彻底调查，并制定详细的 CAPA 计划来整改质量标准。

9 生产线清场不充分，有导致药品混淆的风险

警告信编号： MARCS-CMS 657886

签发时间： 2023-9-5；**公示时间：** 2023-9-12

签发机构： 药品质量业务一处（Division of Pharmaceutical Quality Operations I）

公　　司： Safecor Health，LLC

所在国家/地区： 美国

主　　题： cGMP/成品制剂/掺假（cGMP/Finished Pharmaceuticals/Adulterated）

简　　介： FDA 于 2023 年 3 月对位于马萨诸塞州的药品生产设施进行了检查。在检查中，FDA 指出该公司存在清场不彻底的问题。调查员观察到泡罩包装机上下有各种不同的胶囊和片剂。尽管批记录表明已执行生产线清理，但在泡罩包装机上和周围观察到的片剂不属于当前批次。包装机械上方和下方存在各种药品的片剂和胶囊，表明生产线清场不充分。这种不充分的生产线清场增加了药品混淆的潜在危险。FDA 将此与历史质量事件进行了关联，指出该公司有产品混淆投诉历史，并根据客户投诉进行了内部召回。在该公司的回复中，他们声称操作员已经接受了重新培训，特别针对生产线清场，并在分包装操作中添加了额外的确认步骤。然而，FDA 认为该公司的批记录缺乏充分的详细信息，无法证明生产线清场已经得到有效执行。

本警告信以下部分与本书此前其他警告信内容类似，故略去：前言、cGMP 顾问推荐（cGMP Consultant Recommended）、结论（Conclusion）。

生产线清场不充分

1. Your firm does not adequately inspect the packaging and labeling facilities immediately

before use to assure that all drug products have been removed from the previous operations（21 CFR 211.130（e））.

1. 在使用前，你公司没有充分检查包装和贴标设施，以确保所有药品均已从之前的操作中清除［21 CFR 211.130（e）］。

Your firm operates as a drug manufacturer and repackager. You failed to implement adequate controls to prevent mix-ups, and to assure that all materials not suitable for subsequent operations have been removed. During the inspection, our investigators observed a variety of different capsules and tablets on and under the Commercial Blister Packing Machine "（b）（4）" while packaging a lot of 81mg chewable aspirin tablets. The tablets observed on and around the blister packaging machine did not belong to the current run, despite your batch records indicating that line clearance was performed. The presence of tablets and capsules of various drugs on and under the packaging machinery indicates that line clearance was not adequately performed. Inadequate line clearance increases the risk for potentially dangerous drug product mix-ups.

你公司是一家药品生产商和分包装商。未能实施充分的控制措施来防止混淆，并确保所有不适合后续操作的物料均已被清除。在检查过程中，在包装一批 81mg 阿司匹林咀嚼片时，我们的调查员观察到商用泡罩包装机"（b）（4）"上下有各种不同的胶囊和片剂。尽管你公司的批记录表明已执行生产清场，但在泡罩包装机上和周围观察到的片剂不属于当前批次。包装机械上方和下方存在各种药品的片剂和胶囊，表明生产线清场不充分。生产线清场不充分，会增加潜在的药品混淆的风险。

Notably, your firm has a history of complaints for product mix-ups and has conducted internal recalls upon customer complaints. For example, a drug product, tacrolimus, you repackaged intended to prevent organ transplant rejection contained a vitamin. In another instance, you labeled enoxaparin 80mg, a drug product intended to prevent blood clots, as 30mg strength. We note that you later recalled the tacrolimus drug product, and that your customer returned the mislabeled enoxaparin syringe.

值得注意的是，你公司有产品混淆投诉历史，并根据客户投诉进行了内部召回。例如，你公司分包装的一种药品他克莫司，旨在预防器官移植排斥，其中含有一粒维生素。在另一个例子中，你公司将依诺肝素 80mg（一种旨在预防血栓的药品）标识为 30mg 剂量。我们注意到，你公司后来召回了他克莫司药品，并且你公司的客户退回了标签错误的依诺肝素注射器。

In your response, you state that your operators have been re-trained on line clearance and you have added an additional verification step to your repackaging operations. However, your batch records lack sufficient detail for performing line clearance.

在回复中，你公司声称你们的操作员已经接受了生产线清场方面的重新培训，并且在分包装操作中，你公司添加了额外的确认步骤。但是，你们的批记录缺乏充分的详细信息，来证明执行了生产线清场。

In response to this letter, provide a comprehensive evaluation of packaging and labeling operations, with emphasis on failure modes, capability, and design sufficiency. Provide an analysis including, but not limited to, all human interactions with equipment before, during, and after(e.g., clearance)operations to identify all points with potential human error.

作为对本函的回应，你公司应对包装和标签操作进行全面评估，重点是失效模式、能力和设计充分性。并提供分析，其中包括但不限于操作之前、期间和之后（例如，清场）与设备的所有人为交互，以识别所有潜在人为错误的点。

设备清洁

2. Your firm failed to establish and follow adequate written procedures for cleaning and maintenance of equipment(21 CFR 211.67(b)).

2. 你公司未能建立并遵循适当的设备清洁和维护书面程序 ［ 21 CFR 211.67(b)］。

Your firm lacks adequate cleaning and maintenance procedures for your equipment used to manufacture your drug products. During the inspection, our investigators observed unidentified white powder residue on non-dedicated product contact surfaces of(b)(4) used for packaging tablets that were held to be in "clean status." Furthermore, your 2019 cleaning requalification summary report utilized a "random selection" of drug products without adequate scientific rationale. Inadequate removal of drug residues from manufacturing equipment during cleaning can lead to cross-contamination of drug products subsequently repackaged on the same pieces of equipment.

你公司缺乏充分的用于生产药品的设备的清洁和维护程序。在检查过程中，在用于包装处于"洁净状态"的片剂的（b）（4）非专用产品接触表面上，我们的调查员观察到了不明的白色粉末残留物。此外，你公司 2019 年的清洁再确认总结报告使用了"随机选择"的药品，没有充分的科学论证。在清洁过程中，生产设备中的药品残留清除不充分，这可能会导致随后在同一设备上分包装的药品发生交叉污染。

In your response, you describe your plan to store the "cleaned"(b)(4)in an enclosed cabinet to prevent "dust-like material" from accumulating on the(b)(4). You also state that you are revising your cleaning standard operating procedure(SOP)to include a mandatory cleaning step prior to use. Your response is inadequate because you did not determine the identity of the white powder residue observed on the "clean"(b)(4). You also did not address the adequacy of your cleaning procedures.

在回复中，你公司描述了将"已清洁的"（b）(4）存放在封闭柜中的计划，以防止"灰尘状物料"积聚在（b）(4）上。你公司还声称正在修订清洁标准操作程序（SOP），以纳入使用前的强制清洁步骤。你公司的回复不充分，因为就在"洁净"（b）(4）上观察到的白色粉末残留物，你公司没有对其进行鉴别。也没有解决清洁程序的充分性问题。

In your response to this letter, provide the following:

在你公司对本函的回复中，请提供以下信息：

● Appropriate improvements to your cleaning validation program, with special emphasis on incorporating conditions identified as worst case in your drug manufacturing operation. This should include but not be limited to identification and evaluation of all worst-case:

● 适当改进你公司的清洁验证计划，特别强调将确定为药品生产操作中最差情况的条件纳入其中。这应包括但不限于识别和评估所有最差情况：

○ drugs with higher toxicities

○ 具有较高毒性的药物

○ drugs with higher drug potencies

○ 具有较高药物活性的药物

○ drugs of lower solubility in their cleaning solvents

○ 在清洁溶剂中溶解度较低的药物

○ drugs with characteristics that make them difficult to clean

○ 具有难以清洁特性的药物

○ swabbing locations for areas that are most difficult to clean

○ 最难清洁区域的擦拭位置

○ maximum hold times before cleaning

○ 清洁前的最长存放时间

In addition, describe the steps that must be taken in your change management system before introduction of new manufacturing equipment or a new product.

此外，描述在引入新生产设备或新产品之前，在变更管理系统中必须采取的步骤。

● A summary of updated SOPs that ensure an appropriate program is in place for verification and validation of cleaning procedures for products, processes, and equipment.

● 更新的标准操作程序汇总，确保制定适当的计划来验证和确认产品、工艺和设备的清洁程序。

物料检验

3. Your firm failed to test samples of each component for conformity with all appropriate written specifications for purity, strength, and quality (21 CFR 211.84 (d)(2)).

3. 你公司未能检验每种原辅料的样品，来确认其是否符合所有适当的纯度、规格和质量书面标准［21 CFR 211.84 (d)(2)］。

You use water as a component in your drug products. Your firm failed to test incoming components including (b)(4) water USP and (b)(4) water used to manufacture prescription drug products to determine their identity, purity, strength, and other appropriate quality attributes. During the inspection, you informed investigators that you purchase (b)(4) water USP for use in the manufacture of Lugol's Solution and only perform a visual inspection of the water, no other tests are performed. Pharmaceutical water must be suitable for its intended use, and routinely and adequately tested to ensure ongoing conformance with appropriate chemical and microbiological attributes.

你公司使用水作为药品的原辅料。未能检验进场原辅料，包括（b）（4）USP 水和（b）（4）用于生产处方药产品的水，以确定其鉴别、纯度、规格和其他适当的质量属性。在检查期间，你公司告知调查员，你们购买了（b）（4）水 USP，用于生产卢戈溶液，并且仅对水进行了目检，未进行其他检验。制药用水必须适合其预期用途，并定期进行充分检验，以确保持续符合相应的化学和微生物属性。

In your response you state that you plan to use a contract laboratory to test your component water. Your response is inadequate because you fail to address the full scope and impact of the cGMP deficiencies as well as the associated risks to drug product quality, including batches already in distribution. Your response also lacked adequate information on how you will evaluate the suitability of the contract laboratory to perform testing of your (b)(4) water.

在回复中，你公司声明，你们计划使用委托实验室，来检验你公司的原辅料水。该回应是不充分的，因为你公司未能解决 cGMP 缺陷的全部方面和影响，以及药品质量的相关风险，包括已经流通的批次。你公司的回复也缺乏关于如何评估委托实验室对（b）（4）水进行检验的适宜性的充分信息。

Without adequate testing, you have no assurance that your purchased water meets minimum microbiological and chemical standards suitable for the manufacture of your drug products.

如果没有充分的检验，你公司无法保证购买的水符合适合药品生产的最低微生物和化学标准。

In response to this letter, provide：

在回复本函时，请提供：

● Your microbiological test results for all lots of Lugol's Solution shipped over the past 2 years including during stability studies.

● 过去两年流通的所有批次卢戈溶液的微生物检验结果，包括稳定性研究期间的数据。

● Your microbiological test results of water samples that you used to qualify your water suppliers.

● 你公司用来进行水供应商资质确认的水样微生物检验结果。

● The chemical and microbiological quality control specifications you use to test and release each incoming lot of components for use in manufacturing to ensure USP monograph specifications and appropriate microbial limits.

● 针对每批用于生产目的的进场物料，用于检验和放行的化学和微生物质控标准，确保 USP 专论质量标准和相应的微生物限度。

● A description of how you will test each component lot for conformity with all appropriate specifications for identity, strength, quality, and purity. If you intend to accept any results from your supplier's COA instead of testing each component lot for strength, quality, and purity, specify how you will robustly establish the reliability of your supplier's results through initial validation as well as periodic re-validation. In addition, include a commitment to always conduct at least one specific identity test for each incoming component lot.

● 说明如何检验每个物料批次，确定是否符合有关鉴别、规格、质量和纯度的标准。如果你公司打算接受供应商 COA 的结果，而不是检验每个物料批次的规格、质量和纯度，请说明如何进行初始验证和定期再验证，从而稳健地确定供应商结果的可靠性。此外，还应承诺：对于每个进场原辅料批次，至少进行一个专属鉴别检验。

质量部门

4. Your firm's quality control unit failed to exercise its responsibility to ensure drug products manufactured are in compliance with cGMP, and meet established specifications for identity, strength, quality, and purity (21 CFR 211.22).

4. 你公司的质量控制部门未能履行职责，以确保所生产的药品符合 cGMP 要求，并符合有关鉴别、规格、质量和纯度的既定质量标准（21 CFR 211.22）。

Your quality unit (QU) failed to ensure adequate document control over paper records. For example, our investigators observed partially completed and torn-up manufacturing records for a lot of children's acetaminophen and stacks of loose printed forms on a desk next to the repackaging area. Manufacturing records are not adequately controlled as they can be accessed and printed by employees with access to your firm's (b)(4) site. The use of correction fluid was also observed to make corrections on the daily cleaning log for solid oral dose packaging equipment. Your documentation practices raise concerns about the integrity, authenticity, and reliability of all your data, and quality of your drug products. Document control is essential to maintaining an adequate quality system.

你公司的质量部门（QU）未能确保对纸质记录进行充分的文件控制。例如，对于一批儿童用对乙酰氨基酚，我们的调查员观察到部分已完成并撕毁的生产记录，以及分包装区旁边桌子上有成堆松散的印制表格。生产记录没有得到充分控制，因为有权访问你公司（b）(4)站点的员工可以访问和打印这些记录。我们还观察到你公司员工使用修正液，对固体口服剂量包装设备的日常清洁台账进行修正。你公司的记录实践引起了对所有数据的可靠性、真实性和可靠性以及药品质量的担忧。对于维持适当的质量体系，文件控制至关重要。

Your response is inadequate because while you indicate that training was provided to employees on good documentation practices, you did not conduct a comprehensive review to determine the extent of data integrity issues at your facility.

你公司的回复不充分，因为虽然你们表示已向员工提供了有关良好记录实践的培训，但没有进行全面审查，来确定你公司设施数据可靠性问题的程度。

In response to this letter, provide：

在回复本函时，请提供：

● A comprehensive assessment and remediation plan to ensure your QU is given the authority and resources to effectively function. The assessment should also include, but not be limited to：

● 全面的评估和整改计划，以确保你公司的 QU 获得有效发挥职能的权限和资源。评估还应包括但不限于以下内容：

○ A determination of whether procedures used by your firm are robust and appropriate.

○ 确定你公司使用的程序是否可靠和适当。

○ Provisions for QU oversight throughout your operations to evaluate adherence to appropriate practices.

○ 在整个运营过程中关于 QU 监督的规定，以评估对相应规范的遵守情况。

○ A complete and final review of each batch and its related information before the QU disposition decision.

○ 在 QU 决定处置之前，对每批产品及其相关信息进行完整和最终审查。

○ Oversight and approval of investigations and discharging of all other QU duties to ensure identity, strength, quality, and purity of all products.

○ 监督和批准调查以及履行所有其他 QU 职责，以确保所有产品的鉴别、规格、质量和纯度。

● A complete assessment of documentation systems used throughout your manufacturing and laboratory operations to determine where documentation practices are insufficient. Include a detailed corrective action and preventive action（CAPA）plan that comprehensively remediates your firm's documentation practices to ensure you retain attributable, legible, complete, original, accurate, and contemporaneous records throughout your operation.

● 对整个生产和实验室操作中使用的文档系统进行完整评估，以确定记录实践的不足之处。包括一份详细的 CAPA 计划，全面整改你公司的文件记录实践，以确保在整个运营过程中保存可追溯的、清晰的、完整的、原始的、准确的和同步的记录。

● A comprehensive assessment and CAPA plan for computer system security and integrity. Include a report that identifies vulnerabilities in design and controls, and appropriate remediations for each of your computer systems.

● 针对计算机系统安全性和可靠性的全面评估和 CAPA 计划。包括一份报告，识别设计和控制中的漏洞，以及针对每个计算机系统的相应整改措施。

第七部分

特殊类型的
警告信

1 FDA 检验发现婴幼儿产品存在微生物污染

警告信编号： MARCS-CMS 639545

签发时间： 2023-1-18；**公示时间：** 2023-1-24

签发机构： 药物审评与研究中心 | CDER（Center for Drug Evaluation and Research | CDER）

公　　司： Buzzagogo，LLC

所在国家 / 地区： 美国

主　　题： cGMP/ 成品制剂 / 掺假 / 未批准的新药（cGMP/Finished Pharmaceuticals/Adulterated/Unapproved New Drug）

简　　介： 在 COVID-19 期间，FDA 对进口物品进行取样检验，其中特别强调对手部消毒产品的监管。目前，这种检验方式也继续成为 FDA 检查的替代工具之一，而本警告信则是基于检验所发出的代表之一。基于 FDA 实验室的分析，发现了该公司婴幼儿产品样品被芽孢杆菌污染的情况。根据 FD&C 法案的规定，这种产品被视为掺假，可能会对儿童造成严重的危害风险。因此，FDA 要求该公司提供所有药品批次的样品检验结果汇总，特别关注微生物质量。如果发现检验结果不合格，FDA 要求该公司提供纠正措施，包括通知客户并启动产品召回程序。

本警告信以下部分与本书此前其他警告信内容类似，故略去：未批准的新药（Unapproved New Drugs）、使用委托生产商（Use of Contract Manufacturers）、结论（Conclusion）。

This letter is to advise you that the United States Food and Drug Administration（FDA）has reviewed your product labeling，including on your website at the Internet address https://buzzagogo.com/，in August 2022 and has determined that you take orders there for the product "Allergy Bee Gone for Kids." The claims on your labeling establish that "Allergy Bee Gone for Kids" is an unapproved new drug under section 505 of the Federal Food，Drug，and

Cosmetic Act（FD&C Act），21 U.S.C. 355.

本函旨在告知你公司，FDA 已于 2022 年 8 月审查了你公司的产品标签，包括你们网站上的产品标签（网址为 https://buzzagogo.com/），并确定你公司于网站上接受产品"Allergy Bee Gone for Kids"的订单。你公司的标签上声明"Allergy Bee Gone for Kids"是一种未经 FD&C 法案第 505 条（即 21 U.S.C. 355）规定批准的新药。

In addition, FDA laboratory analysis determined that a sample of your "Allergy Bee Gone for Kids" product was contaminated with bacillus sp., including *B. cereus*, *B. amyloliquefaciens*, *B. atrophaeus*, and others. This contamination is particularly concerning because "Allergy Bee Gone for Kids" is a nasal swab product and directed for use in young children.

此外，FDA 实验室分析确定，你公司的"Allergy Bee Gone for Kids"产品样品被芽孢杆菌污染，包括蜡样芽孢杆菌、解淀粉假单胞菌和萎缩芽孢杆菌等。这种污染尤其令人担忧，因为"Allergy Bee Gone for Kids"是一种鼻擦拭产品，专门用于幼儿。

The results of the FDA laboratory testing of a batch of Allergy Bee Gone For Kids Nasal Swab Remedy demonstrate that this drug product is adulterated within the meaning of section 501（a）（1）of the FD&C Act, 21 U.S.C. 351（a）（1）, in that it consists in whole or in part of any filthy, putrid, or decomposed substance. Introducing or delivering this product for introduction into interstate commerce violates section 301 of the FD&C Act, 21 U.S.C. 331.

FDA 对一批 Allergy Bee Gone For Kids 鼻擦拭药品的实验室检验结果表明，该药品存在 FD&C 法案第 501（a）（1）条［即 21 U.S.C. 351（a）（1）］规定的掺假行为。因为它全部或部分由肮脏、腐烂或分解的物质组成。引入或交付该产品以引入州际贸易违反了 FD&C 法案第 301 条（21 U.S.C. 331）。

Adulteration Violations | 掺假违规情况

FDA laboratory testing of a batch of Allergy Bee Gone For Kids Nasal Swab Remedy drug product（lot 2006491）found that it contained objectionable microbial contamination. The individual sample results from the tested batch spanned between 50 and 770 colony forming units（CFU）/mL for total aerobic microbial count, and between 5 and 70 CFU/mL for total yeast and mold counts. Therefore, this homeopathic drug product is adulterated under section 501（a）（1）of the FD&C Act, in that it consists in whole or in part of any filthy, putrid, or decomposed substance.

FDA 对一批 Allergy Bee Gone For Kids 鼻擦拭药品（批号 2006491）进行实验室检验，发现其中含有有害微生物污染。检验批次中单个样品的需氧微生物总计数为

50~770 个菌落形成单位（CFU）/ml，酵母和霉菌总计数为 5~70 CFU/ml。因此，根据 FD&C 法案第 501（a）（1）条，该顺势疗法药品被视为掺假，因为它全部或部分由肮脏、腐烂或分解的物质组成。

Microorganisms identified included *Bacillus cereus*, *Bacillus amyloliquefaciens*, *Bacillus atrophaeus* and others. *Bacillus cereus* produces a toxin and is pathogenic to humans. The labeling on your product indicates it may be used for children as young as 1 year old. The high bioburden and presence of objectionable microorganisms in conjunction with the route of administration poses a high risk of harm to patients, including children.

鉴别出的微生物包括蜡样芽孢杆菌、解淀粉芽孢杆菌、萎缩芽孢杆菌等。蜡样芽孢杆菌产生毒素，对人类致病。产品上的标签表明它可用于 1 岁以下的儿童。基于高生物负荷和有害微生物的存在以及给药途径，对包括儿童在内的患者将造成很高的危害风险。

During the FDA teleconference on May 24, 2022, you stated that your drug products are manufactured by a contract manufacturer and that your drug products are tested before release by your contract manufacturer. During the call, you agreed to conduct a voluntary recall of the lot currently in U.S. distribution.

在 2022 年 5 月 24 日的 FDA 电话会议上，你公司声称该药品是由合同生产商生产的，并且这些药品在放行前由你公司的合同生产商进行了检验。在通话过程中，你公司同意自愿召回目前在美国流通的批次。

On June 7, 2022, you conducted a voluntary recall of lot 2006491 of Allergy Bee Gone For Kids Nasal Swab Remedy to the consumer level due to potential microbial contamination, as noted on the following FDA website:

https://www.fda.gov/safety/recalls-market-withdrawals-safety-alerts/buzzagogo-inc-issues-voluntary-nationwide-recall-allergy-bee-gone-kids-nasal-swab-remedy-due

2022 年 6 月 7 日，由于潜在的微生物污染，你公司对批次 2006491 的 Allergy Bee Gone For Kids 鼻擦拭药品进行了自愿召回，该召回达到消费者水平，如以下 FDA 网站所述：网址（略，见上）。

In response to this letter, provide:

在回复本函时，请提供：

● The name and address of the contract organizations you are currently using to manufacture and conduct microbiological analysis on Allergy Bee Gone For Kids Nasal Swab Remedy.

● 就你公司目前用于生产 Allergy Bee Gone For Kids 鼻擦拭药品并进行微生物分析的合同组织，提供其名称和地址。

● A comprehensive, independent assessment of the design and control of your firm's manufacturing operations, with a detailed and thorough review of all microbiological hazards.

● 对你公司生产操作的设计和控制进行全面、独立的评估，并对所有微生物危害进行详细、彻底的审查。

● A detailed risk assessment addressing the hazards posed by distributing drug products with potentially objectionable contamination. Specify actions you will take in response to the risk assessment, such as customer notifications and product recalls.

● 详细的风险评估，针对流通具有潜在不良污染的药品所造成的危害。指定你公司将针对风险评估采取的行动，例如客户通知和产品召回。

● Complete investigations into all batches with potential objectionable microbial contamination (e.g., total counts, identification of bioburden to detect objectionable microbes). The investigations should detail your findings regarding the root causes of the contamination.

● 对所有可能存在有害微生物污染的批次进行全面调查（例如，总计数、微生物负荷鉴别以检测有害微生物）。调查应详细说明有关污染根本原因的调查结果。

● Appropriate microbiological batch release specifications (e.g., total counts, identification of bioburden to detect objectionable microbes) for each of your drug products.

● 每种药品的适当微生物批放行质量标准（例如，总计数、微生物负荷鉴别以检测有害微生物）。

● All microbial test methods used to analyze each of your drug products.

● 用于分析你公司每种药品的所有微生物检验方法。

● A summary of results from testing retain samples of all drug product batches within expected period of marketing. You should test all appropriate quality attributes including, but not limited to, microbiological quality (total counts and identification of bioburden to detect any objectionable microbes) of each batch. If testing yields an OOS result, indicate the corrective actions you will take, including notifying customers and initiating recalls.

● 针对效期内所有药品批次的样品，提供检验结果汇总。你公司应检验每批次所有相应的质量属性，包括但不限于微生物质量（总计数和微生物负荷鉴别，以检测任何有害微生物）。如果检验得出 OOS 结果，请指出你公司将采取的纠正措施，包括通知客户和启动召回。

2 记录审查：显示放行前未对成品进行检验

警告信编号： MARCS-CMS 641099

签发时间： 2023-1-19；**公示时间：** 2023-3-14

签发机构： 药品质量业务一处（Division of Pharmaceutical Quality Operations I）

公　　司： B & J Group

所在国家 / 地区： 美国

主　　题： cGMP/ 成品制剂 / 掺假（cGMP/Finished Pharmaceuticals/ Adulterated）

简　　介： FDA 在 COVID-19 暴发初期就开始发布 704（a）（4）记录要求，并于 2021 年发出了第一封与这些要求相关的警告信。目前，704（a）（4）记录要求继续作为 FDA 检查的一种替代工具，而这封警告信则是其中之一的代表性示例。该警告信的对象是负责灌装 OTC 手部消毒剂药品的合同企业。FDA 发现，在产品放行前，该企业没有对成品进行检验。具体来说，对于 FDA 要求提供在美国生产的每种手部消毒剂产品的分析和微生物检验的成品质量标准和检验方法，该企业表示这是"由客户完成"的，并且"我们只是负责灌装"。然而，FDA 指出这一解释并不充分。因为根据 cGMP 的规定，产品所有者和合同生产设施都有责任，其中包括对药品生产的监督和控制，以确保质量，管理风险，并确立原料、物料和成品制剂的安全性。

本警告信以下部分与本书此前其他警告信内容类似，故略去：前言、作为合同商的责任（Responsibilities as a Contractor）、结论（Conclusion）。

Your facility is registered with the United States Food and Drug Administration（FDA or Agency）as a manufacturer of over-the-counter（OTC）drug products，including consumer antiseptic hand rub drug products (also referred to as consumer hand sanitizers). FDA has reviewed the records you submitted in response to our January 25, 2022 and February 9, 2022 request for records and other information pursuant to section 704 (a)(4) of the Federal Food, Drug, and Cosmetic Act (FD&C Act)(21 U.S.C. 374 (a)(4)) for your facility, B & J Group, FEI 3010096700, at 1001 New Ford Mill Road, Morrisville, Pennsylvania.

你公司的设施已在 FDA 注册为非处方（OTC）药品生产商，包括手部消毒药品（也称为手部消毒剂）。FDA 于 2022 年 1 月 25 日和 2022 年 2 月 9 日提出了记录和其他信息要求，你公司为回应提交了记录，对此 FDA 进行了审查。该要求是基于 FD&C 法案第 704（a）（4）条 [21 U.S.C. 374（a）（4）]。你公司的设施为 B & J Group，FEI 3010096700，地址为美国宾夕法尼亚州（具体地址略，见上）.

This warning letter summarizes significant violations of current Good Manufacturing Practice (cGMP) regulations for finished pharmaceuticals. See Title 21 Code of Federal Regulations (CFR), parts 210 and 211 (21 CFR parts 210 and 211).

本警告信总结了对成品制剂 cGMP 法规的严重违规情况。请参阅联邦法规（CFR）第 21 篇第 210 和 211 部分（21 CFR 第 210 和 211 部分）。

Because your methods, facilities, or controls for manufacturing, processing, packing, or holding drugs as described in your response to our 704 (a)(4) request do not conform to cGMP regulations, your drug products are deemed adulterated within the meaning of section 501 (a)(2)(B) of the FD&C Act (21 U.S.C. 351 (a)(2)(B)).

由于你公司在对我们的 704（a）（4）要求的回复中描述的生产、加工、包装或保存药品的方法、设施或控制措施不符合 cGMP 法规，因此你公司的药品被视为掺假，这是基于 FD&C 法案第 501（a）（2）（B）条 [21 U.S.C. 351（a）（2）（B）]。

704(a)(4)Request for Records and Related cGMP Violations
704（a）（4）记录要求和相关 cGMP 违规行为

Following review of records and other information provided pursuant to section 704 (a)(4) of the FD&C Act, significant violations were observed including, but not limited to, the following：

在审查根据 FD&C 法案第 704（a）(4）条提供的记录和其他信息后，我们发现了重大违规情况，包括但不限于以下内容：

成品检验

1. Your firm failed to have, for each batch of drug product, appropriate laboratory determination of satisfactory conformance to final specifications for the drug product, including the identity and strength of each active ingredient, prior to release, and for each batch of drug product required to be free of objectionable microorganisms, appropriate laboratory testing, as necessary(21 CFR 211.165(a) and(b)).

1. 你公司未能对每批药品进行适当的实验室测定，以确保每批药品符合最终质量标准，包括每种原料药的鉴别和规格，在放行前，要求每批药品不含有害微生物，必要时进行适当的实验室检验［21 CFR 211.165(a) 和（ b)]。

Your response to our request for records and other information under section 704(a) (4) indicated that you are a contract filler of OTC hand sanitizer drug products and that you did not test the finished drug products before release. Specifically, in response to our request to provide the finished product specifications and test methods for both analytical and microbiological tests for each hand sanitizer product manufactured for distribution in the United States, you stated that this is "Done by customer" and "We just filled the bottles."

你公司对我们根据第 704(a)(4) 条要求提供记录和其他信息的回复表明，你公司是 OTC 手部消毒剂的合同灌装商，且你公司在放行前没有对成品进行检验。具体来说，为了回应我们要求提供在美国生产的每种手部消毒剂产品的分析和微生物检验的成品质量标准和检验方法，你公司表示这是"由客户完成"的并且"我们只是灌装"。

Owners and contract manufacturing facilities are both responsible for cGMPs, which includes the implementation of oversight and controls over the manufacture of drugs to ensure quality, including managing the risk of and establishing the safety of raw materials, materials used in the manufacturing of drugs, and finished drug products.

产品所有者和合同生产承包商均对 cGMP 负责，其中包括对药品生产实施监督和控制以确保质量，包括管理风险，确立原料、药品生产中所用物料和成品制剂的安全性。

Full release testing, including for identity, strength, and impurities, must be performed prior to drug release and distribution. Without adequate testing, there is no scientific evidence to assure that your drug products conform to appropriate specifications before release.

在药品放行和流通之前必须进行全面的放行检验，包括鉴别、规格和杂质。如果没有充分的检验，就没有科学证据，来确保你公司的药品在放行前符合相应的质量标准。

In response to this letter, provide:

在回复本函时，请提供：

（略）

此处与 FDA 发给 Dunagin Pharmaceuticals Inc. dba Massco Dental 的警告信（编号：MARCS-CMS 644335，即 "3 与非药用产品的共线生产问题"）中有关实验室检验回应的要求类似，故略去。

物料检验

2. Your firm failed to conduct at least one test to verify the identity of each component of a drug product(21 CFR 211.84(d)(1)).

2. 你公司未进行至少一项检验来验证药品每种原辅料的鉴别 [21 CFR 211.84（d）（1）]。

Based on the records and information you provided, you did not demonstrate adequate testing of the identity of incoming components used in the manufacture of your drug products. Specifically, your response stated that raw material identity testing for each lot of each component is "Not Applicable," testing of ethanol or isopropyl alcohol and methanol is "Done by each customer," and testing the potency(assay)of ethanol or isopropyl alcohol used for hand sanitizer is "Not Applicable".

根据你公司提供的记录和信息，没有证明对药品生产中使用的原辅料进行了充分的检验。具体来说，你公司的回复指出，每个原辅料每个批次的原料鉴别检验 "不适用"，乙醇或异丙醇和甲醇的检验 "由每个客户完成"，并且用于手部消毒剂的乙醇或异丙醇活性（测定）检验为 "不适用"。

You manufacture multiple drugs that contain ethanol. The use of ethanol contaminated with methanol has resulted in various lethal poisoning incidents in humans worldwide. See FDA's guidance document *Policy for Testing of Alcohol(Ethanol) and Isopropyl Alcohol for Methanol, Including During the Public Health Emergency(COVID-19)* at: https://www.fda.gov/media/145262/download.

你公司生产多种含有乙醇的药品。在全球范围，使用被甲醇污染的乙醇已导致内多起人类致命中毒事件。请参阅 FDA 指南，酒精（乙醇）和异丙醇检验政策——包括在公共卫生紧急事件（COVID-19）期间的要求，以帮助你公司在生产含有乙醇的药物时满足 cGMP 要求，网址（略，见上）。

In response to this letter, provide:

在回复本函时，请提供：

● A description of how you will test each component lot for conformity with all appropriate specifications for identity, strength, quality, and purity. If you intend to accept any results from your supplier's Certificates of Analysis（COA）instead of testing each component lot for strength, quality, and purity, specify how you will robustly establish the reliability of your supplier's results through initial validation as well as periodic re-validation. In addition, include a commitment to always conduct at least one specific identity test for each incoming component lot.

● 描述如何检验每个原辅料批次是否符合所有适当的鉴别、规格、质量和纯度标准。如果你公司打算接受供应商分析证书（COA）的任何结果，而不是检验每个原辅料批次的规格、质量和纯度，请指定如何通过初步验证和定期再验证来稳健地确保供应商结果的可靠性。此外，还应承诺始终对每个进场批次至少进行一次专属鉴别检验。

未能提供批记录

3. Your firm failed to establish written procedures for production and process control designed to assure that the drug products you manufacture have the identity, strength, quality, and purity they purport or are represented to possess（21 CFR 211.100（a））.

3. 你公司未能建立书面的生产和过程控制程序，旨在确保生产的药品具有其声称拥有的鉴别、规格、质量和纯度［21 CFR 211.100（a）］。

Based on the information you provided, you did not demonstrate that your manufacturing processes are reproducible and controlled to yield a product of uniform character and quality. For example, we asked you to provide a copy of the most recent, completed batch production record for each hand sanitizer product manufactured. You stated in your response that batch production records are "Maintained by customers."

根据你公司提供的信息，没有证明你们的生产工艺是可重现且受控的，无法生产出具有统一特性和质量的产品。例如，我们要求你公司提供生产的每种手部消毒剂产品的最新、完整的批生产记录的副本。你公司在回复中表示批生产记录"由客户维护"。

In response to this letter, provide：

在回复本函时，请提供：

● A complete assessment of documentation systems used throughout your manufacturing and laboratory operations to determine where documentation practices are insufficient.

Include a detailed corrective action and preventive action (CAPA)plan that comprehensively remediates your firm's documentation practices to ensure you retain attributable, legible, complete, original, accurate, contemporaneous records throughout your operation.

● 对整个生产和实验室操作中使用的文档系统进行全面评估，以确定记录实践的不足之处。包括详细的纠正和预防措施（CAPA）计划，全面整改你公司的文件记录实践，以确保在整个运营过程中保存可追溯、清晰、完整、原始、准确、同步的记录。

● A list of all batches of any hand sanitizer drug products distributed by your firm, and a full reconciliation of all material you distributed.

● 你公司流通的手部消毒剂药品所有批次的清单，以及你公司流通的所有物料的完整物料平衡信息。

3 记录审查：显示稳定性数据不充分

警告信编号： MARCS-CMS 633084

签发时间： 2023-1-30；**公示时间：** 2023-1-31

签发机构： 药物审评与研究中心 | CDER（Center for Drug Evaluation and Research | CDER）

公　　司： Fei Fah Medical Manufacturing Pte. Ltd.

所在国家 / 地区： 新加坡

主　　题： cGMP/ 成品制剂 / 掺假（cGMP/Finished Pharmaceuticals/ Adulterated）

简　　介： 该公司已向 FDA 注册为非处方药品制造商。2021 年 5 月，FDA 根据 FD&C 法案第 704（a）(4) 条的记录要求审查了该公司的设施。审查结果显示，该公司缺乏足够的稳定性数据支持其药品的有效期。此外，该公司还未采用稳定性指示方法来确立质量标准或检验杂质、降解物。FDA 指出，该公司的回应并不充分，因为他们只提供了一批药品的两年稳定性数据。此外，该公司计划进行稳定性检验的批次数量不足。除此之外，该公司也未承诺使用稳定性指示方法，来检验稳定性批次中的杂质和降解物，并且还未评估已流通批次中的杂质和降解物。

本警告信以下部分与本书此前其他警告信内容类似，故略去：前言、结论（Conclusion）。

稳定性研究

1. Your firm failed to establish and follow an adequate written testing program designed to assess the stability characteristics of drug products and to use results of stability testing to determine appropriate storage conditions and expiration dates（21 CFR 211.166（a））.

1. 你公司未能遵循适当的书面检验程序，以评估药品的稳定性特征；未能使用稳定性检验结果，来确定适当的储存条件和有效期［21 CFR 211.166（a）］。

Based on the records and information you provided, your firm does not have adequate stability data to support the（b）（4）expiration date assigned to your（b）（4）drug product packaged in（b）（4）g and（b）（4）g glass and plastic containers, respectively. Furthermore, you have not established specifications or tested for impurities or degradants using stability indicating methods.

你公司提供的记录和信息显示，你们没有充分的稳定性数据来支持指定给你公司包装的（b）（4）药品效期，这些产品包装在玻璃和塑料容器中。此外，你公司未使用稳定性指示方法，来确立质量标准或检验杂质、降解物。

Your response is inadequate. You only provided two years of stability data for one batch of（b）（4）drug product. Further, the number of batches you intend to place on stability is insufficient. Also, you did not commit to testing your stability batches for impurities and degradants using stability indicating methods, nor evaluate impurities and degradants in distributed batches.

你公司的回应不够充分。仅提供了一批（b）（4）药品的两年稳定性数据。此外，你公司打算进行稳定性检验的批次数量不充分。没有承诺使用稳定性指示方法，来检验稳定性批次中的杂质和降解物，也没有评估已流通批次中的杂质和降解物。

In response to this letter, provide：

在回复本函时，请提供：

（略）

此处与 FDA 发给 Cosmobeauti Laboratories & Manufacturing Inc. 的警告信（编号：MARCS-CMS 657682，即 "12 批生产记录存在倒记问题"）中有关稳定性研究的回应要求部分的内容类似，故略去。

检验方法

2. Your firm failed to establish laboratory controls that include scientifically sound and appropriate specifications, standards, sampling plans, and test procedures designed to assure that components, drug product containers, closures, in-process materials, labeling, and drug products conform to appropriate standards of identity, strength, quality, and purity（21 CFR 211.160（b））.

2. 你公司未能建立实验室控制措施，其中包括科学合理且适当的质量规定、标准、取样计划和检验程序，以确保物料、药品容器、密封件、中间体、标签和药品符合相关规定，即鉴别、规格、质量和纯度的标准［21 CFR 211.160（b）］。

Based on the records and information you provided, your firm failed to demonstrate the suitability of test methods for（b）（4）drug product and its active pharmaceutical ingredients（API）and to establish appropriate release specifications for impurities. For example, your test method for assay of（b）（4）and（b）（4）APIs in（b）（4）finished product was not validated.

根据你公司提供的记录和信息，未能证明（b）（4）药品及其原料药（API）检验方法的适用性，也未能建立适当的杂质放行质量标准。例如，你公司对（b）（4）成品中（b）（4）和（b）（4）API 进行测定的检验方法未经验证。

Your response is inadequate. Even after repeated requests you failed to provide a validation or qualification report for assay of（b）（4）and（b）（4）. In the absence of a method validation or qualification report from you or your contract testing laboratory, there is no assurance that your test method is suitable. In addition, you failed to establish specifications for impurities in your drug product and commit to testing for impurities at release.

你公司的回应不够充分。即使在多次要求后，仍未能提供（b）（4）和（b）（4）测定的验证或确认报告。如果你公司或你们的委托检验实验室无法提供方法验证或确认报告，则无法保证该检验方法是合适的。此外，你公司未制定药品中杂质的质量标准并承诺在放行时检测杂质。

Drug product batches must be tested for identity, strength, quality, and purity prior to release. Testing is an essential part of ensuring that the drug products you manufacture conform to all predetermined quality attributes and are appropriate for their intended use, including impurities. Without adequate testing, you lack basic data to support that each drug product batch conforms to appropriate specifications before release.

药品批次在放行前，必须进行鉴别、规格、质量和纯度检验。为确保你公司生产的药品符合所有预先确定的质量属性并适合其预期用途（包括杂质），检验是重要组成部分。如果没有充分的检验，你公司就缺乏基本数据，来确保每个药品批次在放行前符合相应的质量标准。

For general principles and approaches that FDA considers appropriate elements of method validation, see FDA's guidance document, *Analytical Procedures and Methods Validation for Drugs and Biologics* at: https://www.fda.gov/media/87801/download.

有关 FDA 认为适当的方法验证要素的一般原则和方法，请参阅 FDA 指南，药品和生物制品的分析程序和方法验证，网址（略，见上）。

In response to this letter, provide:

在回复本函时，请提供：

● A comprehensive, independent assessment of your laboratory practices, procedures, methods, equipment, documentation, and analyst competencies. Based on this review, provide a detailed plan to remediate and evaluate the effectiveness of your laboratory system.

● 对你公司的实验室实践、程序、方法、设备、文件和分析人员能力进行全面、独立的评估。在此审查的基础上，提供一个详细的计划来整改和评估实验室系统的有效性。

● A list of chemical and microbial specifications, including test methods, used to analyze each lot of your drug products before a lot disposition decision.

● 在做出批处置决定之前，用于分析每批药品的化学和微生物质量标准（包括检验方法）的清单。

○ An action plan and timelines for conducting full chemical and microbiological testing of retain samples to determine the quality of all batches of drug product distributed to the United States that are within expiry as of the date of this letter.

○ 行动计划和时间表：对留样进行全面的化学和微生物检验，对于流通给美国的所有效期内（本函发出之日计）药品批次，确定其质量。

○ A summary of all results obtained from testing retain samples from each batch. If such testing reveals substandard quality drug products, take rapid corrective actions, such as notifying customers and product recalls.

○ 所有批次的留样检验汇总。如果此类检验表明药品质量不合格，请迅速采取整改措施，例如通知客户和产品召回。

● A method validation report for assay of（b）（4）and（b）（4）APIs in your（b）（4）drug product and evidence that the test method is suitable for its intended use.

● （b）（4）药品中（b）（4）和（b）（4）API 测定的方法验证报告，以及检验方法适合其预期用途的证据。

物料检验

3. Your firm failed to conduct at least one test to verify the identity of each component of a drug product. Your firm also failed to validate and establish the reliability of your component supplier's test analyses at appropriate intervals（21 CFR 211.84（d）（1）and 211.84（d）（2））.

3. 你公司未进行至少一项检验来确认药品中每种原辅料的鉴别。也未能在适当的时间间隔内，验证和确定你公司的物料供应商检验分析的可靠性［21 CFR 211.84（d）（1）和（2）］。

Based on the records and information you provided, you did not provide sufficient evidence demonstrating that you adequately test all your incoming raw materials, including API and other components. You relied on your supplier's certificate of analysis（COA）in lieu of testing each component lot for purity, strength, identity, and quality. You also did not establish a supplier qualification program to assess（i.e., initially and periodically）the reliability of your suppliers' test results for these attributes.

根据你公司提供的记录和信息，没有充分的证据证明你公司对所有进场原料（包括 API 和其他原辅料）进行了充分检验。你公司依靠供应商的分析证书（COA），来代替检验每个原辅料批次的纯度、规格、鉴别和质量。你公司也没有建立供应商确认计划（即初始和定期确认），来评估这些属性检验结果的可靠性。

Your response is inadequate. You stated that samples of all raw materials, including excipients, will be sent to an external laboratory for analysis. It is not clear that you committed to conducting full testing for each lot of raw material and you did not describe a plan for supplier qualification.

你公司的回应不够充分。你们表示，包括辅料在内的所有原料的样品将被送往外部实验室进行分析。目前尚不清楚，你公司是否承诺对每批原料进行全面检验，也没有描述供应商确认计划。

In response to this letter, provide:

在回复本函时，请提供：

● A comprehensive review of your material system to determine whether all suppliers of components, containers, and closures, are each qualified and the materials are assigned appropriate expiration or retest dates. The review should also determine whether incoming material controls are adequate to prevent use of unsuitable components, containers, and closures.

● 对你公司的物料系统进行全面、独立的审查，以确定所有物料、容器和密封件的供应商是否均有资质，并为物料指定适当的有效期或复验期。审查还应确定进场物料控制是否足以防止使用不适当的物料、容器和密封件。

● The chemical and microbiological quality control specifications you use to test and release each incoming lot of components for use in manufacturing.

● 针对每批用于生产目的的进场物料，用于检验和放行的化学和微生物质控标准。

● A description of how you will test each component lot for conformity with all appropriate specifications for identity, strength, quality, and purity. If you intend to accept any results from your supplier's COA instead of testing each component lot for strength, quality, and purity, specify how you will robustly establish the reliability of your supplier's results through initial validation as well as periodic re-validation. In addition, include a commitment to always conduct at least one specific identity test for each incoming component lot.

● 说明如何检验每个批次，确定其是否符合有关鉴别、规格、质量和纯度的标准。如果你公司打算接受供应商 COA 的结果，而不是检验每个物料批次的规格、质量和纯度，请说明如何进行初始验证和定期再验证，从而稳健地确定供应商结果的可靠性。此外，还应承诺：对于每个进场原辅料批次，至少进行一个专属鉴别检验。

● A summary of your program for qualifying and overseeing contract facilities involved in any cGMP activities.

● 你公司对参与任何 cGMP 活动的外包设施进行确认和监督计划的汇总。

Repeat Observations | 重复观察到的违规行为

While the violations summarized above were based on FDA's recent review of your response to our records request and Observation Letter, FDA also reviewed data from past inspections of your facility. In inspections conducted in March 2013 and December 2015, FDA noted similar cGMP findings regarding the lack of adequate stability data to support a（b）（4）expiry of your（b）（4）drug product. These repeated failures demonstrate that executive management oversight and control over the manufacture of drugs is inadequate.

虽然上述违规情况是基于 FDA 最近对你公司基于我们的记录要求和观察函的回复进行的审查，但 FDA 还审查了你公司设施过去检查的数据。在 2013 年 3 月和 2015 年 12 月进行的检查中，FDA 注意到类似的 cGMP 调查结果，即缺乏充分的稳定性数据来支持（b）（4）药品的（b）（4）效期。这些重复的不合格表明，行政管理层对药品生产的监督和控制并不充分。

4 记录审查：显示未进行原料鉴别检验

警告信编号： MARCS-CMS 669407

签发时间： 2023-11-15；**公示时间：** 2023-11-21

签发机构： 药物审评与研究中心 | CDER（Center for Drug Evaluation and Research | CDER）

公　　司： Xiamen Wally Bath Manufacture Co., Ltd.

所在国家 / 地区： 中国

主　　题： cGMP/ 成品制剂 / 掺假（cGMP/Finished Pharmaceuticals/Adulterated）

简　　介： 这家位于中国厦门的工厂已在美国 FDA 注册为非处方药品制造商。根据 FD&C 法案第 704（a）（4）条，FDA 于 2022 年提出了记录和其他信息的要求。经审查发现，根据其提供的记录和信息，该公司无法证明检验了用于生产药品的进场原料，以确定其鉴别。具体来说，当 FDA 询问其是否进行原料鉴别检验时，该公司表示通过检查供应商的分析证书来鉴别原料。此外，没有对所有进场批次的乙醇进行甲醇检测，也没有提供公司用于生产药品的乙醇中允许的甲醇含量的质量标准，对此该公司表示依赖供应商的分析证书。此外，FDA 还发现该公司在成品检验和稳定性研究方面存在重大缺陷。

本警告信以下部分与本书此前其他警告信内容类似，故略去：前言、cGMP 顾问推荐（cGMP Consultant Recommended）、结论（Conclusion）。

物料检验

1. Your firm failed to conduct at least one test to verify the identity of each component of a drug product（21 CFR 211.84（d）（1））.

1. 你公司未进行至少一项检验来验证药品中每种原辅料的鉴别［21 CFR 211.84（d）（1）］。

Based on the records and information you provided, you have not demonstrated that you are testing incoming raw materials, used to manufacture your drug products, to determine their identity. Specifically, when we requested whether you perform raw material identity testing, you stated that you identify the raw material by checking the certificate of analysis (COA) from the supplier. In addition, you did not test for methanol on all incoming lots of ethanol or provide your firm's specification (or limit) for allowable methanol content in ethanol used to manufacture your drug products, such as ROADPRO Hand Sanitizer, for distribution in the United States. You stated you rely on the supplier's COA.

根据你公司提供的记录和信息，不能证明你公司检验了用于生产药品的进场原料，以确定其鉴别。具体来说，当我们询问你公司是否进行原料鉴别检验时，你们表示通过检查供应商的分析证书（COA）来鉴别原料。此外，你公司没有对所有进场批次的乙醇进行甲醇检测，也没有提供你公司用于生产药品（例如在美国流通的 ROADPRO 手部消毒剂）的乙醇中允许的甲醇含量的质量标准（或限度）。说明你公司依赖供应商的 COA。

Component testing is fundamental to quality. Without adequate testing, you do not have scientific evidence that your raw materials conform to appropriate specifications before use in the manufacture of your drug products.

物料检验是质量的基础。如果没有充分的检验，你公司就没有科学证据，来证明你们的原料在用于药品生产之前符合相应的质量标准。

You manufacture drugs that contain ethanol. The use of ethanol contaminated with methanol has resulted in various lethal poisoning incidents in humans worldwide. See FDA's guidance document *Policy for Testing of Alcohol (Ethanol) and Isopropyl Alcohol for Methanol* at: https://www.fda.gov/media/173005/download.

你公司生产含有乙醇的药品。在全球范围内，使用被甲醇污染的乙醇已导致多起人类致命中毒事件。请参阅 FDA 指南，酒精（乙醇）和异丙醇检验政策——包括在公共卫生紧急事件（COVID-19）期间的要求，网址（略，见上）。

In response to this letter, provide the following for all drug products imported to the United States prior to and after our 704 (a)(4) request:

作为对本函的回应，针对我们 704（a）（4）要求之前和之后进口到美国的所有药品，请提供以下信息:

● The chemical and microbiological quality control specifications you use to test and release each incoming lot of component for use in manufacturing.

● 针对每批用于生产目的的进场物料，用于检验和放行的化学和微生物质控标准。

● A description of how you will test each component lot for conformity with all appropriate specifications for identity, strength, quality, and purity. If you intend to accept any results from your supplier's COA instead of testing each component lot for strength, quality, and purity, specify how you will robustly establish the reliability of your supplier's results through initial validation as well as periodic re-validation. In addition, include a commitment to always conduct at least one specific identity test for each incoming component lot.

● 说明如何检验每个批次，确定其是否符合有关鉴别、规格、质量和纯度的标准。如果你公司打算接受供应商 COA 的结果，而不是检验每个物料批次的规格、质量和纯度，请说明如何进行初始验证和定期再验证，从而稳健地确定供应商结果的可靠性。此外，还应承诺：对于每个进场原辅料批次，至少进行一个专属鉴别检验。

● A summary of results obtained from testing all components to evaluate the reliability of the COA from each component manufacturer. Include your standard operating procedure (SOP) that describes this COA validation program.

● 一份从所有物料检验获得的结果汇总，以评估每个物料生产商的 COA 的可靠性。包括描述此 COA 验证计划的程序。

● A summary of your program for qualifying and overseeing contract facilities that test the drug products you manufacture.

● 你公司对检验生产药品的外包设施进行确认和监督计划的汇总。

成品检验

2. Your firm failed to have, for each batch of drug product, appropriate laboratory determination of satisfactory conformance to final specifications for the drug product, including the identity and strength of each active ingredient, prior to release (21 CFR 211.165 (a)).

2. 你公司未能在放行前对每批药品进行适当的实验室测定，以确保其符合药品的最终质量标准，包括每种原料药的鉴别和规格［21 CFR 211.165（a）］。

Based on the records and information you provided, you did not demonstrate that you adequately test your OTC finished drug products prior to release for distribution to the United States. Specifically, in response to our request to provide release specifications of

U.S. products and the test methods used to evaluate them, you provided finished product specifications that included only test results from "(b)(4)" with microbial specifications.

根据你公司提供的记录和信息，没有证明你公司在向美国流通之前对非处方药成品进行了充分检验。具体来说，为了回应我们提供美国产品的放行质量标准和用于评估它们的检验方法的要求，你公司提供了成品质量标准，其中仅包括"（b）（4）"的检验结果和微生物质量标准。

Full release testing, including identity, strength, and impurities, must be performed prior to drug product release and distribution. Without adequate testing, there is no scientific evidence to assure that your drug products conform to appropriate specifications before release.

在药品放行和流通之前必须进行全面的放行检验，包括鉴别、规格和杂质。如果没有充分的检验，就没有科学证据，来确保你公司的药品在放行前符合相应的质量标准。

In response to this letter, provide the following for all drug products imported to the United States prior to and after our 704(a)(4) request：

作为对本函的回应，针对我们 704（a）（4） 要求之前和之后进口到美国的所有药品，请提供以下信息：

● A list of chemical and microbial specifications, including test methods, used to analyze each batch of your drug products before a batch disposition decision.

● 在做出批处置决定之前，用于分析每批药品的化学和微生物质量标准（包括检验方法）的清单。

○ An action plan and timelines for conducting full chemical and microbiological testing of retain samples to determine the quality of all batches of drug product distributed to the United States that are within expiry as of the date of this letter.

○ 行动计划和时间表：对留样进行全面的化学和微生物检验，对于流通到美国的所有效期内（本函发出之日计）的药品批次，确定其质量。

○ A summary of all results obtained from testing retain samples from each batch. If such testing reveals substandard quality drug products, take rapid corrective actions, such as notifying customers and product recalls.

○ 每批样品留样检验结果的汇总。如果此类检验发现药品质量不合格，请迅速采取纠正措施，例如通知客户和产品召回。

稳定性研究

3. Your firm failed to establish and follow an adequate written testing program designed to assess the stability characteristics of drug products and to use results of stability testing to determine appropriate storage conditions and expiration dates（21 CFR 211.166（a））.

3. 你公司未能遵循适当的书面检验程序，以评估药品的稳定性特征；未能使用稳定性检验结果，来确定适当的储存条件和有效期 [21 CFR 211.166（a）]。

You did not provide adequate stability data to demonstrate that the chemical properties of your drug products remain acceptable throughout the labeled expiry period. Specifically, you reported that the expiry period assigned and applied to your hand sanitizer products is（b）（4）. However, you provided only 13-week stability data to support the（b）（4）expiry period.

你公司没有提供充分的稳定性数据，来证明药品的化学性质在标签有效期内仍然可以接受。具体来说，你公司报告指定并适用于手部消毒剂产品的有效期是（b）（4）。但是，你公司仅提供了 13 周的稳定性数据，来支持（b）（4）有效期。

In addition, your stability data does not include testing for identity and strength. Therefore, the data does not demonstrate that the drug's active ingredient is stable throughout its shelf life. Also, the information provided does not include microbiological stability data.

此外，你公司的稳定性数据不包括鉴别和规格检验。因此，这些数据并不能证明该药品的原料药在其整个有效期内是稳定的。此外，所提供的信息不包括微生物稳定性数据。

Without appropriate stability studies, you do not have scientific evidence to support whether your drug products meet established specifications and retain their quality attributes through their labeled expiry.

如果没有适当的稳定性研究，你公司就没有科学证据，来支持你们的药品是否符合既定质量标准并在标签有效期内保持其质量属性。

In response to this letter, provide the following for all drug products imported to the United States prior to and after our 704（a）（4）request:

作为对本函的回应，请针对我们 704（a）（4）要求之前和之后进口到美国的所有药品提供以下信息：

● A comprehensive, independent assessment and CAPA plan to ensure the adequacy of your stability program. Your remediated program should include, but not be limited to:

● 全面、独立的评估和 CAPA 计划，以确保你公司的稳定性计划是充分的。整改计划应包括但不限于以下内容：

○ Stability indicating methods

○ 稳定性指示方法

○ Stability studies for each drug product in its marketed container–closure system before distribution is permitted

○ 在流通之前，对市售容器密闭系统中的每种药品进行稳定性研究

○ An ongoing program in which representative batches of each product are added each year to the program to determine if the shelf–life claim remains valid

○ 持续进行的计划，每年将每种产品的代表性批次添加到其中，以确定有效期声明是否仍然有效

○ Detailed definition of the specific attributes to be tested at each station（timepoint）

○ 每个点（时间点）要检验的特定属性的详细定义

● All procedures that describe these and other elements of your remediated stability program.

● 针对稳定性整改计划的这些以及其他元素，其所有相关的描述性程序。

5 未能提供信息

警告信编号： MARCS-CMS 663495

签发时间： 2023-8-3；**公示时间：** 2023-8-8

签发机构： 药物审评与研究中心 | CDER（Center for Drug Evaluation and Research | CDER）

公　　司： Sangleaf Pharm., Co. Ltd.

所在国家 / 地区： 韩国

主　　题： 未能提供信息（Failure to Provide Information）

简　　介： 这是 FDA 向一家注册为非处方药品生产商的公司发出警告信，指控其未回应 FDA 的记录要求。该公司被指涉嫌生产含有易受二甘醇和乙二醇污染原辅料的药品，并未对 FDA 关于记录和信息的要求做出任何回应。尽管 FDA 多次尝试与公司联系，但均未获得回复。警告信中还指出，使用二甘醇和乙二醇污染的原辅料已导致全球多起致命中毒事件。在 FDA 未确认公司符合生产规范和其他要求之前，可能会暂停批准其作为药品生产商的新申请，同时还可能对该公司生产的药品进行扣留或拒绝入境。此外，FDA 还将该公司生产的所有药品列入进口警报。该公司被要求在 15 个工作日内书面回复，提供信息以供 FDA 考虑。

Your firm was registered with the United States Food and Drug Administration（FDA or Agency）as a manufacturer of over-the-counter（OTC）drug products, including toothpaste for children. Ingredients of the drugs registered as manufactured at your firm include ingredients susceptible to Diethylene Glycol（DEG）and Ethylene Glycol（EG）substitution. A review of import records showed multiple shipments of drug products into the United States which declared Sangleaf Pharm., Co., Ltd., as the drug manufacturer. On December 14, 2022, the FDA sent an electronic request for records and other information pursuant to section 704（a）（4）of the Federal Food, Drug, and Cosmetic Act（FD&C Act）, 21 U.S.C. 374（a）（4）, to the contact e-mail address provided in your registration file. This request went unanswered. A second request was sent via e-mail on January 11, 2023, followed by an attempted contact by telephone with your registered U.S. Agent on January 26, 2023, regarding this matter. The Agency sent a follow-up written request for such records and other information on January 27, 2023. Delivery to you was confirmed by the shipper, but you failed to respond to these attempted communications or otherwise provide the requested records or other information. Pursuant to section 704(a)(4), FDA's request and follow-up communication included a sufficient and clear description of the records sought.

你公司已在 FDA 注册为非处方（OTC）药品（包括儿童牙膏）生产商。你公司生产的注册药品原辅料包括容易被二甘醇（DEG）和乙二醇（EG）污染的原辅料。对进口记录的审查显示，多批药品运往美国，宣称 Sangleaf Pharm., Co., Ltd. 为药品生产商。2022 年 12 月 14 日，FDA 根据 FD&C 法案第 704(a)(4) 条、21 U.S.C. 374(a)(4) 发出了一份电子要求至你们的注册文件中提供的电子邮件地址，要求提供记录和其他信息。这一要求没有得到回复。第二次要求于 2023 年 1 月 11 日通过电子邮件发出，随后于 2023 年 1 月 26 日尝试通过电话与你公司的美国注册代理人取得联系，讨论此事。FDA 于 2023 年 1 月 27 日发出了一份后续书面要求，要求提供此类记录和其他信息。代理人已确认向你公司传达，但你们未能回应这些尝试的沟通，或以其他方式提供所要求的记录或其他信息。根据第 704(a)(4) 条，FDA 的要求和后续沟通包括了对所需记录的充分且清晰的描述。

It is a prohibited act under section 301(e) of the FD&C Act(21 U.S.C. 331(e)) to refuse to permit access to or copying of any record as required by section 704(a).

根据 FD&C 法案第 301(e) 条［21 U.S.C. 331(e)］，拒绝访问或复制第 704(a) 条要求的任何记录属于禁止行为。

The use of ingredients contaminated with DEG or EG has resulted in various lethal poisoning incidents in humans worldwide. See FDA's guidance document *Testing of Glycerin, Propylene Glycol, Maltitol Solution, Hydrogenated Starch Hydrolysate, Sorbitol Solution, and Other High-Risk Drug Components for Diethylene Glycol and Ethylene Glycol* to help you meet the current good manufacturing practice(cGMP)requirements when manufacturing drugs containing ingredients at high-risk for DEG or EG contamination at https://www.fda.gov/media/167974/download.

在全球范围内，使用受 DEG 或 EG 污染的原辅料已导致多起人类致命中毒事件。请参阅 FDA 指南，甘油、丙二醇、麦芽糖醇溶液、氢化淀粉水解物、山梨醇溶液和其他高风险药品原辅料中二甘醇和乙二醇的检验，以帮助你公司在生产含有 DEG 或 EG 污染风险原辅料的药品时，满足 cGMP 要求，请访问网址（略，见上）。

Because your firm failed to respond to the section 704(a)(4) records requests and associated communication attempts, we have no indication of the level of quality assurance for drugs registered as manufactured at your facility.

由于你公司未能回应第 704（a）（4）条记录要求和相关沟通尝试，因此我们无法获悉你公司生产的注册药品的质量水平。

Until FDA is able to confirm compliance with cGMP and other applicable requirements, we may withhold approval of any new applications or supplements listing your firm as a drug manufacturer. In addition, shipments of articles manufactured at Sangleaf Pharm., Co., Ltd., 4 Sagimakgol-ro, 62 Beon-gil, Jungwon-gu, Seongnam Gyeonggi, 13210 South Korea, into the United States that appear to be adulterated or misbranded are subject to being detained or refused admission pursuant to section 801（a）（3）of the FD&C Act, 21 U.S.C. 381（a）（3）.

在 FDA 能够确认符合 cGMP 和其他适用要求之前，我们可能会拒绝批准将你公司列为药品生产商的新申请或补充申请。此外，在 Sangleaf Pharm., Co., Ltd.（地址略，见上）生产的物品运往美国时，这些物品被视为掺假或标识错误，根据 FD&C 法案第 801（a）（3）条，也即 21 U.S.C. 381（a）（3），可能会被扣留或拒绝入境。

FDA placed all drugs and drug products manufactured by your firm on Import Alert 66-79 on March 30, 2023.

FDA 于 2023 年 3 月 30 日将你公司生产的所有药品列入进口警报 66-79。

After you receive this letter, respond to this office in writing within 15 working days. In response to this letter, you may provide information for our consideration as we continue to assess your activities and practices, and/or submit a request to schedule an FDA inspection.

收到此函后，请在 15 个工作日内以书面形式回复本办公室。在回复本函时，你公司可以提供信息供我们考虑，因为我们将继续评估你公司的活动和实践，和（或）提出安排 FDA 检查的要求。

6　拒绝提供对记录的访问和复制

警告信编号： MARCS-CMS 664934

签发时间： 2023-9-18；**公示时间：** 2023-9-26

签发机构： 药物审评与研究中心 | CDER（Center for Drug Evaluation and Research | CDER）

公　　司： Zhao Qing Longda Biotechnology Co. Ltd.

所在国家/地区： 中国

主　　题： 拒绝提供对记录的访问和复制（Refusal to Provide Access to and Copying of Records）

简　　介： 这家国内企业在美国 FDA 注册为非处方药品生产商，近日因未能回应 FDA 的记录请求而受到指控。FDA 审查了进口记录后发现，该企业多批药品运往美国，并宣称自己是这些药品的制造商。2023 年，FDA 向该公司发送了电子记录和信息请求至其提供的联系电子邮件地址，但遗憾未得到回复。随后的请求同样未获得回应。直到最近，该公司回复称"不准备允许 FDA 审计和检查"。根据 FD&C 法案第 301（e）条，拒绝允许访问或复制第 704（a）条记录要求属于禁止行为。由于该公司未能回应第 704（a）（4）条记录请求和相关沟通尝试，FDA 无法获悉该公司生产药品的质量保证水平。因此，FDA 已于 2023 年 8 月将该公司生产的所有药品列入进口警报中。

　　Your firm was registered with the United States Food and Drug Administration（FDA or Agency）as a manufacturer of over-the-counter（OTC）drug products，including toothpaste for children. Ingredients of the drugs registered as manufactured at your firm include ingredients susceptible to Diethylene Glycol（DEG）and Ethylene Glycol（EG）substitution. A review of import records showed multiple shipments of drug products into the United States，which declared Zhao Qing Longda Biotechnology Co. Ltd.，as the drug manufacturer. On March 17，2023，the FDA sent an electronic request for records and other information pursuant to section 704（a）（4）of the Federal Food，Drug，and Cosmetic Act（FD&C Act），

21 U.S.C. 374（a）（4）, to the contact email address provided in your registration file. This request went unanswered. Second and third requests were sent via email on April 6 and April 18, 2023. On April 19, 2023, you responded stating that you were "not prepared to allow the FDA to audit and inspect" your firm. The Agency sent a follow-up written request for such records and other information on April 28, 2023, to your registered address on file; however, we received a delivery failure notification. Pursuant to section 704（a）（4）, FDA's request and follow-up communications included a sufficient and clear description of the records sought.

你公司已在 FDA 注册为非处方（OTC）药品（包括儿童牙膏）生产商。你公司生产的注册药品原辅料包括容易被二甘醇（DEG）和乙二醇（EG）污染的原辅料。进口记录审查显示，多批药品被运往美国，宣称肇庆龙达生物科技有限公司为药品生产商。2023 年 3 月 17 日，FDA 根据 FD&C 法案第 704（a）（4）条、21 U.S.C. 374（a）（4）发出了一份电子要求至注册文件中提供的电子邮件联系地址，要求提供记录和其他信息。这一要求没有得到回复。第二次和第三次要求于 2023 年 4 月 6 日和 4 月 18 日通过电子邮件发出。2023 年 4 月 19 日，你公司回复称"不准备允许 FDA 审计和检查"。FDA 于 2023 年 4 月 28 日向你公司备案的注册地址发出了一份后续书面要求，要求提供此类记录和其他信息；然而，我们收到了送件失败的通知。根据第 704（a）（4）条，FDA 的要求和后续沟通包括了对所寻求记录的充分且清晰的描述。

It is a prohibited act under section 301（e）of the FD&C Act（21 U.S.C. 331（e））to refuse to permit access to or copying of any record as required by section 704（a）.

根据 FD&C 法案第 301（e）条［21 U.S.C. 331（e）］，拒绝允许访问或复制第 704（a）条要求的任何记录属于禁止行为。

The use of ingredients contaminated with DEG or EG has resulted in various lethal poisoning incidents in humans worldwide. See FDA's guidance document *Testing of Glycerin, Propylene Glycol, Maltitol Solution, Hydrogenated Starch Hydrolysate, Sorbitol Solution, and Other High-Risk Drug Components for Diethylene Glycol and Ethylene Glycol* to help you meet the current good manufacturing practice（cGMP）requirements when manufacturing drugs containing ingredients at high-risk for DEG or EG contamination at https://www.fda.gov/media/167974/download.

在全球范围内，使用受 DEG 或 EG 污染的原辅料已导致多起人类致命中毒事件。请参阅 FDA 指南，甘油、丙二醇、麦芽糖醇溶液、氢化淀粉水解物、山梨醇溶液和其他高风险药品原辅料中二甘醇和乙二醇的检验，以帮助你公司在生产含有 DEG 或 EG 污染风险原辅料的药品时，满足 cGMP 要求，请访问网址（略，见上）。

Because your firm failed to respond to the section 704（a）（4）records requests and associated communication attempts, we have no indication of the level of quality assurance for drugs registered as manufactured at your facility.

由于你公司未能回应第 704（a）（4）条记录要求和相关沟通尝试，因此我们无法获悉你公司生产的注册药品的质量保证水平。

Until FDA is able to confirm compliance with cGMP and other applicable requirements, we may withhold approval of any new applications or supplements listing your firm as a drug manufacturer. In addition, shipments of articles manufactured at Zhao Qing Longda Biotechnology Co. Ltd., No. 20 Yingbin Road, Gaoxin District, Zhaoqing Guangdong, 526238 China into the United States that appear to be adulterated or misbranded are subject to being detained or refused admission pursuant to section 801（a）（3）of the FD&C Act, 21 U.S.C. 381（a）（3）.

在 FDA 能够确认你公司符合 cGMP 和其他适用要求之前，我们可能会拒绝批准将你公司列为药品生产商的新申请或补充申请。此外，肇庆龙达生物科技有限公司（地址略，见上）生产的物品运往美国，将被视为掺假或标识错误，根据 FD&C 法案第 801（a）（3）条，也即 21 U.S.C. 381（a）（3），可能会被扣留或拒绝入境。

FDA placed all drugs and drug products manufactured by your firm on Import Alert 66-79 on August 29, 2023.

FDA 于 2023 年 8 月 29 日将你公司生产的所有药品列入进口警报 66-79。

After you receive this letter, respond to this office in writing within 15 working days. In response to this letter, you may provide information for our consideration as we continue to assess your activities and practices, and/or submit a request to schedule an FDA inspection.

收到此函后，请你公司在 15 个工作日内以书面形式回复本办公室。在回复本函时，可以提供信息供我们考虑，因为我们将继续评估你公司的活动和实践，和（或）提出安排 FDA 检查的要求。